Contemporary Medical Imaging

Series Editor: U. Joseph Schoepf

For further volumes:
http://www.springer.com/series/7687

James G. Ravenel
Editor

Lung Cancer Imaging

Humana Press

Editor
James G. Ravenel
Department of Radiology
Medical University of South Carolina
Charleston, SC, USA

ISBN 978-1-4939-4068-4 ISBN 978-1-60761-620-7 (eBook)
DOI 10.1007/978-1-60761-620-7
Springer New York Heidelberg Dordrecht London

Printed on acid-free paper

Humana Press is a brand of Springer
Springer is part of Springer Science+Business Media (www.springer.com)

This book is dedicated to the memory of Carolyn E. Reed, M.D. (1950–2012). Carolyn epitomized the principles of patient care and humanism that is so often lost in today's world of technology. A thoracic surgeon by trade, her primary focus was on doing what was right for each individual patient and was at the heart of the multidisciplinary thoracic oncology practice at the Medical University of South Carolina. Her goal was simple: to ensure that everyone came together to render the best possible evidence-based treatment for each patient. She touched the lives of so many nurses, physicians, and patients and her spirit lives on through the memories and skill of those she trained.

Foreword

Lung cancer is the paradigm disease of the first 2 decades of the twenty-first century. It was once seen as a single, monolithic, self-inflicted entity, nearly always caused by smoking, and usually viewed by patients (and often their families and their physicians) as a death knell at the time of diagnosis.

Today we know much more about lung cancer and almost always have more options to provide to patients with the disease. Tobacco exposure is still recognized as the leading cause worldwide. In the United States more lung cancer cases occur in former smokers than current smokers. Smoking cessation programs are working and, happily, there are fewer new smokers as well. At the same time, an increasing number of never-smokers with lung cancer are part of our more textured and deeply scientific appreciation of the range of entities that fall squarely under the lung cancer rubric.

Among significant developments in lung cancer diagnosis and treatment:

- Data from large and well-constructed screening trials have shown that the risk of death from lung cancer can be reduced by approximately 20 % when multiyear CT screening is applied to carefully defined, higher risk patient populations.
- The iterative emergence of more probing, sensitive, imaging technologies—CT scanning, magnetic resonance imaging, and the still quite early technology of PET and PET/CT—has allowed us to better understand the apparent distribution of disease and apportion therapy recommendations accordingly.
- Improvements in minimally invasive staging, e.g., image-guided transthoracic tissue acquisition, thoracoscopic diagnosis and staging, and esophageal or endobronchial ultrasound assessments of nodal involvement, have allowed more accurate pathologic staging to guide surgical interventions, multimodality treatment approaches, and sequencing of systemic management.
- Adjuvant chemotherapy can significantly improve survival for patients in selected disease settings. Evidence-based recommendations improve post-operative care. Improved systemic therapies significantly prolong survival in patients with advanced stage disease.
- Improved therapeutic radiation technologies, such as image driven target volume determinations, 3D treatment planning, IMRT, respiratory gating, and stereotactic brain or body radiosurgery, enhance efficacy, decrease

radiation-related toxicities, and expand the utility of radiation for both palliative management and potentially curative interventions.

- Interventional radiology now offers radiofrequency ablation of specific lesions as a beneficial addition to the therapeutic armamentarium.
- Several chemotherapy combinations appear about equally active. Each has been shown to provide overall survival benefits compared to prior systemic therapy standards. In addition, oncogene science and the recognition of molecular drivers of lung cancer proliferation are the bedrock of our new capacity for targeted therapy with its breathtaking rapidity of effect and durability of response in the majority of individuals who receive treatment based on their tumor's molecular profile.
- Early introduction of palliative care as a component of systemic management for patients with advanced disease has been shown to improve quality of life and may actually contribute to prolonged survival.

Quality staging continues to be the principal driver for the selection of the best lung cancer care regimen for every individual patient. As a result, "tissue remains the issue." Pathologists play the central role in tissue handling and assessment. Initially, they utilize the traditional histopathologic classification of lung cancer, dividing the "monolith" into small cell, adeno-, large cell, and squamous cell subgroups. While inter- and even intra-observer reproducibility of subgroup designation is far from perfect, clinical decision making can be driven by these sub-histology designations. For example, pemetrexed and bevacizumab are considered "contra-indicated" for patients with advanced lung cancer of the squamous cell type based on either poorer activity (pemetrexed vs. gemcitabine) or increased toxicity (increased hemorrhagic risk among patients with squamous cell subtype treated with bevacizumab). At the same time basic research and patient-tumor tissue-based translational science investigations have revealed striking new and actionable information about critical molecular drivers (biomarkers), further defining lung cancer subgroups and directing clinical management with "targeted therapy." Even patterns of molecular marker evolution after initial therapy can now be ascertained and used to direct salvage therapy recommendations, making repeat tissue acquisition yet another new element of our current lung cancer paradigm.

Another critical piece of this new lung cancer paradigm is an intensely interactive, collaborative, multidisciplinary team approach. When present in an ongoing way, it allows patients and their cancer care providers to receive and to deliver the best that committed care providers and medical science together can offer. Each patient's experience with their disease and their therapy is distinct. What seems clear to one specialist may become more textured and seen differently when reviewed and discussed in the multidisciplinary setting.

- Primary care clinicians practice their art and separate the less common but more threatening scenarios from the more common but self-limited or less threatening chronic entities with which they are most often dealing. This type of triage is not easy, but it is key.
- Imaging specialists, thoracic surgeons, and pulmonary medicine physicians work together to correlate underlying risks and current physiology, assess new signs and symptoms of disease, and radiographic findings to

determine the imperative for a diagnostic intervention vs. careful observation.

- Tissue acquirers (radiologists, pulmonologists, and thoracic surgeons), tissue assessors (surgical and molecular pathologists), and therapy providers (physicians, nurses, and other professionals) driven by both the art of medicine and the available data must discuss (and optimally meet) together on a regular basis. Such patient by patient, multidisciplinary discussions insure that optimal therapy directing information can be acquired with maximized efficiency and minimized patient risk. Multi-specialty collaborations to define timing and type of iterative assessments for response status and restaging are also critical parts of the continuum of optimized care.

In this textbook on lung cancer, Dr. Ravenel and his contributing authors, many who are now or have been on the faculty at the Medical University of South Carolina, have built on their own deep understanding of the lung cancer continuum, fashioned in no small part by their active participation as a multidisciplinary thoracic oncology team, to provide a superbly well-informed, clinically focused, user-friendly, and up-to-date data source for every constituency interested in or touched by this paradigm disease of these first 2 decades of the twenty-first century.

Charleston, SC, USA Mark R. Green, MD

Preface

Despite all the advances in knowledge and detection, lung cancer remains the leading cause of cancer deaths in the United States. I would be remiss if I did not mention the devastating effects that tobacco has had. However, even if quit rates improve and better yet fewer people take up the smoking habit, we are still left with a long lag time of risk. Although lung cancer appears to have plateaued for men, tobacco-related cancer deaths continue to climb in women. As we have improved our ability to diagnose and treat the disease, it remains that the majority of people diagnosed with the disease will not be curable at the time of detection. Screening over time may change the equation, but even with screening, we will still be left with a large population of people with incurable lung cancer.

My paternal grandfather succumbed to lung cancer in the late 1950s; I was robbed of the opportunity to meet him. Many others, alike, struggle with the loss of friends and relatives to lung cancer. Screening and treatment unfortunately are not enough. If we are to truly put a dent in lung cancer deaths, it will take a coordinated approach of tobacco control, education, and smoking cessation.

For over a decade, I have been privileged to work in a multidisciplinary thoracic oncology setting to discuss difficult cases with dedicated thoracic oncologists, pulmonologists, pathologists, thoracic surgeons, and radiation oncologists. I have seen this not only optimize the care of individuals but also improve each and every team member's knowledge. This flow of information across specialties is critical in tailoring therapy. It is from this experience that I undertook this book in hopes that the wisdom and pearls learned in such a setting could help those who may not have easy access to a multidisciplinary care team. Many of the authors are colleagues and friends from the Thoracic Tumor Board at the Medical University of South Carolina.

While a group of specialists often guide the care for lung cancer patients in large institutions, it is often a general radiologist, general practitioner, and internist in smaller communities who are on the front line of the diagnosis and initial discussions. In many cases, these can be the most difficult and trying days for both physician and patient. It is my hope that this book can provide a guide to the diagnosis, staging, and management of lung cancer that can aid in these initial discussions and help patients understand the following steps and what to expect when they come for treatment.

While the focus of this book is on lung cancer, the disease, we must never forget that on the other side of the diagnosis there is a person with hopes, fears, and dreams. They often are scared and confused. There is a family who wants their loved one to be cared for, to be listened to. For all the new technology, procedures, and drugs described, these must be seen as aids to care for the patient and not a replacement for the eyes, ears, and touch. I would like to end with the final two paragraphs of Dr. Carolyn Reed's Presidential Address at the 54th Annual Meeting of the Southern Thoracic Surgical Association:

> We have to realize when technology is a hindrance, not a help. Tests, machines, and procedures cannot supplant listening, experience, and intuitiveness.
>
> Patient versus customer, technology versus touch, organ versus soul: where has humanism gone? It has not gone. Humanism is why we chose medicine and why young people enter medical school. We cannot let the light flicker, but must keep the beacon bright. If each one of us keeps the individual patient as the primary focus, and if we remember that medicine will always be an art as well as a science, humanism can never be lost. [1]

Charleston, SC, USA James G. Ravenel, MD

Reference

1. Reed CE. Patient versus consumer, technology versus touch: where has humanism gone? Ann Thorac Surg. 2008;85:1511–4.

Contents

Contributors

Anthony J. Alberg, PhD, MPH Department of Public Health Sciences, Medical University of South Carolina, Charleston, SC, USA

Cancer Prevention and Control Program, Hollings Cancer Center, Medical University of South Carolina, Charleston, SC, USA

Sanjeev Bhalla, MD Department of Radiology, Barnes-Jewish Hospital, St. Louis, MO, USA

James Brashears, MD Ranier Cancer Center, Tukwila, WA, USA

Aqeel A. Chowdhry, MD Department of Radiology, Radiology/South Pointe Hospital, Cleveland Clinic, Cleveland, OH, USA

S. Lewis Cooper, MD Department of Radiation Oncology, Medical University of South Carolina, Charleston, SC, USA

Kristopher W. Cummings, MD Department of Radiology, Barnes-Jewish Hospital, St. Louis, MO, USA

Chadrick E. Denlinger, MD Division of Cardiothoracic Surgery, Department of Surgery, Medical University of South Carolina, Charleston, SC, USA

Mostafa M. Fraig, MD Division of Anatomic Pathology, Department of Pathology and Pulmonary Medicine, University of Louisville, Louisville, KY, USA

J. David Godwin, MD Department of Radiology, University of Washington, Seattle, WA, USA

Mario Gomez, MD Pulmonary and Sleep Center of the Valley, Weslaco, TX, USA

Jeffrey P. Kanne, MD Department of Radiology, University of Wisconsin School of Medicine and Public Health, Madison, WI, USA

Hiren J. Mehta, MD Division of Pulmonary Medicine, Medical University of South Carolina, Charleston, SC, USA

Tan-Lucien H. Mohammed, MD, FCCP Department of Radiology C5-XR, Virginia Mason Medical Center, Seattle, Washington, USA

James G. Ravenel, MD Department of Radiology, Medical University of South Carolina, Charleston, SC, USA

Ernest M. Scalzetti, MD Department of Radiology, SUNY Upstate Medical University, Syracuse, NY, USA

Clayton J. Shamblin, MD Department of Internal Medicine, Division of Pulmonary and Critical Care, Allergy and Sleep Medicine, Medical University of South Carolina, Charleston, SC, USA

Anand Sharma, MD Department of Radiation Oncology, Medical University of South Carolina, Charleston, SC, USA

Carol A. Sherman, MD Division of Hematology/Oncology, Department of Medicine, Medical University of South Carolina, Charleston, SC, USA

Keisuke Shirai, MD Division of Hematology/Oncology, Department of Medicine, Medical University of South Carolina, Charleston, SC, USA

Gerard A. Silvestri, MD, MS Department of Internal Medicine, Division of Pulmonary and Critical Care, Allergy and Sleep Medicine, Medical University of South Carolina, Charleston, SC, USA

George R. Simon, MD Department of Thoracic/Head & Neck Medical Oncology, MD Anderson Cancer Center, Houston, TX, USA

Lee Wheless, BS Department of Public Health Sciences and Hollings Cancer Center, Medical University of South Carolina, Charleston, SC, USA

Epidemiology of Lung Cancer

1

Lee Wheless, James Brashears,
and Anthony J. Alberg

Lung cancer is the leading cause of cancer death in the United States, claiming an estimated 157,300 victims in 2010 [1]. Lung cancer was a rare disease in 1900 but has been propelled to epidemic proportions due largely to cigarette smoking. In 1950, three separate studies were published that suggested cigarette smoking was associated with increased risk of lung cancer [2–4]. This and subsequent research revealed a clear dose–response relationship between amount of cigarettes smoked and lung cancer incidence, offering further proof of its association with the dramatic increase in lung cancer rates seen during the 1900s [5]. Since then, an ever-expanding body of evidence continues to identify cigarette smoking as the single most important cause of lung cancer [6–8].

L. Wheless, B.S.
Department of Public Health Sciences and Hollings Cancer Center, Medical University of South Carolina, Charleston, SC, USA

J. Brashears, M.D.
Ranier Cancer Center, Tukwila, WA, USA

A.J. Alberg, Ph.D., M.P.H. (✉)
Department of Public Health Sciences, Medical University of South Carolina, 68 President Street, Charleston, SC 29425, USA

Cancer Prevention and Control Program, Hollings Cancer Center, Medical University of South Carolina, 68 President, Charleston, SC 29425, USA
e-mail: alberg@musc.edu

Patterns of Occurrence

Incidence

In the United States, since 1992, the age-adjusted incidence rates (per 100,000) of lung cancer have gradually declined from 67.0 to 54.6 in 2008 [9]. In 2010, there were an estimated 222,520 new cases of lung cancer, which accounted for approximately 15 % of all new cancer diagnoses in the United States [1]. From 1984 to 2008, the age-adjusted incidence rate (per 100,000) in men decreased from 102.1 to 70.2. This decrease can largely be attributed to the decreased smoking prevalence in men that began in the mid-1960s. After steadily increasing up until the mid-1990s, female age-adjusted incidence rates (per 100,000) have leveled off to remain between 50 and 52 for the past 15 years with no evidence yet of a decline.

Survival

Lung cancer is the leading cause of cancer mortality among both males and females. The 5-year relative survival rate for lung cancer has improved only slightly during the past decades, increasing from 13.5 % in 1985–1989 to 16.3 % in 2001–2007. Five-year survival depends heavily on the stage at diagnosis, ranging from 50.1 % for local disease, to 21.3 % for regional spread, and 2.8 % for distant disease [10]. More than half of all new lung cancers

J.G. Ravenel (ed.), *Lung Cancer Imaging*, Contemporary Medical Imaging,
DOI 10.1007/978-1-60761-620-7_1, © Springer Science+Business Media New York 2013

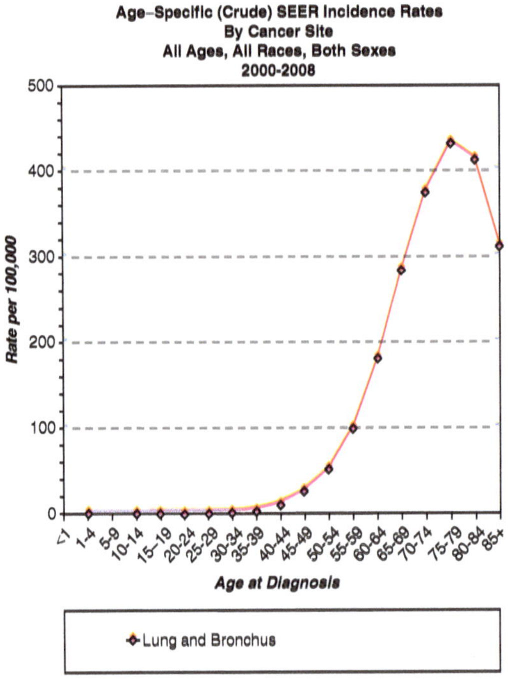

Fig. 1.1 Age group-specific lung cancer incidence in SEER 17 registries. Cancer sites include invasive cases only, unless otherwise noted. Incidence source: SEER 17 areas (San Francisco, Connecticut, Detroit, Hawaii, Iowa, New Mexico, Seattle, Utah, Atlanta, San Jose-Monterey, Los Angeles, Alaska Native Registry, rural Georgia, California excluding SF/SJM/LA, Kentucky, Louisiana, and New Jersey). Rates are per 100,000. Datapoints were not shown for rates that were based on less than 16 cases (from Surveillance, Epidemiology, and End Results (SEER) Program [http://www.seer.cancer.gov] SEER*Stat Database: Mortality—All COD, Aggregated With State, Total U.S. (1969–2007), National Cancer Institute, DCCPS, Surveillance Research Program, Cancer Statistics Branch, released April 2011. Underlying mortality data provided by NCHS [http://www.cdc.gov/nchs])

are diagnosed with metastatic disease, resulting in the poor overall survival rate. Other factors are strongly associated with survival, with poorer prognoses seen among patients who are older, male, and African-American [10, 11].

Age

Lung cancer is rare among those younger than 45 years of age, but incidence increases thereafter, with rates of 272 per 100,000 or higher for all age groups 65 and older (Fig. 1.1) [9]. With the aging of those born during the baby boom following World War II, more Americans will be in these high-incidence age groups. This will likely result in an increase in the absolute number of lung cancer cases, even if the relative rate continues to decline.

Race and Ethnicity

The patterns of incidence and survival by race and ethnicity make lung cancer an important area for disparities research. The rates among women are similar for both African-Americans and European-Americans, but African-American males have consistently experienced a greater burden of lung cancer than European-American males [9]. In 1980, age-adjusted lung cancer incidence among African-American males was 55 % greater than that among European-American males. This disparity narrowed to 47.4 % in 2008 (Fig. 1.2). African-American males have also experienced a greater mortality from lung cancer, with the largest disparity in rates being 42 % greater than European-American males in 1990, which decreased to 19.2 % in 2008 [12]. The racial disparity in mortality reflects not just the differences in incidence but also poorer survival among African-American males and females, even after controlling for stage at diagnosis.

The persistent racial disparity remains a major cause for concern. Research that allows risk to be compared between different racial or ethnic groups can help delineate why the risk among African-American men is so high. Results of the Multiethnic Cohort Study showed that even after controlling for number of cigarettes smoked, African-Americans had an increased lung cancer risk compared to European Americans [13]. Historical differences in smoking prevalence do not explain all of the higher risks seen in African-Americans compared to European Americans [14].

Sex

The present epidemic of lung cancer in the USA began in males. In the late 1920s, the number of cases increased sharply, paralleling the

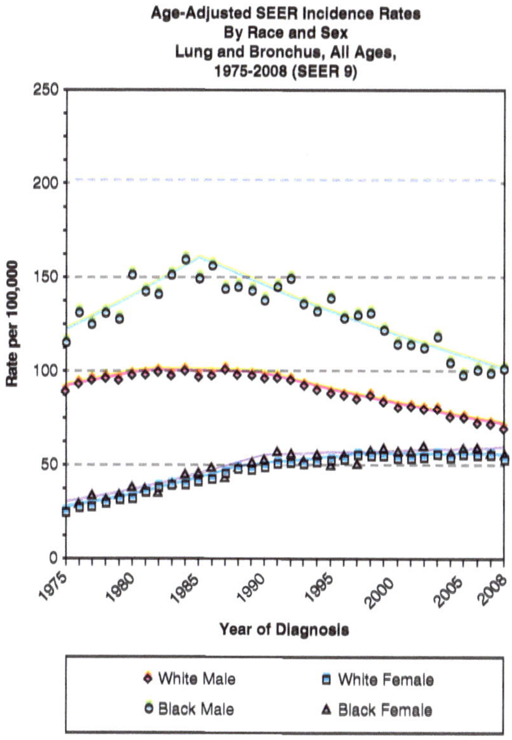

Fig. 1.2 Age-adjusted lung cancer mortality rates by gender, 1975–2008. Cancer sites include invasive cases only, unless otherwise noted. Incidence source: SEER nine areas (San Francisco, Connecticut, Detroit, Hawaii, Iowa, New Mexico, Seattle, Utah, and Atlanta). Rates are per 100,000 and are age adjusted to the 2000 US Std Population (19 age groups Census P25-1130). Regression lines are calculated using the Joinpoint Regression Program Version 3.5, April 2011, National Cancer Institute (from Surveillance, Epidemiology, and End Results (SEER) Program [http://www.seer.cancer.gov] SEER*Stat Database: Mortality—All COD, Aggregated With State, Total U.S. (1969–2007), National Cancer Institute, DCCPS, Surveillance Research Program, Cancer Statistics Branch, released April 2011. Underlying mortality data provided by NCHS [http://www.cdc.gov/nchs])

popularization of smoking among men that had started 2 decades earlier. Among women, the significant increase in smoking prevalence lagged behind men by approximately 30 years. As a result, lung cancer rates in women did not begin its striking upward trend until the 1960s [9]. The peak rates for women will never approach those for men, but the epidemic in women has not yet shown clear evidence that it is subsiding; rather, mortality rates have remained relatively constant since the mid-1990s (Fig. 1.3). Incidence rates among younger age groups have declined in both men and women for several decades. As these birth cohorts with reduced risk of lung cancer age, they should produce a substantial decrease in incidence among both sexes.

Susceptibility to lung cancer based on gender has been explored. Studies from the late 1980s and early 1990s concluded that male sex was a poor prognostic indicator for late-stage lung cancer (as reviewed in [15]), generating interest in finding a biologic explanation. More recent evidence, however, has shown a marked narrowing of the gender gap, and models predict an eventual closing [16]. One study proposed that compared to males, female smokers are more likely to develop lung cancer but less likely to die from it [17]. Currently, there is no consensus on whether there is an inherent difference in lung cancer susceptibility between men and women.

Socioeconomic Status

Low socioeconomic status (SES) is associated with increased lung cancer risk [18–20]. This association persists even after adjustment for cigarette smoking [21]. Educational level is also inversely associated with lung cancer incidence and mortality rates [1, 20]. SES is associated with a number of factors that play a role in lung cancer risk, such as smoking, diet, and exposures to lung carcinogens in both the workplace and home. An improved understanding of the complex interrelationships between SES and other lung cancer risk factors will provide guidance for how to address the social disparity in an effective manner.

Histopathology

Lung cancer occurs in four major types as classified by light microscopy: adenocarcinoma, squamous cell carcinoma, large cell carcinoma, and small cell carcinoma. All four of these types are caused by tobacco smoking [22]. For prognostic purposes, diagnoses are often simplified to either small cell (about 15 % of lung cancers) or non-small cell (about 85 %) [1]. The reason for this

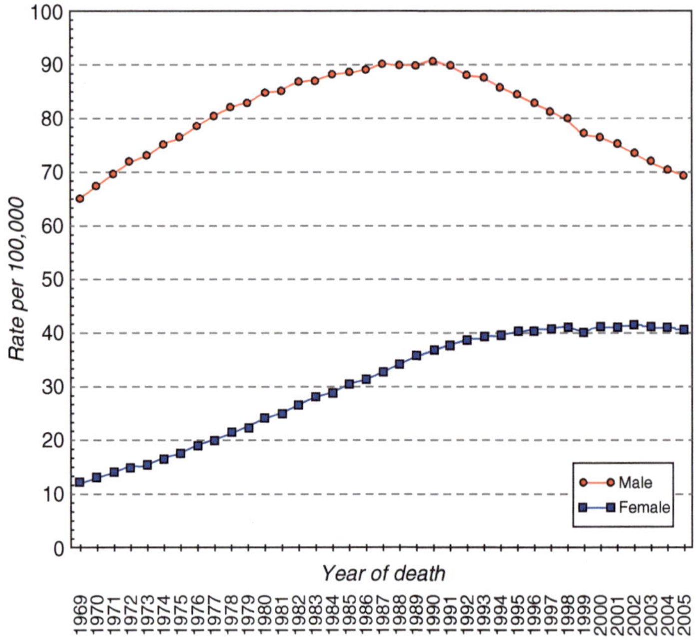

Fig. 1.3 Age-adjusted lung cancer mortality rates by gender (from Surveillance, Epidemiology, and End Results (SEER) Program [http://www.seer.cancer.gov] SEER*Stat Database: Mortality—All COD, Aggregated With State, Total U.S. (1969–2007), National Cancer Institute, DCCPS, Surveillance Research Program, Cancer Statistics Branch, released April 2011. Underlying mortality data provided by NCHS [http://www.cdc.gov/nchs])

classification is that small cell has an inferior survival and different treatment paradigms than non-small cell lung cancer and often does not present until the later stages of disease.

The histologic characteristics of lung cancer in developed countries, including the United States, have changed in recent decades. Adenocarcinoma has become more common, whereas squamous cell carcinoma has declined. For radiologic diagnoses, this shift is notable because adenocarcinoma tends to arise more peripherally and squamous cell carcinoma more centrally [23]. Consensus has not been achieved on a definitive explanation for the cause for the shift to adenocarcinoma, but the central hypothesis focuses on the changing cigarette, with its concomitant change in smoking topography, leading to greater depth of inhalation [22, 24]. Early analyses of gene expression profiles of tumor cells tended to cluster by histologic subtype, thus giving no further prognostic value beyond what is determined by light microscopy [25]. More recent discoveries have indicated a combination of clinical and genomic features that can provide better estimates of risk [26] and prognosis [27].

Modifiable Risk Factors

The majority of lung cancers are caused by environmental exposures. Strategies to limit or prevent these exposures have led directly to the sharp decrease in incidence and mortality of lung cancer beginning in the early 1990s. In addition to anti-smoking campaigns, many jurisdictions have adopted laws to protect nonsmokers from exposure to secondhand smoke (SHS). Awareness of the dangers of both radon and asbestos has also led to testing and strict regulations surrounding exposure.

Cigarette Smoking

Cigarette smoking is the single greatest cause of lung cancer, accounting for approximately 85 % of all lung cancer deaths [1]. Individual risk depends on the age of initiation, number of years smoked, number of cigarettes per day, as well as individual susceptibility. On average cigarette smokers experience an approximately

20-fold increased risk of lung cancer compared to never smokers. Few environmental exposures carry such a great risk for disease. Patterns of occurrence for lung cancer have closely mirrored the trends for smoking, with lung cancer incidence rates lagging by about 2 decades [28]. Lung cancer mortality rates have shown tight associations with smoking in statistical models adjusting for population characteristics. An incredibly large and high-quality body of evidence documents the irrefutable role of tobacco smoking in causing lung cancer.

Lung cancer risk increases with number and frequency of cigarettes smoked in a dose–response relationship [29]. The duration of smoking carries a greater effect than the amount smoked, as shown by Doll and Peto [5, 29]. They found that tripling the amount of cigarettes smoked per day led to a tripling in risk, whereas a tripling in the duration of smoking led to a 100-fold increase in lung cancer risk [29]. For this reason, there has been particular attention given to the dangers of smoking initiation among youths. Individuals who begin smoking at earlier ages are likely to continue smoking and to become heavy smokers [30]. They are also more likely to develop lung cancer at an earlier age. Programs that delay the onset of smoking in a population could reduce the duration of smoking and hence lung cancer rates.

Epidemiologic studies have found only a slight decrease in lung cancer risk among those who smoked filtered or high-tar cigarettes compared to those who smoked unfiltered or low-tar cigarettes, respectively (reviewed in [11]). In addition, cigarettes with lower tar and nicotine content are on the market, but these cigarettes have not resulted in reduced risk of lung cancer [31].

Not only does cigarette smoking itself lead to an enormous increase in lung cancer risk, but it also acts synergistically with many other risk factors. One study examined the effects of emphysema, hay fever, family history of lung cancer, bleomycin sensitivity of tumor cells, pack-year smoking history, asbestos exposure, and wood dust exposure on lung cancer risk [32]. Among smokers, having five or more of these risk factors increased the risk of lung cancer by 17-fold compared to smokers experiencing no additional risk factors, with a significant trend for increasing number of risk factors. These effects were not observed in nonsmokers, suggesting that smoking may interact with these other factors to cause lung cancer.

Other Forms of Smoking

All forms of tobacco smoking are associated with an increased risk of lung cancer. Pipe and cigar smoking are causally associated with lung cancer, incurring substantially elevated risks compared to never smokers [33, 34]. These forms of tobacco smoking pose less risk for lung cancer compared to cigarettes, but this is not due to the smoke being less harmful, but rather due to lower frequency of pipe and cigar smoking and a shallower depth of inhalation [1, 33, 34]. Although notable progress has been achieved in controlling cigarette consumption, the use of cigars has increased by about 150 % since 1993 [1].

With respect to smoking non-tobacco products, the effect of smoking marijuana cigarettes on lung cancer risk has also been studied. Marijuana is the most commonly used illicit drug in the United States, and its smoke contains many of the same carcinogens as does tobacco smoke, but marijuana smoking has consistently not been associated with any change in lung cancer risk [35, 36].

Smoking Trends

In the United States, smoking prevalence decreased from 42 % in 1965 to 21 % in 2008, resulting in a reduction of lung cancer incidence and mortality rates that continues today [1]. An estimated 45 million Americans currently smoke cigarettes. The prevalence of smoking among high school students has also fallen from 36 % in 1997 to 20 % in 2007. These decreases were seen regardless of race or gender, a trend which should help to eliminate the racial and gender disparities as this cohort ages [37]. Smoking rates tend to decrease with increasing years of education, with only 9 % of college graduates being smokers in 2008.

Smoking Cessation

Smoking cessation at any time decreases an individual's risk of lung cancer, regardless of age, race, gender, or pack-year history [30, 38]. The individual decrease in risk is influenced by the smoking history and the duration of abstinence. As the period of abstinence increases, the risk of lung cancer decreases. Even after decades of abstinence, however, lung cancer risk remains elevated compared to never smokers, underscoring the importance of preventing the initiation of smoking [38, 39].

Physicians play a crucial role in helping patients to stop smoking. Clinical guidelines have been developed based on the "5 As": (1) Ask if a patient smokes, (2) Assess willingness to quit, (3) Advise to quit, (4) Assist with quitting, and (5) Arrange follow-up [40]. The current clinical practice guidelines recommend that all patients be screened for tobacco use [41]. Depending on the patient's willingness and ability to quit, the physician role may range from simple counseling to prescribing medications. For a comprehensive discussion of the available therapies, see the 2008 Update to the Clinical Practice Guideline for Treating Tobacco Use and Dependence [41].

The benefits of smoking cessation reach far beyond lung cancer risk. Tobacco smoking has also been associated with many other malignancies, including cancer of the oropharynx, larynx, esophagus, stomach, pancreas, bladder, kidney, and myeloid leukemia [1]. Smoking is also a major cause of cardiovascular disease, stroke, chronic bronchitis, and emphysema. All current smokers would experience enormous health benefits from smoking cessation.

Smoking Prevention and Control

Any steps to reduce tobacco use will help prevent lung cancer. According to the Surgeon General, there are four main goals of comprehensive tobacco control: (1) preventing initiation of tobacco use among youth, (2) promoting quitting in all smokers, (3) eliminating the public's exposure to SHS, and (4) identifying and eliminating disparities in tobacco use and conditions arising from its use [42]. Estimates indicate that tobacco control programs prevented nearly 150,000 lung cancer deaths between 1991 and 2003 [16].

Secondhand Smoke Exposure

Tobacco smoke contains more than 4,000 chemicals, including at least 50 documented carcinogens [1]. Unlike active smokers, passive smokers inhale these compounds mostly unfiltered. In 1986, a report from the Surgeon General outlined the evidence that SHS was causally associated with lung cancer risk [43]. In 2006, the Surgeon General concluded that there is no safe level of exposure to SHS [44]. SHS causes approximately 3,000 lung cancer deaths annually in the United States [1].

Compared to active smokers, passive smokers are exposed to lower doses of carcinogens. For this reason, passive smoking carries less of a risk for lung cancer than active smoking. Meta-analyses have found a 25–30 % increased risk of lung cancer among nonsmokers whose spouses were smokers [45, 46].

Occupational and Environmental Exposures

Occupational groups are often heavily exposed to chemicals and other workplace-specific agents. Examination of these groups has led to the identification and characterization of numerous carcinogens. Of the cancers associated with these occupational exposures, lung cancer is the most common [47]. It is estimated that 9–15 % of all lung cancer cases are caused by exposures other than tobacco [11]. Although this represents a small proportion of cases compared to cigarette smoking, occupational exposures remain an important cause of lung cancer. Exposures to the metals nickel, arsenic, and chromium are all associated with greatly increased risk of lung cancer [48]. In the United States and other developed countries, however, exposure to these carcinogens has been greatly reduced, minimizing the impact of exposure to carcinogens in the workplace on the overall burden of lung cancer.

Asbestos

Asbestos is the general term for a number of fibrous, naturally occurring silica-based minerals. Known for centuries to be resistant to heat and fire, it was used heavily in insulation, roofing, flooring, and brake pads. Although evidence in the first decade of the 1900s suggested a link between asbestos and lung cancer, its association with mesothelioma was not formally described until around 1940 [49, 50]. Today, asbestos exposure is known to cause this rare malignancy of the pleura.

Early investigations estimated that asbestos exposure resulted in a tenfold increased risk of lung cancer [51]. Associations of similar magnitude have subsequently been observed among insulation workers [52, 53]. The increased lung cancer risk associated with asbestos exposure follows a dose–response gradient [54]. Asbestos exposure and smoking are both independent risk factors for lung cancer. When combined, they have a synergistic effect, increasing the risk above what would be obtained by simply adding the risks from both [55], possibly due to smoking increasing the retention of asbestos fibers in the lung [56].

Radiation

Epidemiologic studies have shown that lung cancer is associated with ionizing radiation in a dose-dependent, non-threshold fashion; that is, even the smallest dose can increase the risk of lung cancer. With the widespread use of noninvasive imaging modalities, concern has been raised regarding the association of lung cancer exposure to low-dose radiation typically found with CT scans, nuclear medicine, and fluoroscopic studies. Separating the additional risk posed by low dosage, such as that received from imaging studies, from background risk has been difficult [57, 58]. Large studies of the atomic bomb survivors in Japan, however, have provided clear evidence of an association between lung cancer and low-dose ionizing radiation [59, 60].

Two types of radiation are relevant to lung cancer: low-linear energy transfer (LET) radiation (e.g., X-rays and gamma rays) and high LET (e.g., neutrons and alpha particles). High-LET radiation produces a higher density of radiation that, for equivalent doses, produces more biological damage than low-LET radiation [61]. Both high- and low-LET radiation can cause direct cytotoxicity as well as bystander effects in neighboring cells, leading to chromosomal instability [62, 63]. Risk from both types has been quantified by studying cohorts with exposures greater than what would be experienced by the general population. These risk models are then used to assess the risk conveyed to the population.

High LET: Radon

Radon is an inert gas produced naturally in the decay series of uranium. Two of the decay products emit alpha particles that can damage DNA. Studies of underground uranium miners with very high levels of radon exposure have shown that these decay products cause lung cancer [64]. Radon may be the earliest identified occupational hazard. For centuries, miners along the Czech–German border developed "Mountain Sickness," a fatal condition marked by chronic cough, dyspnea, and chest pain [65]. With careful clinical examination and anatomical pathology, the disease was determined to be lung cancer. In the early twentieth century, radium and its decay product radon, a radioactive gas, were identified. Subsequent research proved this to be a cause of lung cancer among miners [64]. Due to an interaction with cigarette smoking, the risk of lung cancer due to radon exposure is markedly higher in smokers [64, 66].

Beyond occupational exposures, radon is an important public health concern as it is a commonly occurring airborne pollutant. It contributes more than one-half of all background radiation exposure in the United States, accounting for 2.0 mSv of the average annual effective dose per person of 3.6 mSv [67]. Formed from underground rocks, radon gas seeps into basements of buildings and decays to a microscopic solid that sticks to dust particles that can then be inhaled and deposited in the respiratory tract.

There, radon progeny emits alpha particles that may have carcinogenic effects on nearby cells. Average indoor levels of exposure are about 37 Bq/m^3 but may be much higher in poorly ventilated basements and in certain areas of the country, such as the Colorado Plateau. One study found that every 100 Bq/m^3 increase in radon concentration is estimated to increase the relative risk for lung cancer by 8–16 % [68]. In 1999, the US National Research Council Committee on the Biological Effects of Ionizing Radiation concluded that radon in homes posed a significant risk of lung cancer [64]. Their model estimated risk in a linear, non-threshold manner. Evidence that even a single hit by an alpha particle can cause permanent damage to a cell supports this non-threshold model. This robust risk model coupled with a mechanistic understanding of the role of radon in lung carcinogenesis indicates that surveillance of radon exposures in homes is an important primary prevention strategy.

Low LET: X-Rays and Gamma Rays

Information about low-LET radiation has come from three main populations: Japanese survivors of the atomic bomb, patients treated with radiation, and people in occupations with radiation exposure [11]. Studies in Japan have shown that even a single large dose of radiation, such as that experienced from the atomic bomb, is sufficient to increase the risk of lung cancer. The excess risk in these atomic bomb survivors did not appear immediately, but rather was observed only after they had reached the ages at which lung cancer most commonly occurs [69].

Lung cancer risk in patients treated with radiation for a number of medical conditions has also been evaluated. In contrast to the single, high dose experienced by atomic bomb survivors, these patients received several much smaller doses staggered over time. Studies of tuberculosis patients treated with radiation therapy suggest that this pattern of exposure carries little risk, if any [70, 71]. Radiation therapy for breast cancer [72, 73] and Hodgkin lymphoma [74], however, has in several studies been found to increase risk of lung cancer. Combining radiation therapy with chemotherapy had an additive effect on risk, while smoking multiplied the effect of radiation therapy.

Of importance to physicians, particularly radiologists, is quantifying the risk posed by small doses of radiation encountered in therapeutic and diagnostic procedures. X-rays and nuclear medicine contribute approximately 80 % of all man-made radiation exposures [67]. A study looking specifically at radiology technicians between 1983 and 1998 found no statistically significant increase in lung cancer risk [75]. After controlling for smoking, age, and race/ethnicity, the only group identified with excess risk was those who had 24 or more practice X-rays (Relative Risk 1.8; 95 % CI 1.1–2.9). In a larger study of individuals having multiple occupational X-rays, there was a similar trend. Compared to those who received 1–10 lifetime X-rays, those who received >40 lifetime X-rays had double the risk of lung cancer [76]. This increase raises concerns about the potential risk of repeated CT scans, such as for screening. Still, a study in patients with cystic fibrosis who had annual lung CT scans resulted in an estimate of the excess total risk of all cancers to be less than 0.5 % [77]. Continued surveillance of those who receive multiple CT scans and other radiologic studies will provide a better understanding of the potential risks.

Air Pollution

The average adult breathes about 10,000 L of air every day, making airborne carcinogens of even the lowest concentrations relevant to lung cancer [78]. Outdoor air can contain a number of hazardous agents, many of which are generated by the combustion of fossil fuels. Diesel exposures, often studied in the trucking industry, have consistently been observed to increase lung cancer risk by 20–40 % [79–81].

Particulate matter has also been examined as a potential lung cancer risk factor. A study of six US cities found an approximately 40 % increase in risk of lung cancer mortality rate (mortality rate ratio range 0.8–2.3) in urban environments with the highest concentration of fine particles compared to the city with the lowest concentration [82]. The data from the American Cancer

Society's Cancer Prevention Study II showed that each 10 g/m^3 increase in concentration of fine particles carried an increased lung cancer risk of 14 % [83]. Another study identified traffic as a source of carcinogenic air pollution and observed an association with lung cancer risk [84].

In many developed nations, indoor air pollution has been considerably reduced in recent years. Asbestos may remain an indoor exposure risk; however, its concentrations are generally very low [85]. In developing nations, a major concern for indoor air pollution has been the use of solid fuels, specifically coal, for heating and cooking. One study showed that compared to stoves without vents, the simple addition of a chimney to the stove decreased lung cancer risk by greater than 40 % [86]. Another study revealed that burning coal for cooking and heating was associated with greater lung cancer risk than burning biomass [87].

Diet and Physical Activity

Lifestyle factors other than cigarette smoking, such as diet and exercise, have been extensively investigated for a potential role in influencing lung cancer risk. In a review on this topic, the evidence was judged to be either "convincing" or "probable" that lung cancer was inversely associated with intake of non-starchy vegetables, fruits, and foods containing compounds such as carotenoids, selenium, quercetin, and calcium [88]. There has also been interest in the potential protective effects of specific fruits and vegetables; for example, higher intakes of cruciferous vegetables, which contain isothiocyanates, have been consistently inversely associated with lung cancer risk [89].

On the other hand, the evidence was judged to be "probable" that consumption of red meat, processed meat, butter, and foods containing animal fat was associated with increased lung cancer risk. Elevated concentrations of arsenic in drinking water are also associated with increased lung cancer risk [90].

With respect to physical activity and lung cancer, the World Cancer Research Fund review judged the evidence to be "probable" that increased physical activity is inversely associated with lung cancer risk [88]. Consistent with this conclusion, a meta-analysis of leisure-time activity observed that both moderate and high levels of physical activity were associated with a 13–30 % decrease in lung cancer risk [91]. Further investigation will be required to elucidate the mechanisms of action whereby physical activity reduces the risk of lung cancer.

Host Factors

History of Lung Disease

Preexisting lung disease may increase the risk for lung cancer. The association has been difficult to characterize, as common risk factors for both acquired lung disease and lung cancer make it a complex issue.

Chronic Obstructive Pulmonary Disease

There is substantial evidence relating chronic obstructive pulmonary disease to lung cancer. However, the fact that cigarette smoking is the major cause of both diseases makes it difficult to distinguish if COPD is truly a lung cancer risk factor or rather if the co-occurrence of both conditions is due to the shared risk factor of cigarette smoking. To address this issue, studies have been conducted in individuals who never smoked. In one such study, emphysema (hazard ratio 1.66) and the combination of emphysema and chronic bronchitis (hazard ratio 2.44) were associated with increased risk of lung cancer mortality [92]. Chronic bronchitis by itself, however, was not significantly associated. A study looking at smokers concluded that the presence of chronic bronchitis or emphysema increased the risk for developing lung cancer by 29 %, independent of smoking history [93]. The fact that lung cancer risk remains elevated in both smokers and nonsmokers supports the hypothesis that COPD is a risk factor for lung cancer.

Tuberculosis

Since the mid-1800s, it has been hypothesized that tuberculosis may be associated with lung cancer [94]. Currently, the evidence shows that tuberculosis patients have an increased risk of lung cancer, but it is uncertain whether the increased risk can be attributed to tuberculosis or rather characteristics of tuberculosis patients, such as high smoking prevalence, that place them at increased lung cancer risk [95–98].

Genetic Susceptibility

The increased risk generated by a family history of lung cancer indicates the potential for genetic predisposition [99]. Varying degrees of susceptibility also help explain why only a minority of smokers ever develop lung cancer. In a large study of nonsmokers, the association between family history and lung cancer risk was strongest for those aged 40–59 years, suggesting that genetics may play a larger role in earlier onset cancers [100].

Even with the vast majority of lung cancers caused by smoking, only a minority of smokers develop lung cancer [64]. This makes it important to understand the determinants of interindividual susceptibility. Characterizing genetic profiles that enhance lung cancer susceptibility will help identify individuals at greatest risk. Identifying the specific germ-line genetic variants or somatic genetic mutations associated with lung cancer would aid in characterizing the sequence of molecular events that lead to carcinogenesis. Such discoveries hold the potential for finding novel targets for therapy.

Current efforts at finding genetic markers with diagnostic and prognostic significance have focused on single-nucleotide polymorphisms (SNP) in a number of genes, including those in pathways related to DNA repair, inflammation, and carcinogen metabolism [101–103]. Due to the enormous sample sizes required for appropriately powered genetic studies, few candidate SNPs have been validated by replication studies focused on any form of cancer. A large meta-analysis combining the evidence from studies of greater than 1,000 SNPs in all of the DNA repair pathways found only two that showed "strong credibility" to be causally associated with cancer. Both of these polymorphisms, found in the XRCC1 and ERCC2 genes, were associated with lung cancer risk [104]. It remains to be determined how the identification of these genetic variants will translate to lung cancer diagnosis and treatment.

Chemoprevention

Another area of inquiry has focused on identifying chemopreventive agents for lung cancer that could be taken as a primary prevention strategy. We provide a few examples: β-carotene, selenium, and lipoxygenase inhibitors such as aspirin and statins. Based on evidence from observational epidemiologic studies, the provitamin A carotenoid β-carotene was once thought to be a promising agent for the chemoprevention of lung cancer. The Carotene and Retinol Efficiency Trial (CARET), a large, double-blind, placebo-controlled randomized study examined the effectiveness of β-carotene and retinol (vitamin A) supplementation in lung cancer prevention for those at high risk (smokers, former smokers, and former asbestos workers). This study was closed early after detecting a statistically significant 28 % increase in lung cancer [105]. Similarly, the Alpha Tocopherol β-Carotene (ATBC) Cancer Prevention Study, another large randomized clinical trial, also found an elevated incidence of lung cancer among smokers with β-carotene supplementation [106]. Currently, beta-carotene supplementation is not recommended for lung cancer prevention and is contraindicated in those with a history of smoking [107].

Selenium has anticancer properties, perhaps due to its essential role in the antioxidant enzyme glutathione peroxidase or an anti-inflammatory effect by blocking the 5-lipoxygenase pathway [108]. A clinical trial of nonmelanoma skin cancer patients observed as a secondary outcome that selenium supplementation was inversely associated with lung cancer risk [109, 110]. Currently, a trial is enrolling patients with previously resected stage I non-small cell lung cancer to determine if selenium supplementation can reduce the risk of second primary lung cancers (ECOG-5597). This trial aims to complete the data collection period by November 2014. The Selenium and Vitamin E Cancer Prevention Trial (SELECT) reported no effect of selenium supplementation by itself or in conjunction with vitamin E on lung cancer incidence or mortality [111].

The evidence from cohort studies of the association between aspirin use and lung cancer has been suggestive of an inverse association, but this has not been true in all studies [112]. Other nonsteroidal anti-inflammatory drugs (NSAIDs) have also been studied. One case–control study found NSAIDs other than aspirin to provide a modest reduction in lung cancer risk [113], whereas other case–control studies of COX-2-selective inhibitors found a more pronounced effect [114].

A potential protective role of statins on lung cancer risk has been explored. Most studies found no significant difference in risk of lung cancer between users and nonusers of statins [115]. A large nested case–control study, however, found a strong inverse association between statin use for greater than 6 months duration and lung cancer [116]. With the widespread use of statins in the USA, a more definitive assessment of the potential impact of statins on lung cancer risk is needed.

Conclusion

Lung cancer continues to be the leading cause of cancer death in the United States and in developed nations worldwide. The prevention, diagnosis, and treatment of lung cancer will continue to be of major importance in the coming decades [117]. Primary prevention strategies that prevent exposure to risk factors such as cigarette smoke, asbestos, and radon hold promise for continuing to achieve reductions in the population burden of lung cancer. Preventive efforts contributing to this trend extend from the arena of public policy down to individual behavior modification. By far the most central strategy needs to be continued emphasis on prevention of initiation and cessation of smoking.

References

1. American Cancer Society. Cancer facts and figures 2010. Atlanta: American Cancer Society; 2010.
2. Doll R, Hill AB. Smoking and carcinoma of the lung; preliminary report. Br Med J. 1950;2(4682): 739–48.
3. Levin ML, Goldstein H, Gerhardt PR. Cancer and tobacco smoking; a preliminary report. J Am Med Assoc. 1950;143(4):336–8.
4. Wynder EL, Graham EA. Tobacco smoking as a possible etiologic factor in bronchiogenic carcinoma; a study of 684 proved cases. J Am Med Assoc. 1950;143(4):329–36.
5. Doll R, Peto R. Cigarette smoking and bronchial carcinoma: dose and time relationships among regular smokers and lifelong non-smokers. J Epidemiol Community Health. 1978;32(4):303–13.
6. Doll R, Hill AB. Lung cancer and other causes of death in relation to smoking; a second report on the mortality of British doctors. Br Med J. 1956;2: 1071–81.
7. U.S. Public Health Service. Smoking and health. Report of the Advisory Committee to the surgeon general. US Department of Health, Education, and Welfare, Public Health Service, Center for Diseases Control. PHS publication no. 1103. Washington, DC: GPO; 1964.
8. White C. Research on smoking and lung cancer: a landmark in the history of chronic disease epidemiology. Yale J Biol Med. 1990;63(1):29–46.
9. US National Cancer Institute. Surveillance, Epidemiology, and End Results (SEER) Program. SEER*Stat Database: incidence—SEER 9 Regs Limited-Use, Nov 2007 Sub (1973–2008), National Cancer Institute, DCCPS, Surveillance Research Program, Cancer Statistics Branch, released April 2011, based on the November 2010 submission.
10. US National Cancer Institute. Surveillance, Epidemio logy, and End Results (SEER) Program (http://www.seer.cancer.gov) SEER*Stat Database: incidence—SEER 17 Regs Limited-Use+Hurricane Katrina impacted Louisiana cases, Nov 2010 Sub (1973–2007 varying), National Cancer Institute, DCCPS, Surveillance Research Program, Cancer Statistics Branch, released April 2011, based on the November 2010 submission.
11. Alberg AJ, Samet JM. Epidemiology of lung cancer. Chest. 2003;123(1 Suppl):21S–49S.
12. US National Cancer Institute. Surveillance, Epidemio logy, and End Results (SEER) Program (http://www.seer.cancer.gov) SEER*Stat Database: mortality—all COD, aggregated with state, total U.S. (1969–2007), National Cancer Institute, DCCPS, Surveillance Research Program, Cancer Statistics Branch, released April 2011. Underlying mortality data provided by NCHS http://www.cdc.gov/nchs.

13. Haiman CA, Stram DO, Wilkens LR, et al. Ethnic and racial differences in the smoking-related risk of lung cancer. N Engl J Med. 2006;354(4):333–42.
14. Pinsky PF. Racial and ethnic differences in lung cancer incidence: how much is explained by differences in smoking patterns? (United States). Cancer Causes Control. 2006;17(8):1017–24.
15. Belani CP, Marts S, Schiller J, Socinski M. Women and lung cancer: epidemiology, tumor biology, and emerging trends in clinical research. Lung Cancer. 2007;55(1):15–23.
16. Thun MJ, Jemal A. How much of the decrease in cancer death rates in the United States is attributable to reductions in tobacco smoking? Tob Control. 2006;15(5):345–7.
17. International Early Lung Cancer Action Program Investigators, Henschke CI, Yip R, Miettinen OS. Women's susceptibility to tobacco carcinogenesis and survival after diagnosis of lung cancer. JAMA. 2006;296(2):180–4.
18. Mao Y, Hu J, Ugnat AM, Semenciw R, Fincham S. Canadian cancer registries epidemiology research group. Socioeconomic status and lung cancer risk in Canada. Int J Epidemiol. 2001;30(4):809–17.
19. Li K, Yu S. Economic status, smoking, occupational exposure to rubber, and lung cancer: a case-cohort study. J Environ Sci Health C Environ Carcinog Ecotoxicol Rev. 2002;20(1):21–8.
20. van Loon AJ, Goldbohm RA, Kant IJ, Swaen GM, Kremer AM, van den Brandt PA. Socioeconomic status and lung cancer incidence in men in The Netherlands: is there a role for occupational exposure? J Epidemiol Community Health. 1997;51(1):24–9.
21. Ekberg-Aronsson M, Nilsson PM, Nilsson JA, Pehrsson K, Löfdahl CG. Socio-economic status and lung cancer risk including histologic subtyping—a longitudinal study. Lung Cancer. 2006;51(1):21–9.
22. Toh C-K, Gao F, Lim WT, et al. Differences between small-cell lung cancer and non-small-cell lung cancer among smokers. Lung Cancer. 2007;56(2):161–6.
23. Travis WD, Brambilla E, Müller-Hermelink HK, Harris CC, editors. World Health Organization Classification of Tumours: Pathology and Genetics of tumours of the Lung, Pleura, Thymus and Heart. Lyon: IARC Press; 2004.
24. Govindan R, Page N, Morgensztern D, et al. Changing epidemiology of small-cell lung cancer in the United States over the last 30 years: analysis of the surveillance, epidemiologic, and end results database. J Clin Oncol. 2006;24(28):4539–44.
25. Sun Z, Yang P. Gene expression profiling on lung cancer outcome prediction: present clinical value and future premise. Cancer Epidemiol Biomarkers Prev. 2006;15(11):2063–8.
26. Beane J, Sebastiani P, Whitfield TH, et al. A prediction model for lung cancer diagnosis that integrates genomic and clinical features. Cancer Prev Res (Phila). 2008;1(1):56–64.
27. Director's Challenge Consortium for the Molecular Classification of Lung Adenocarcinoma, Shedden K, Taylor JM, et al. Gene expression-based survival prediction in lung adenocarcinoma: a multi-site, blinded validation study. Nat Med. 2008;14(8):822–7.
28. Samet JM. Lung cancer. In: Greenwald P, Kramer BS, Weed DL, editors. Cancer prevention and control. New York, NY: Marcel Dekker, Inc.; 1995. p. 561–4.
29. Peto R. Influence of dose and duration of smoking on lung cancer rates. IARC Sci Publ. 1986;74: 23–33.
30. US Department of Health and Human Services (US-DHHS). Smoking and health: a national status report. Washington, DC: US Government Printing Office; 1987.
31. Alberg AJ, Ford JG, Samet JM, American College of Chest Physicians. Epidemiology of lung cancer: ACCP evidence-based clinical practice guidelines (2nd edition). Chest. 2007;132(3 Suppl):29S–55S.
32. Wu X, Lin J, Etzel CJ, et al. Interplay between mutagen sensitivity and epidemiological factors in modulating lung cancer risk. Int J Cancer. 2007;120(12): 2687–95.
33. Smoking and Tobacco Control Monograph 9. Cigars: health effects and trends. NIH publication no. 98–4302. Bethesda, MD: U.S. Department of Health and Human Services, National Institutes of Health (NIH), National Cancer Institute; 1998.
34. Boffetta P, Pershagen G, Jöckel KH, et al. Cigar and pipe smoking and lung cancer risk: a multicenter study from Europe. J Natl Cancer Inst. 1999;91(8): 697–701.
35. Mehra R, Moore BA, Crothers K, Tetrault J, Fiellin DA. The association between marijuana smoking and lung cancer. Arch Intern Med. 2006;166(13): 1359–67.
36. Hashibe M, Straif K, Tashkin DP, Morgenstern H, Greenland S, Zhang ZF. Epidemiologic review of marijuana use and cancer risk. Alcohol. 2005;35(3): 265–75.
37. American Cancer Society. Cancer prevention & early detection facts & figures 2007. Atlanta: American Cancer Society; 2007.
38. US Department of Health and Human Services. The health benefits of smoking cessation. A report of the surgeon general [DHHS publication number 90–8416]. Washington, DC: U.S. Government Printing Office, US Department of Health and Human Services; 1990.
39. Hrubec Z, McLaughlin JK. Former cigarette smoking and mortality among U.S. veterans: a 26-year follow-up, 1954–1980. In: Burns D, Garfinkel L, Samet JM, editors. Changes in cigarette-related disease risks and their implication for prevention and control. Bethesda, MD: U.S. Government Printing Office; 1997. p. 501–30.
40. Fiore M, Bailey W, Cohen S. Treating tobacco use and dependence. Clinical practice guideline. Rockville, MD: US Department of Health and Human Services. Public Health Service; 2000.
41. Clinical Practice Guideline Treating Tobacco Use and Dependence 2008 Update Panel, Liaisons, and

Staff. A clinical practice guideline for treating tobacco use and dependence: 2008 update. A U.S. Public Health Service report. Am J Prev Med. 2008;35(2):158–76.
42. Centers for Disease Control and Prevention (US). Best practices for comprehensive tobacco control programs—August 1999. Atlanta: Department of Health and Human Services, Centers for Disease Control and Prevention, National Center for Chronic Disease Prevention and Health Promotion, Office on Smoking and Health; 1999.
43. US Department of Health and Human Services. The health consequences of involuntary smoking: a report of the surgeon general. DHHS publication no. (CDC) 87–8398. Washington, DC: U.S. Government Printing Office; 1986.
44. US Department of Health and Human Services. The health consequences of involuntary exposure to tobacco smoke: a report of the surgeon general. Washington, DC: US Department of Health and Human Services, Centers for Disease Control and Prevention, National Center for Chronic Disease and Prevention and Health Promotion, Office of Smoking and Health; 2006.
45. Boffetta P. Involuntary smoking and lung cancer. Scand J Work Environ Health. 2002;28 Suppl 2:30–40.
46. Taylor R, Cumming R, Woodward A, Black M. Passive smoking and lung cancer: a cumulative meta-analysis. Aust N Z J Public Health. 2001;25(3):203–11.
47. Doll R, Peto R. The causes of cancer: quantitative estimates of avoidable risks of cancer in the United States today. J Natl Cancer Inst. 1981;66(6):1191–308.
48. Alberg AJ, Yung R, Strickland PT, Nelson J. Respiratory cancer and exposure to arsenic, chromium, nickel and polycyclic aromatic hydrocarbons. Clin Occup Environ Med. 2002;2:779–801.
49. Lynch KM, Smith WA. Pulmonary asbestosis: V. A report of bronchial carcinoma and epithelial metaplasia. Am J Cancer. 1939;36(4):567–73.
50. Wedler HW. Asbestosis and pulmonary carcinoma (asbestose und lungenkrebs). Bull Hyg. 1944;19:362.
51. Doll R. Mortality from lung cancer in asbestos workers. Br J Ind Med. 1955;12(2):81–6.
52. Selikoff IJ, Churg J, Hammond EC. Asbestos exposure and neoplasia. JAMA. 1964;188(1):22–6.
53. Selikoff IJ, Hammond EC, Seidman H. Mortality experience of insulation workers in the United States and Canada, 1943–1976. Ann N Y Acad Sci. 1979;330:91–116.
54. Newhouse ML, Berry G. Patterns of mortality in asbestos factory workers in London. Ann N Y Acad Sci. 1979;330:53–60.
55. Wraith D, Mengersen K. Assessing the combined effect of asbestos exposure and smoking on lung cancer: a Bayesian approach. Stat Med. 2007;26(5):1150–69.
56. Churg A, Stevens B. Enhanced retention of asbestos fibers in the airways of human smokers. Am J Respir Crit Care Med. 1995;151(5):1409–13.
57. MacMahon B. Some recent issues in low-exposure radiation epidemiology. Environ Health Perspect. 1989;81:131–5.
58. Boice Jr JD. Studies of atomic bomb survivors. Understanding radiation effects. JAMA. 1990; 264(5):622–3.
59. Pierce DA, Sharp GB, Mabuchi K. Joint effects of radiation and smoking on lung cancer risk among atomic bomb survivors. Radiat Res. 2003;159(4):511–20.
60. Preston DL, Shimizu Y, Pierce DA, Suyama A, Mabuchi K. Studies of mortality of atomic bomb survivors. Report 13: solid cancer and noncancer disease mortality: 1950–1997. Radiat Res. 2003; 160(4):381–407.
61. Hendee WR. Estimation of radiation risks. BEIR V and its significance for medicine. JAMA. 1992;268(5):620–4.
62. Prise KM, Folkard M, Michael BD. Bystander responses induced by low LET radiation. Oncogene. 2003;22(45):7043–9.
63. Hall EJ, Hei TK. Genomic instability and bystander effects induced by high-LET radiation. Oncogene. 2003;22(45):7034–42.
64. Institute of Medicine. Health effects of exposure to radon (BEIR VI). Washington, DC: National Academy Press, National Research Council (NRC), Committee on Health Risks of Exposure to Radon, Board on Radiation Effects Research, Commission on Life Sciences; 1999.
65. Pirozynski M. 100 years of lung cancer. Respir Med. 2006;100(12):2073–84.
66. Lubin JH, Boice Jr JD, Edling C, et al. Lung cancer in radon-exposed miners and estimation of risk from indoor exposure. J Natl Cancer Inst. 1995;87(11): 817–27.
67. National Research Council of the National Academies, Committee to Assess Health Risks from Exposure to Low Levels of Ionizing Radiation. Health risks from exposure to low levels of ionizing radiation BEIR VII-phase 2. Washington, DC: The National Academies Press; 2005.
68. Schmid K, Kuwert T, Drexler H. Radon in indoor spaces: an underestimated risk factor for lung cancer in environmental medicine. Dtsch Arztebl Int. 2010;107(11):181–6.
69. Shimizu Y, Kato H, Schull WJ. Studies of the mortality of A-bomb survivors. 9. Mortality, 1950–1985: part 2. Cancer mortality based on the recently revised doses (DS86). Radiat Res. 1990;121(2):120–41.
70. Davis FG, Boice Jr JD, Hrubec Z, Monson RR. Cancer mortality in a radiation-exposed cohort of Massachusetts tuberculosis patients. Cancer Res. 1989;49(21):6130–6.
71. Howe GR. Lung cancer mortality between 1950 and 1987 after exposure to fractionated moderate-dose-rate ionizing radiation in the Canadian fluoroscopy cohort study and a comparison with lung cancer mortality in the atomic bomb survivors study. Radiat Res. 1995;142(3):295–304.
72. Prochazka M, Hall P, Gagliardi G, et al. Ionizing radiation and tobacco use increases the risk of a

subsequent lung carcinoma in women with breast cancer: case-only design. J Clin Oncol. 2005;23(30):7467–74.
73. Kaufman EL, Jacobson JS, Hershman DL, Desai M, Neugut AI. Effect of breast cancer radiotherapy and cigarette smoking on risk of second primary lung cancer. J Clin Oncol. 2008;26(3):392–8.
74. Lorigan P, Radford J, Howell A, Thatcher N. Lung cancer after treatment for Hodgkin's lymphoma: a systematic review. Lancet Oncol. 2005;6(10):773–9.
75. Rajaraman P, Sigurdson AJ, Doody MM, et al. Lung cancer risk among US radiologic technologists, 1983–1998. Int J Cancer. 2006;119(10):2481–6.
76. Boffetta P, Mannetje A, Zaridze D, et al. Occupational X-ray examinations and lung cancer risk. Int J Cancer. 2005;115(2):263–7.
77. de González AB, Kim KP, Samet JM. Radiation-induced cancer risk from annual computed tomography for patients with cystic fibrosis. Am J Respir Crit Care Med. 2007;176(10):970–3.
78. National Research Council. Epidemiology and air pollution. Washington, DC: National Academy Press, National Research Council (NRC), Commission on Life Sciences, Board on Toxicology and Environmental Health Hazards, Committee on the Epidemiology of Air Pollutants; 1985. p. 1–224.
79. Laden F, Hart JE, Eschenroeder A, Smith TJ, Garshick E. Historical estimation of diesel exhaust exposure in a cohort study of U.S. railroad workers and lung cancer. Cancer Causes Control. 2006;17(7):911–9.
80. Davis ME, Smith TJ, Laden F, et al. Driver exposure to combustion particles in the U.S. trucking industry. J Occup Environ Hyg. 2007;4(11):848–54.
81. Garshick E, Laden F, Hart JE, et al. Lung cancer and vehicle exhaust in trucking industry workers. Environ Health Perspect. 2008;116:1327–32.
82. Dockery DW, Pope III CA, Xu X, et al. An association between air pollution and mortality in six U.S. cities. N Engl J Med. 1993;329(24):1753–9.
83. Pope III CA, Thun MJ, Namboodiri MM, et al. Particulate air pollution as a predictor of mortality in a prospective study of U.S. adults. Am J Respir Crit Care Med. 1995;151(3 Pt 1):669–74.
84. Raaschou-Nielsen O, Bak H, Sørensen M, et al. Air pollution from traffic and risk for lung cancer in three Danish cohorts. Cancer Epidemiol Biomarkers Prev. 2010;19(5):1284–91.
85. Health Effects Institute. Asbestos in public and commercial buildings: a literature review and a synthesis of current knowledge. Cambridge, MA: Health Effects Institute, Asbestos Research Committee, Literature Review Panel; 1991.
86. Lan Q, Chapman RS, Schreinemachers DM, Tian L, He X. Household stove improvement and risk of lung cancer in Xuanwei, China. J Natl Cancer Inst. 2002;94(11):826–35.
87. Kleinerman RA, Wang Z, Wang L, et al. Lung cancer and indoor exposure to coal and biomass in rural China. J Occup Environ Med. 2002;44(4):338–44.
88. World Cancer Research Fund/American Institute for Cancer Research. Food, nutrition, physical activity, and the prevention of cancer: a global perspective. Washington, DC: AICR; 2007.
89. Lam TK, Gallicchio L, Lindsley K, et al. Cruciferous vegetable consumption and lung cancer risk: a systematic review. Cancer Epidemiol Biomarkers Prev. 2009;18(1):184–95.
90. Celik I, Gallicchio L, Boyd K, et al. Arsenic in drinking water and lung cancer: a systematic review. Environ Res. 2008;108(1):48–55.
91. Tardon A, Lee WJ, Delgado-Rodriguez M, et al. Leisure-time physical activity and lung cancer: a meta-analysis. Cancer Causes Control. 2005;16(4):389–97.
92. Turner MC, Chen Y, Krewski D, Calle EE, Thun MJ. Chronic obstructive pulmonary disease is associated with lung cancer mortality in a prospective study of never smokers. Am J Respir Crit Care Med. 2007;176(3):285–90.
93. Littman AJ, Thornquist MD, White E, Jackson LA, Goodman GE, Vaughan TL. Prior lung disease and risk of lung cancer in a large prospective study. Cancer Causes Control. 2004;15(8):819–27.
94. Cicenas S, Vencevicius V. Lung cancer in patients with tuberculosis. World J Surg Oncol. 2007;5:22.
95. Aoki K. Excess incidence of lung cancer among pulmonary tuberculosis patients. Jpn J Clin Oncol. 1993;23(4):205–20.
96. Ramanakumar AV, Parent ME, Menzies D, Siemiatycki J. Risk of lung cancer following nonmalignant respiratory conditions: evidence from two case–control studies in Montreal, Canada. Lung Cancer. 2006;53(1):5–12.
97. Wu AH, Fontham ET, Reynolds P, et al. Previous lung disease and risk of lung cancer among lifetime nonsmoking women in the United States. Am J Epidemiol. 1995;141(11):1023–32.
98. Brenner AV, Wang Z, Kleinerman RA, et al. Previous pulmonary diseases and risk of lung cancer in Gansu province, China. Int J Epidemiol. 2001;30(1):118–24.
99. Matakidou A, Eisen T, Houlston RS. Systematic review of the relationship between family history and lung cancer risk. Br J Cancer. 2005;93(7):825–33.
100. Schwartz AG, Yang P, Swanson GM. Familial risk of lung cancer among nonsmokers and their relatives. Am J Epidemiol. 1996;144(6):554–62.
101. Shields PG. Molecular epidemiology of smoking and lung cancer. Oncogene. 2002;21(45):6870–6.
102. Berwick M, Vineis P. Markers of DNA repair and susceptibility to cancer in humans: an epidemiologic review. J Natl Cancer Inst. 2000;92(11):874–97.
103. Robles AI, Linke SP, Harris CC. The p53 network in lung carcinogenesis. Oncogene. 2002;21(45):6898–907.
104. Vineis P, Manuguerra M, Kavvoura FK, et al. A field synopsis on low-penetrance variants in DNA repair genes and cancer susceptibility. J Natl Cancer Inst. 2009;101(1):24–36.

105. Omenn GS, Goodman GE, Thornquist MD, et al. Effects of a combination of beta carotene and vitamin A on lung cancer and cardiovascular disease. N Engl J Med. 1996;334(18):1150–5.
106. The effect of vitamin E and beta carotene on the incidence of lung cancer and other cancers in male smokers. The Alpha-Tocopherol, Beta Carotene Cancer Prevention Study Group. N Engl J Med. 1994;330(15):1029–35.
107. Gallicchio L, Boyd K, Matanoski G, et al. Carotenoids and the risk of developing lung cancer: a systematic review. Am J Clin Nutr. 2008;88(2): 372–83.
108. Jackson MI, Combs Jr GF. Selenium and anticarcinogenesis: underlying mechanisms. Curr Opin Clin Nutr Metab Care. 2008;11(6):718–26.
109. Clark LC, Combs GF, Turnbull BW, et al. Effects of selenium supplementation for cancer prevention in patients with carcinoma of the skin. JAMA. 1996; 276(24):1957–63.
110. Mahabir S, Spitz MR, Barrera SL, Beaver SH, Etzel C, Forman MR. Dietary zinc, copper and selenium, and risk of lung cancer. Int J Cancer. 2007;120(5): 1108–15.
111. Lippman SM, Klein EA, Goodman PJ, et al. Effect of selenium and vitamin E on risk of prostate cancer and other cancers: the selenium and vitamin E cancer prevention trial (SELECT). JAMA. 2009; 301(1):39–51.
112. Bosetti C, Gallus S, La Vecchia C. Aspirin and cancer risk: an updated quantitative review to 2005. Cancer Causes Control. 2006;17(7):871–88.
113. Hernández-Díaz S, García Rodríguez LA. Nonsteroidal anti-inflammatory drugs and risk of lung cancer. Int J Cancer. 2007;120(7):1565–72.
114. Harris RE, Beebe-Donk J, Alshafie GA. Cancer chemoprevention by cyclooxygenase 2 (COX-2) blockade: results of case control studies. Subcell Biochem. 2007;42:193–212.
115. Setoguchi S, Glynn RJ, Avorn J, Mogun H, Schneeweiss S. Statins and the risk of lung, breast, and colorectal cancer in the elderly. Circulation. 2007;115(1):27–33.
116. Khurana V, Bejjanki HR, Caldito G, Owens MW. Statins reduce the risk of lung cancer in humans: a large case–control study of US veterans. Chest. 2007;13(5):1282–8.
117. Jemal A, Ward E, Hao Y, Thun M. Trends in the leading causes of death in the United States, 1970–2002. JAMA. 2005;294(10):1255–9.

Classification of Lung Tumors

2

Mostafa M. Fraig

Background

The first classification of lung tumors was published in 1967 by the International Association for the Study of Lung Cancer under the auspices of the World Health Organization. It was updated for the first time in 1981. The third edition of the same classification was published in 1997. The last published WHO classification was in 2004.

The WHO adopts a policy of making any classification based on methods and criteria that are easy to apply and reproduce in any setting anywhere in the world. For histopathologic diagnosis, hematoxylin and eosin (H&E)-stained histologic sections are the standard type of morphology that is followed for classification. The role of ancillary studies such as immunohistochemistry or molecular markers should be to confirm not to make the diagnosis. Differentiation along the epithelial vs. mesenchymal types of tissue would serve as a basis to differentiate most carcinomas from sarcomas. Within the epithelial category, carcinomas would be distinguished according to their further differentiation along glandular or squamous lineage. Undifferentiated carcinoma with neuroendocrine differentiation is reserved for small carcinoma with specific clinical and molecular implications. Combined or mixed differentiation could also occur [1]. The majority of tumors in the lung are carcinomas (90–95 %), with the remainder 5 % representing bronchial carcinoid and 2–5 % representing mesenchymal or other miscellaneous tumors [2].

Adenocarcinoma

This is a malignant epithelial tumor with glandular formation or mucin production. It is the most common type of lung cancer, especially in women and nonsmokers. The glandular differentiation could take the forms of acinar, papillary, solid, or micropapillary formations.

On imaging the tumor could present as a speculated nodule, ground-glass opacities or pneumonia-like picture, or multiple nodules with central lucency (Cheerios pattern). Grossly the tumors are soft white-tan with close proximity to the pleural surface or with pleural puckering when the pleura is involved by the tumor or the tissue reaction around it. Areas of necrosis could be seen as well as carbon pigments if the patient has been a smoker.

The lesion starts as a small precancerous lesion known as atypical adenomatous hyperplasia (AAH) where atypical cells with early molecular genetic aberration similar to those in adenocarcinoma in situ (AIS) appear in the lung. Their size is usually less than 5 mm in diameter

M.M. Fraig, M.D. (✉)
Division of Anatomic Pathology, Department of Pathology and Pulmonary Medicine, University of Louisville, 530 S. Jackson Street, Louisville, KY 40202, USA
e-mail: m.fraig@louisville.edu

J.G. Ravenel (ed.), *Lung Cancer Imaging*, Contemporary Medical Imaging,
DOI 10.1007/978-1-60761-620-7_2, © Springer Science+Business Media New York 2013

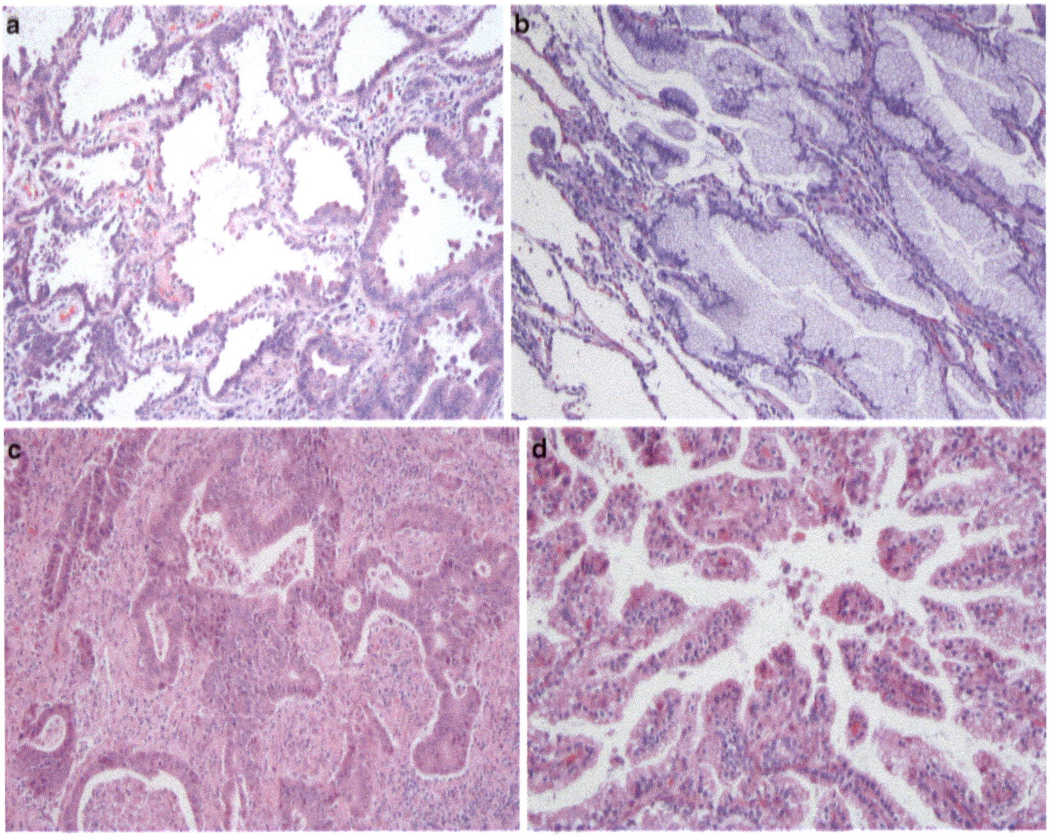

Fig. 2.1 Adenocarcinoma of the lung starts as (**a**) adenocarcinoma in situ (AIS) where the tumor cells line the pre-existing alveolar space in a lepidic pattern similar to birds sitting on a line or a fence. In (**b**) the same pattern is seen but with mucin-secreting cells in mucinous adenocarcinoma. (**c**) Invasive adenocarcinoma, acinar type where the tumor cells invade in a dense scar formed by a collagenous matrix and inflammatory cells representing the host response. The tumor cells assume a glandular pattern or form acini. (**d**) Papillary carcinoma is a variant of adenocarcinoma where the tumor cells form papillary fronds and tufts devoid of fibrovascular cores

and could be encountered in resected lungs for any other reason, and they are considered as "field effect." Microscopically the tumor could present with a "lepidic pattern," an expression used to describe birds sitting on a fence, where the tumor cells line the alveolar spaces without invading or invoking much of host response (Fig. 2.1a). The majority of patients with adenocarcinoma are smokers, but the occurrence of well-differentiated adenocarcinoma, AIS, is common in nonsmokers. This type of adenocarcinoma of the non-mucinous type is considered an AIS, as the prognosis of these tumors is considered 100 % survival at 5 years on complete resection. Once the tumor invades, and as long as the focus of invasion is less than 5 mm, the prognosis is still close to 100 % survival at 5 years. In the latter case, the tumor is called adenocarcinoma with minimal invasion (AMI). Any invasion beyond 5 mm makes the tumor an invasive adenocarcinoma [3]. The tumor formerly known as mucinous bronchioloalveolar carcinoma is now called mucinous adenocarcinoma as these tumors have a different presentation and immunohistochemical and molecular profile than AIS. These tumors can present as a multifocal disease, pneumonia-like pattern or as a solitary irregular area of consolidation on imaging studies. They are characterized by a copious amount of secreted mucin which patients often cough out.

The cells usually have enlarged nuclei with irregular nuclear contours but are basally located with an abundant amount of columnar cytoplasm (Fig. 2.1b). They differ from non-mucinous type in their reactivity to CK20 and variable staining with CK7, which is consistently positive in AIS. They have a variable staining for TTF-1 which is also usually positive in AIS. Mucinous adenocarcinoma has high level of Kras mutations as it is also associated with history of smoking. For those reasons, the biology and prognosis of mucinous adenocarcinoma are thought to represent a different entity from AIS even though they were previously lumped together under the term bronchioloalveolar carcinoma.

The subtyping of adenocarcinoma is based on the predominant pattern (acinar (Fig. 2.1c), solid with mucin production, papillary (Fig. 2.1d), and micropapillary), and these carry with them an increasing risk of worse prognosis, respectively [4].

Mucinous adenocarcinoma should always be differentiated from metastatic counterparts from other organs such as the breast, pancreas, and colon in addition to gynecologic tumors with similar morphology. Reactivity to such organ-specific markers as CDX2, in cases of metastatic colorectal carcinoma, is helpful in this regard.

By immunohistochemistry, adenocarcinomas react positively to thyroid transcription factor (TTF-1) in about 80 % of cases. Another marker is napsin A, which stains surfactant-producing cells as it also stains other tumors from the kidney, thyroid, and others. [5]. These two markers are very useful in differentiating poorly differentiated adenocarcinoma from poorly differentiated squamous cell carcinoma, along with other markers for squamous cell differentiation as p63 and/or CK5/6. Mucin stain can also be used as a cheap and quick method in identifying intracellular mucin secretion and as a proxy for glandular differentiation.

At the molecular level, adenocarcinomas express higher frequency of Kras mutation, especially in smokers (30 %). The revolutionary discovery of Epithelial Growth Factor Receptor (EGFR) mutation in patients with adenocarcinoma (especially women nonsmokers from Asian origin) and the introduction of tyrosine kinase inhibitor chemotherapy made it imperative to identify patients with adenocarcinoma and to test these patients for the mutation [6]. Other mutations such as EML 4-ALK mutation which is encountered less frequently than EGFR ones opened the door for more molecular testing and targeted therapy to these patients.

Squamous Cell Carcinoma

This is the second most common carcinoma in the lung. It is characterized by squamous differentiation with keratinization and formation of intercellular bridges corresponding to desmosomes on the ultrastructural level.

Over 90 % of squamous cell carcinoma occur in smokers. They are usually preceded by squamous metaplasia and dysplasia of the bronchial lining epithelium before progressing to squamous cell carcinoma in situ and finally into invasive squamous cell carcinoma. The tumor is usually centrally located; however, peripherally located tumors occur in a minority of cases.

On imaging, the central location of the tumor and proximity to relatively large bronchi and bronchioles are associated with obstruction and occlusion with the resultant collapse or atelectasis of lung segments distal to the tumor. These tumors could also extend to the hilar or mediastinal lymph nodes appearing as masses in those areas. Squamous cell carcinoma is the most common tumor to cavitate resulting in a thick-walled cavity with areas of central lucency. Grossly, the tumor is white or grey with black carbon pigments throughout. They may show necrotic center with stellate-shaped periphery. There may be central necrosis or polypoid growth pattern, especially when the tumor extends into the bronchial lumen.

Microscopically, the tumor shows keratin formation, the amount of which is proportionate to the degree of differentiation, more-differentiated tumor having more keratinization. The cells have large dark nuclei and a moderate amount of waxy eosinophilic cytoplasm. When the cells show cytoplasmic clearing, this would indicate clear

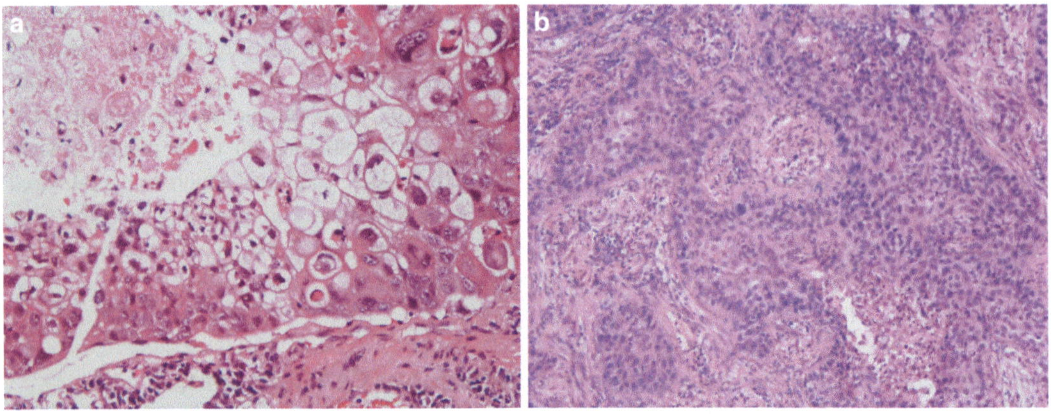

Fig. 2.2 Squamous cells carcinoma: (**a**) tumor cells with dark nuclei growing in sheets with thick cytoplasm and clear cell change in some of the cells. (**b**) Poorly differentiated squamous cell carcinoma where the tumor cells grow in sheets without keratin pearls but the same type of thick waxy cytoplasm

cell change, and the name clear cell variant is used (Fig. 2.2a). Sometimes the cells have a smaller amount of cytoplasm with dark and amphophilic color and peripheral palisading similar to that of basal cell carcinoma of the skin, which invoked the name basaloid variant of squamous cell carcinoma (Fig. 2.2b). When the cells still get smaller but with distinct borders, prominent nucleoli, and intercellular bridges, small cell variant is rendered in the diagnosis. This needs to be distinguished from small cell carcinoma or combined small cell carcinoma and squamous cell carcinoma based on the presence or absence of neuroendocrine differentiation.

Immunohistochemistry is very helpful in differentiating poorly differentiated squamous cell carcinoma from other types of carcinomas. Squamous cell carcinoma is usually positive for pancytokeratin, high molecular weight cytokeratin, and CEA. Two specific markers that are frequently used in practice for squamous differentiation are p63 and CK5/6. A more specific clone of p63 came into use recently and is known as p40.

On the molecular level, squamous cell carcinoma harbors EGFR, in about 84 % of cases. Expression of Her-2/neu is more frequent in adenocarcinoma but rare in squamous cell carcinoma as is the case with Kras activation [2].

Small Cell Carcinoma

This malignant epithelial tumor is characterized by small cells (2 times the size of a resting lymphocyte) with scant cytoplasm, ill-defined borders, granular chromatin, and absent or inconspicuous nucleolus. Extensive necrosis is usually present and mitotic activity is high. The cells exhibit nuclear molding where the nuclei are set together as a cobblestone pattern. The tumor shows a central location as in squamous cell carcinoma with early spread to hilar or mediastinal lymph nodes. The tumor spreads early to distant locations in the liver, adrenal glands, bone marrow, and possibly brain. It is frequently associated with superior vena cava obstruction and paraneoplastic syndrome.

On imaging, the tumor is usually associated with lung obstruction, atelectasis, and collapse of lung segments. Early spread to regional lymph nodes could manifest as hilar or mediastinal masses.

Grossly the tumors are white-tan, soft, and friable. Extensive areas of necrosis could be noted within the tumor. A minority of tumors (about 5 %) may present as solitary pulmonary nodules.

Microscopically the tumor presents as sheet-like growth with small nuclei and very scant

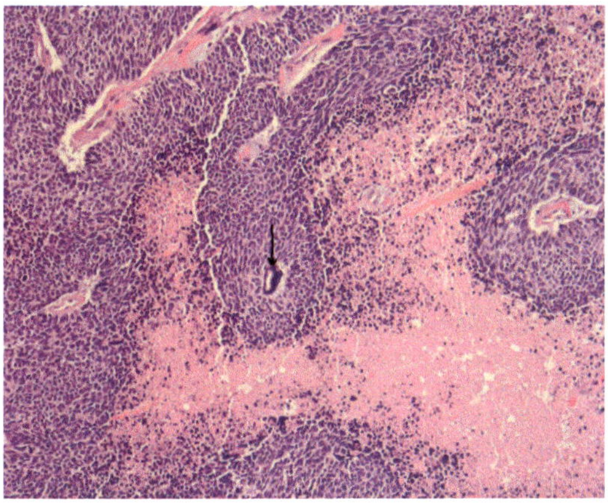

Fig. 2.3 Small cell carcinoma: small cells growing in sheets with nuclear molding and extensive areas of necrosis and Azzopardi effect (*arrow*). The cells have a scant amount of cytoplasm and no or inconspicuous nucleoli

amounts of cytoplasm around them. The chromatin is finely granular with absent or inconspicuous nucleoli. The mitotic activity is very high and extensive areas of necrosis could be seen. The smearing of loose DNA material around the walls of blood vessels is known as Azzopardi effect (Fig. 2.3). The combination of small cell carcinoma with other types of non-small cell carcinomas could be encountered. For this diagnosis to be made, there should be at least 10 % of the other components along with the small cell tumor.

By immunohistochemistry, small cell carcinoma is positive for neuroendocrine markers such as CD56, chromogranin A, and synaptophysin in a majority of cases. Less than 10 % of all small cell carcinoma are negative for all neuroendocrine markers. This possibility makes the diagnosis a morphologic one. On the other hand, other non-small cell carcinoma such as adenocarcinoma and large cell carcinoma could express one or more of the neuroendocrine markers. Small cell carcinoma is also positive for TTF-1 in up to 90 % of cases.

Small cell carcinoma should be differentiated from other neuroendocrine tumors as well as small round blue cell tumors. The neuroendocrine category includes large cell neuroendocrine carcinoma, atypical carcinoid, and typical carcinoid. In cases of carcinoid tumors, the mitotic activity is much lower (less than 10/2 mm^2) with lack of areas of necrosis and the presence of organoid pattern. Large cell neuroendocrine carcinoma usually shows prominent nucleoli and more abundant cytoplasm than that of small cell carcinoma; otherwise, the areas of necrosis and the immunohistochemical profile would be similar. Small round blue cell tumors such as primitive neuroectodermal tumors (PNET) are mitotically active than small cell carcinomas, and they mark for CD99 and not for cytokeratin or TTF-1. Merkel cell carcinoma, when it is metastatic to the lung, can be difficult to distinguish from small cell carcinoma on morphology alone. Positivity for CK20 and lack of TTF-1 positivity are helpful in distinguishing these two tumors from each other.

On the molecular level, small cell carcinoma is usually associated with a higher rate of p53 mutation than other non-small cell carcinomas as well as amplification of MYC and methylation of caspase-8, a key antiapoptotic gene.

Large Cell Carcinoma

Large cell carcinoma is an undifferentiated carcinoma that lacks either squamous or glandular differentiation on light microscopic evaluation. It has been used as a diagnosis by exclusion or a wastebasket group. In the era of targeted chemotherapy, this group of carcinoma is expected to decrease significantly in number as more testing is being performed to classify this group to either a squamous or adenocarcinoma category.

These tumors usually present anywhere in the lung and share similar gross pathologic characteristics with other lung cancers. Microscopically the cells are large (larger than two resting lymphocytes), and they grow in sheets with no specific configuration to suggest either squamous or glandular differentiation. The nuclei are large and vesicular with prominent nucleoli. Mitotic activity is usually high and areas of tumor necrosis could be seen Fig. 2.4.

A specific subtype of large cell carcinoma is large cell neuroendocrine carcinoma which is characterized by cells growing in organoid

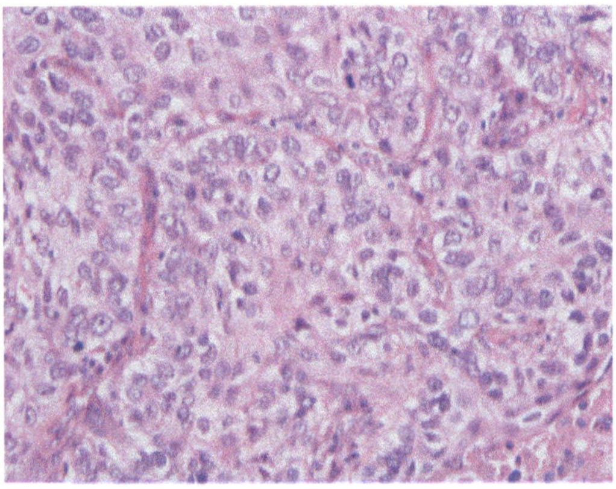

Fig. 2.4 Large cell carcinoma is a poorly differentiated carcinoma with no noticeable differentiation, either glandular or squamous, but grows in sheet with pleomorphic nuclei and a fair amount of cytoplasm

nesting, trabecular or rosette-like, and palisading patterns. The cells have an amphophilic cytoplasm, and the nuclei have prominent nucleoli as opposed to small cell carcinoma. Areas of tumor necrosis and high mitotic count are also characteristic features of this tumor. The tumor cells react positively to neuroendocrine markers such as chromogranin A, synaptophysin, and CD56.

References

1. Travis WD, Brambilla E, Muller-Hermelin HK, et al. Pathology and genetics. Tumours of the lung, pleura, thymus and heart. Lyon, France: IARC; 2004.
2. Hussain AN. Robbins and Cotran pathologic basis of disease. 8th ed. Philadelphia: Saunders Elsevier; 2010. p. 677–737.
3. Travis WD, Brambilla E, Noguchi M, et al. International Association for the Study of Lung Cancer/American Thoracic Society/European Respiratory Society International Multidisciplinary Classification of Lung Adenocarcinoma. J Thorac Oncol. 2011;6(2):244–85.
4. Noguchi M, Morikawa A, Kawasaki M, et al. Small adenocarcinoma of the lung. Histologic characteristics and prognosis. Cancer. 1995;15:2844–52.
5. Bishop JA, Sharma R, Illei PB. Napsin A and thyroid transcription factor-1 expression in carcinomas of the lung, breast, pancreas, colon, kidney, thyroid and malignant mesothelioma. Hum Pathol. 2010;41:20–5.
6. Paez GJ, Janne PA, Lee JC, Tracy S, Greulich H, et al. EGFR mutations in lung cancer: correlation with clinical response to Gefitinib therapy. Science. 2004;304: 1497–500.

Screening for Lung Cancer

3

James G. Ravenel

With the results of the National Lung Screening Trial (NLST) showing a reduction in lung cancer mortality of 20 % when comparing chest CT to chest radiography, a new dawn has broken in the fight against lung cancer [1]. Until this news, there was no proven method for early detection of lung cancer, and the primary tool was the difficult proposition of smoking cessation. While smoking cessation reduces the risk of developing lung cancer, up to 50 % of newly diagnosed lung cancers occur in former smokers [2]. In addition, once diagnosed, the burden of lung cancer on the healthcare system is tremendous with an estimated cost of treating lung cancer in the United States in 2004 of $9.6 billion dollars [3]. All of this points to a need for effective early detection and treatment that can save both lives and costs. While the NLST confirms the scientific basis of screening, there are certainly questions about feasibility and cost that still dominate the policy discussion (Table 3.1).

J.G. Ravenel, M.D. (✉)
Department of Radiology, Medical University of South Carolina, 96 Jonathan Lucas St Room 211, P. O. Box 250322, Charleston, SC 29425, USA
e-mail: ravenejg@musc.edu

Biases Inherent in Screening Studies

Important in understanding the screening debate are the various biases that occur in screening studies. Numerous prospective nonrandomized trials (everyone in the trial gets a CT) were performed in the preceding decade. While they can provide essential information on efficacy of detection, stage distribution, nodule characteristics, and inform management, they are limited by lead time, length time, and overdiagnosis bias, which limit the ability to detect a mortality benefit, the true measure of screening efficacy [4].

Lead time bias results from the earlier detection of a disease which leads to longer time from diagnosis to death and an apparent survival advantage, but does not truly impact the date of death. If you take two identical patients with identical tumors and apply screening to one, the screened individual will have earlier diagnosis and longer survival after diagnosis and yet succumbs to the disease on the same day as the unscreened individual. Length time bias relates to the relative aggressiveness of tumors. In a screened group, indolent tumors are more likely to be detected, while aggressive tumors are more likely to be symptom detected. This means indolent tumors will be overrepresented in a screened population and result in the appearance of a survival benefit compared with symptom-detected tumors. Overdiagnosis bias, the most extreme form of length time bias, is where the disease is

J.G. Ravenel (ed.), *Lung Cancer Imaging*, Contemporary Medical Imaging,
DOI 10.1007/978-1-60761-620-7_3, © Springer Science+Business Media New York 2013

Table 3.1 Criteria for effective screening

1.	The disease has serious consequences
2.	Screening population has a high prevalence of detectable preclinical disease
3.	Screening test detects little pseudo-disease (overdiagnosis)
4.	Screening test has high accuracy for detecting preclinical disease
5.	Screening test detects disease before the critical point
6.	Screening test causes little morbidity
7.	Screening test is affordable and available
8.	Treatment exists
9.	Treatment is more effective when applied before symptomatic detection
10.	Treatment is not too risky or toxic

detected and considered "cured." Under this scenario, however, if the disease had not been detected at all, it would never have caused symptoms, thus providing the illusion of a cure where none was needed.

This is not to say, however, that inherent biases do not occur in randomized control trials (RCT). In prospective RCT the intervention arm (in the case of lung cancer, CT) is compared to a control arm that consists of usual care. In each case participants are followed for a number of years after the intervention with reduction in disease-specific mortality as the end point of the following period. While randomization should lead to both arms of the trial containing similar populations, crossover of patients from the control arm to the intervention arm (e.g., a subject in the chest X-ray arm gets a CT outside the trial) can confound the results, potentially reducing the disease-specific mortality of the control arm and narrowing the screening benefit.

There are two other biases inherent in RCTs that need to be accounted for: sticky diagnosis and slippery linkage [5]. Sticky diagnosis refers to the increased likelihood of disease detection in the screened population. This means that the target disease has a higher likelihood of being listed as the "cause of death" even if not truly related. Thus, the apparent disease-specific mortality of the screened disease will be artificially increased. It is therefore important to have an independent review of deaths to assign appropriate causation in an RCT. Slippery linkage refers to the possibility that the downstream results of screening may lead to mortality without being attributed to the target disease itself. For example, a screen-detected nodule undergoes wedge resection and ultimately proves to be benign. If the subject subsequently dies from complications related to the procedure, for example, myocardial infarct, then the death would not be attributed to lung cancer. Thus, while the screening test and subsequent evaluation directly contribute to outcome, because death is not considered "lung cancer related" and not assigned to death due to the target disease, the value of screening may be overestimated. For this reason, a corollary end point to disease-specific mortality is all-cause mortality [5].

Screening with Chest Radiographs: A Historical Perspective

Radiographic screening for lung cancer dates back to the 1950s. The Philadelphia Pulmonary Neoplasm Research Project performed periodic photofluorogram screening on over 6,000 male volunteers with disappointing results. Although survival was slightly better in the screen-detected cancers vs. symptom-detected cancers, screen-detected cancers had the same outcome regardless of the time from the previous negative study [6]. At about the same time, the North London study randomized over 50,000 men, ages 40–64, to biannual chest X-rays over 3 years or chest X-rays at the beginning and end of the 3-year period. More cancers were detected in the study group (101 vs. 77), and the 5-year survival rate was better (15 % vs. 6 %), although this was not statistically significant [7]. The study also suffered from problems with randomization, as there were statistically more ex-smokers in the screened group and more participants aged 60–64 in the control group [8] (Table 3.2).

Observational nonrandomized trials of chest radiograph screening have showed promise. Case-control series of chest radiographs for lung cancer screening have been performed in Japan owing to the large amount of available data from

Table 3.2 Results of chest X-ray randomized control trials

			Baseline screen	Repeat screening	Lung cancer mortality
Study site	Study arm	Sample size	Cancers, no.	Cancers, no.	Per 1,000 person-years
London 1960–1964	All	55,034	51	177	2.2
	Intervention	29,723	31	101	2.1
	Control	25,311	20	76	2.4
Mayo 1971–1983	All	10,933	91	366	NR
	Intervention	4,618[a]	NA	206	3.2
	Control	4,593[a]	NA	160	3.0
Czechoslovakia 1976–1980	All	6,364	18	66	NR
	Intervention	3,172[a]	NA	39	3.6
	Control	3,174[a]	NA	27	2.6
MSKCC 1974–1982	All	10,040	53	235	NR
	Intervention	4,968	30	114	2.7[b]
	Control	5,072	23	121	2.7[b]
Johns Hopkins 1973–1982	All	10,386	79	396[c]	NR
	Intervention	5,226	39	194	3.4[b]
	Control	5,161	40	202	3.8[b]
PLCO 1993–2001 (All)	All	154,901	NR	3,316[d]	NR
	Intervention	77,445	NR	1,696[d]	1.4
	Control	77,456	NA	1,620[d]	1.4
PLCO 1993–2001 (NLST cohort)	All	30,321	NR	1,038[d]	NR
	Intervention	15,183	NR	518[d]	3.6
	Control	15,138	NA	520[d]	3.8

NA not available, *NR* not reported
[a]Randomization subsequent to baseline screen. Sample size of the study arms does not equal with the number of the total enrollees
[b]Randomization prior to baseline screen. Total number of deaths may include prevalence cases
[c]Includes 379 cancers detected during screening period and 17 cancers detected after the end of screening
[d]Cumulative cancers diagnosed

tuberculosis control programs. The first trial reported from Osaka estimated a 28 % reduction in mortality and better survival for those in the screen-detected group compared to those in the Osaka Cancer Registry [9]. Four more recent case-control series show an estimated mortality reduction between 30 and 60 % [10–13]. Pooling the data of these four prefectures resulted in an estimated mortality reduction of 44 % [14]. In Japan, however, lung cancer in females is a disease of nonsmokers, and female smoking-related cases were excluded to facilitate matching controls [10, 13]. In addition, a high proportion of male never-smokers were present in the Miyagi screening study.

In Varese, Italy, 2,444 heavy smokers were screened with chest radiography annually for 3 years. In the Varese trial, 16 cancers were detected during the prevalence screen, 31 % stage I, and seven cancers were detected during the two incidence screens, 71 % stage I [15]. The Turku Study in Finland studied 93 men out of 33,000 who had lung cancer detected on a one-time screen and compared them to those detected by symptoms or serendipitously noted on chest radiograph performed for other purposes. Screen-detected cases tended to be of an earlier stage and thus resectable (37 % vs. 19 %), and a 5-year survival was better in the screen-detected group (19 % vs. 10 %) [16].

Taken all together, the nonrandomized studies performed in Europe and Japan would seemingly give credence to an advantage to screening with chest radiographs. As pointed out previously, however, the biases present in the design of these studies make it impossible to definitively attribute the apparent benefit to screening. In fact this benefit could not be replicated in randomized controlled trials discussed below.

There have been a number of RCTs performed relative to chest radiograph. However, in all of these studies, the control group underwent some form of screening, though less frequently than the intervention arm. The Erfurt, Germany study was a nonrandomized trial with 41,000 males in the intervention group, who underwent biannual chest X-rays, and 102,000 males in the control group, who had chest X-rays every 18 months. The intervention group had a higher rate of cancers detected (9 % vs. 6.5 %), a higher resection rate (28 % vs. 19 %), and better 5-and 10-year survival. However, there was no difference in lung cancer or all-cause mortality [17].

The Czech Study on Lung Cancer Screening initially screened all participants with a chest X-ray and sputum analysis. After 19 prevalence cancers were excluded, 6,345 were randomized to either semiannual chest X-rays and sputum analysis for 3 years or a chest X-ray and sputum analysis at the end of the 3-year period. Both groups then received annual chest X-rays at 1-year intervals from years 4 through 6. Initial reports were promising, with earlier stage and more "curative" resections in the intervention arm [18]. Despite the fact that the lung cancer in the screened group was of earlier stage, almost 3 times as likely to be resectable, and had a better 5-year survival from time of diagnosis, there were actually more lung cancer deaths in the intervention arm, all-cause mortality was greater in the intervention arm, and smoking-related deaths were greater in the interventional arm [19]. In essence, there was no mortality benefit to screening nor did conclusions change with extended follow-up [20].

Under the auspices of the National Cancer Institute, three separate screening trials were performed in the USA during the 1970s [21]. Two of these studies, the Johns Hopkins study [22] and the Memorial Sloan-Kettering [23] study, enrolled over 10,000 males each into an intervention group who received annual chest X-rays and sputum cytology every 4 months and a control group receiving only an annual chest X-ray. While there was a slight benefit to sputum cytology at the prevalence screen, all-cause mortality was the same in both groups [24–26]. The results led to the conclusion that sputum cytology does not significantly improve the yield of chest X-ray screening.

The Mayo Lung Project randomized 10,933 participants into an intervention arm of chest X-ray and sputum cytology every 4 months and a control arm of "usual care" for 6 years [27]. Ninety-one prevalence cancers were detected with over 50 % postsurgical stage I or II and 5-year survival of 40 %. Prevalence cases tended to be of a more well-differentiated histology [28], and complete resection could be performed in twice as many screening participants compared to a previous cohort of over 1,700 patients. By the end of the trial, 206 lung cancers had been detected in the screening arm and 160 in the control arm. Although screen-detected cancers were more resectable (54 % vs. 30 %), there was no stage shift and no statistically significant difference between the groups in lung cancer mortality [29, 30]. With follow-up out to 20 years, no benefit could be detected in the screened group [31].

The latest trial of chest radiographs was performed by the Prostate, Lung Colorectal, and Ovarian (PLCO) trial [32]. As part of this study, 154,901 subjects were randomized to either 4 years of annual PA chest radiograph or usual care. Across the trial, incidence of lung cancer and lung cancer mortality did not differ significantly. As the large group included many subjects who were not "at risk" for lung cancer, a subset analysis was performed on subjects who would meet NLST criteria which included over 30,000 subjects. Although underpowered to detect a 20 % mortality reduction, there were similar number of lung cancers detected (518 intervention arm; 520 usual care) and slightly greater lung cancer deaths in the usual care arm (316 intervention arm; 334 usual care). Cumulative lung cancer mortality rates (per 10,000 person-years) were 36.1 in the intervention arm and 38.3 in the usual care arm (RR, 0.94; 95 % CI, 0.81–1.10). In essence even in the high-risk group, a statistically significant mortality benefit could not be clearly demonstrated for chest radiography.

Potential Harms Inherent in CT Screening

In general, the radiation dose risk/benefit ratio of CT favors performing CT in symptomatic individuals; however, there are some concerned that this will not be the case for lung cancer screening (criteria 6). Unlike the breast, the lung remains a radiosensitive organ well into the 6th and 7th decades of life and thus has the potential for developing a radiation-induced cancer. Brenner has suggested that annual CT screening resulting in a lung organ dose of 5 mGy from age 50 to 75 would increase the number of expected lung cancers by 5 %, and thus, the mortality benefit would need to exceed 5 % [33]. These risks could be mitigated by starting screening later or increasing time between screens. A risk/benefit analysis performed on the Italung screening trial concluded that there was benefit based on an expected mortality benefit of screening of 20–30 % and that excess mortality from screening would be closer to 1 % [34]. The discrepancy may in part be due to their calculations being based on total body dose rather than organ-specific dose. While this shows that the risk of radiation should not be a significant issue if there is a statistically significant mortality benefit to screening, it also suggests that in the absence of a mortality benefit, screening may not be neutral, but harmful.

While therapy for early stage lung cancer is good, it is not benign (criteria 10). In the ACOSOG Z0030 trial, the mortality for lobectomy by experienced thoracic surgeons was 1 % and complications occurred in 37 %. However, in the community at large, perioperative mortality (within 30 days) was 4.5–7.6 % for lobectomy depending on surgeon expertise [35, 36] and 4.9 % for a wedge resection [36], the operation performed if a nodule was shown to be benign at surgery. It is important to realize that the superiority of CT for the detection of abnormalities is not in question; however, CT identifies many smaller, "indeterminate" nodules, the majority of which will eventually turn out to be benign, but represent a diagnostic dilemma at the time of screening. While it has been suggested that with careful CT follow-up, PET imaging, and transthoracic needle biopsy, benign nodules will not be resected, evidence shows that even in experienced hands, 20 % of surgeries performed on screen-detected nodules are for benign disease [37].

Screening for Lung Cancer: Computed Tomography in Nonrandomized Trials

In the late 1990s, data began to emerge from nonrandomized trials of CT for the early detection of lung cancer in asymptomatic individuals. The most extensive early experience was in Japan with the three trials, Anti-Lung Cancer Association (ALCA) [38], Hitachi Employee's Health Insurance Group (Hitachi) [39], and Matsumoto Research Centre (Matsumoto) [40, 41]. These studies utilized older CT technology with 10 mm collimation for the CT scans. Two studies, ALCA and Matsumoto, included sputum cytology in the screening regimen, and screening was performed at 6-month intervals in ALCA. A total of 72 lung cancers were detected during the prevalence screen (0.4 %), 57 of which were stage IA (79.1 %). At the same time, noncalcified nodules were present in 2,564 (17 %, range 5–26 %) individuals. A total of 7,891 follow-up examinations have been reported in the ALCA study with 19 additional cancers detected, 15 stage IA (78.9 %). One incidence screen has been reported in the Hitachi study in 5,568 individuals with four additional detected lung cancers, three stage IA. In total, 8,303 incidence screens have been reported over 2 years in the Matsumoto study with a total of 37 cancers detected, 32 stage IA (86.5 %). A major consideration in the Japanese trials is that screening was made available at a younger age, usually 40, and that smoking history was not a requirement for participation (nonsmokers accounted for 14 % of the ALCA study, 38 % for Hitachi, and 53 % in Matsumoto). Thus, it is unclear that these results can be generalized to usual screening cohorts. This early data also set the stage for nonrandomized trials in Europe and the USA (Table 3.3).

Table 3.3 Results of selected nonrandomized CT screening trials

		Baseline screen				Annual repeat screening			
Study site	Date of publication	Patients screened, no.	Abnormal results no. (% of total)	Malignancies detected, no. (% of total)	Detected malignancies, stage 1, %	Patients screened, no.	Newly identified abnormal results, no. (% of total)	Detected malignancies, no. (% of total)	Detected malignancies, stage 1, %
Cornell University, United States (ELCAP)	1999, 2001	1,000	233 (23)	27 (2.70)	81	1,184	63 (5)	7 (0.59)	85
Matsumoto Research Center	2001	5,483	676 (12)	22 (0.40)	100	8,303	518 (6)	34 (0.41)	86
Hitachi Health Care Center	2001	8,546	NR	35 (0.41)	97	7,434	NR	7 (0.09)	100
Anti-Lung Cancer Association	2002	1,611	186 (11.5)	14 (0.87)	77	7,891	721 (9.1)	22 (0.28)	82
Milan, Italy	2003	1,035	199 (19)	11 (1.1)	55	996	99 (10)	11	91
Mayo Clinic, United States	2005	1,520	782 (51)	31 (2.0)	58	5,609 (est)	847 (15)	35 (0.20)	49
I-ELCAP	2006	31,567	4,186 (13)	405 (1.3)	86	27,456	1,460 (5)	74 (0.3)	86
Pittsburgh, USA	2008	3,642	1,477 (41)	53 (1.5)	60	3,423	1,450[a] (42)	27	33
Toronto, Canada	2009	3,352	600 (18)	44 (1.3)	73	2,686	NR (9–14)	21	48

NR not reported
[a]New or changed nodules

The International Early Lung Cancer Action Project (I-ELCAP) represents the most extensive nonrandomized trial to date. The nonrandomized International Early Lung Cancer Action Project (I-ELCAP) reported on over 31,000 prevalence screens and over 27,000 annual screens. From these subjects, they found 85 % with clinical stage I lung cancer resulting in a 10-year survival of 88 % for the stage I group. The percentage of stage I cancers and survival were much higher than traditionally reported for lung cancer [42]. In a related study, the authors found a statistically significant relationship between tumor size and tumor stage at smaller sizes. This trend was most pronounced with solid nodules [43]. However, survival is not a sufficient marker for mortality benefit, and without meticulous follow-up of all participants, the lung cancer mortality rate for their entire population cannot be known [44]. To illustrate this, in previous nonrandomized studies, lung cancer mortality rate estimates for the original ELCAP and Mayo CT screening study were estimated at 5.5 and 4.1 per 1,000 person-years, respectively, and are similar to the lung cancer mortality rates in both arms of the Mayo Lung Project (3.9 and 4.4 per 1,000 person-years) [45].

Screening for Lung Cancer: Computed Tomography in Randomized Trials

Two European randomized trials have produced somewhat disappointing results (Table 3.4). The Danish Lung Cancer Screening Trial (DLCST) randomized 4,104 subjects ages 50–70 with a least a 20-pack-year smoking history to five annual CT screenings or no screening [46]. There were 69 total cancers (detection rate 0.70 %) detected in the screened group compared with 24 in the control arm over the 5 years of imaging; however, late-stage tumors were similar in both arms, and no difference in lung cancer mortality between arms could be ascertained [47]. The DANTE study randomized 2,472 subjects ages 60–75 with at least a 20-pack-year smoking history to either CT screening or annual medical examination [48]. All participants had chest radiographs and sputum cytology at baseline. At 3-year follow-up similar to DLCST, there were more cancers detected in the CT group; however, the number of late-stage cancers was similar. The largest European screening trial, NELSON, is ongoing. This study which is closely aligned with the DLCST randomized over 15,000 subjects ages 50–75 who were current or former smokers who quit within 10 years who smoked at least a half pack of cigarettes for 30 years [49]. As designed the study has 80 % power to detect a 25 % mortality benefit. Final results from this study are expected around 2016.

The National Lung Screening Trial Screening for Lung Cancer

Trial Design

The NLST is the largest randomized CT trial performed and the only one so far to show a statistically significant mortality benefit (see below). The study began in late 2002 and accrued over 50,000 medically fit subjects between the ages of 55 and 75 who had at least a 30-pack-year history and were either currently smoking or had quite within the last 15 years to randomize 1:1 between annual CT for 3 years and annual frontal chest radiograph [1, 50]. Chest radiographs were chosen as the control arm due to the contemporaneous PLCO trial on the grounds that if the PLCO showed a mortality benefit for chest radiograph (it subsequently did not), then the control arm would remain valid [1]. The study was designed with 90 % power to detect a 20 % mortality benefit with CT. Technical parameters for CT are listed in Table 3.5.

Across both arms studies were well matched for age, race, gender, education, and smoking status. However, compared to the US Census-derived Tobacco Use Supplement, subjects in the NLST tended to be younger, better educated, and less likely to be smoking currently [51]. The latter fact raises questions about how generalizable the NLST experience will be to the entire US population.

Table 3.4 CT results of selected randomized controlled trials

		Baseline screen				Annual repeat screening			
Study site	Date of publication	Patients screened, no.	Abnormal results no. (% of total)	Malignancies detected, no. (% of total)	Detected malignancies, stage 1, %	Patients screened, no.	Newly identified abnormal results, no. (% of total)	Detected malignancies, no. (% of total)	Detected malignancies, stage 1, %
LSS feasibility	2005	1,660	332 (20)	30 (1.8)	53	1,398	361 (26)	8 (0.6)	25
DANTE Milan, Italy	2008, 2009	1,276	199 (16)	28 (2.2)	57	2,336 (est)	152 (6.5)	32	66
DLSCT	2009	2,052	331 (16)	17 (0.8)	53	NR	NR	NR	NR
Italung, Florence, Italy	2009	1,613	426 (30)	20 (1.2)	55	NR	NR	NR	NR
NLST	2011	26,309	7,191 (27)	297 (1.1)	54	48,817	10,955 (22)	423 (0.8)	59

Table 3.5 CT technical parameters in NLST

Positioning	Supine; arms over head
Inspiration	Suspended maximal
Voltage (kVp)	120–140
Tube current (mAs)	40–60
Collimation	≤2.5 mm
Reconstruction interval	1–2.5 mm
Reconstruction algorithm	Soft (lung optional)

Trial Results

Before the end of data collection, it became apparent that the 20 % mortality benefit for CT screening had been met and the results were released. In total 442 lung cancer deaths occurred in the chest radiograph arm compared with 354 in the CT arm resulting in a 20.3 % reduction in lung cancer-specific mortality and providing a scientific basis for CT screening [52]. In order to prevent one lung cancer death, the data shows that you would need to screen 300 subjects. An ancillary result was that all-cause mortality was significantly lower in the CT-screened group although the reasons for this are currently not clear. It should be noted that over 27 % of all subjects had at least one suspicious nodule detected on the baseline screening and that 39 % of CT arm participants had at least one suspicious nodule detected during the study. Of these, fewer than 4 % were ultimately proven to represent malignancy.

Future Directions

The exciting results have led to numerous organizations adopting guidelines for screening. Prior to widespread adoption, however, a multitude of issues need to be addressed. These include optimization of the target population, implementation of a standard screening CT protocol, and further understanding of risks associated with incidental findings and standardizing evaluation. From a public policy standpoint, cost efficacy needs to be determined, barriers to screening will need to be overcome, and the setting of care for screened individuals needs to be addressed [53].

Target Population

Currently data supports the screening of individuals 55–74 with at least a 30-pack-year smoking history. Inevitably, however, it leads to the question of what to do with individuals who lie just outside these windows. Both the National Comprehensive Cancer Network and American Association for Thoracic Surgery support with lower available evidence the inclusion of subjects over 50 or having slightly lesser smoking history (greater than 20 pack-years) [54, 55]. Screening this population should trigger an individual appraisal of the risks and benefits.

Screening Standardization

There are numerous screening protocols from the various trials that need to be harmonized. As such, imaging techniques, quality assurance, and radiation dose should be standardized across screening sites. In doing this it will be easier to optimize size and volume reporting as well as developing standards for nodule follow-up. Consideration also needs to be given to standardizing the reporting lexicon and definitions of positive screen results.

Cost-Effectiveness

While public policy in the United States has never utilized these estimates to decide on which healthcare interventions should be offered to the population, most cost-effectiveness ratios of accepted test and therapies in medicine cluster in the range of $10,000–$100,000 per quality-adjusted life years (QALY) [56]. Studies based on pre-NLST data have come to wildly different cost estimates ranging from $2,500 dollars per life year gained [57] to $116,300 for current smokers, $558,600 for quitting smokers, and $2,322,700 for former smokers [58]. Other models show more modest results with a range from $10,000 to $60,000 QALY depending on the prevalence of cancer and the estimate of lead time and overdiagnosis bias [59, 60].

Cost-efficacy data derived from the NLST is still pending and should provide a more direct measure of cost efficacy.

Barriers to Screening

The American public generally supports screening for cancer. In one study, 87 % thought that cancer screening was almost always a good idea [61]. Moreover, most are not dissuaded by false-positive results. In the same study, 38 % had experienced at least one false positive, yet the vast majority were still glad they had the test. However, unlike screening for breast, cervix, colon, or prostate, lung cancer screening targets a population with a specific poor health habit—cigarette smoking—and it is not clear whether this target group (smokers) as a whole values screening. Compared to nonsmokers, smokers are significantly more likely to be male, non-white, and less educated; report poor health status; or identify a usual source of healthcare [62]. Compared to nonsmokers, smokers also tend to have a nihilistic view of lung cancer and are less likely to believe that early detection would result improved survival. The implications is that there may be substantial obstacles to widespread screening of the at risk population.

Setting of Care

While it is likely that most screening discussions will occur within physician offices, a case can be made given the complexities of issues surrounding screenings, follow-up of result, and healthcare needs of tobacco users. In this regard multidisciplinary screening centers that bring together resources surrounding the care for smokers and ex-smokers are desirable [63]. The clinic could then provide a one-stop approach for the detection of pulmonary abnormalities, assessment of lung function, and need for smoking cessation counseling. They may also alleviate some of the anxiety surrounding screening by providing contemporaneous evaluation and discussion of CT results [64]. Most importantly, effective tobacco control will prevent more lung cancer deaths than CT screening will [65], and therefore, screening should not occur within a vacuum.

Managing Screen-Detected Nodules (<10 mm)

While a pulmonary nodule has been traditionally defined as a focal pulmonary opacity <3 cm on chest radiograph, the advent of widespread CT use and screening studies have identified many small nodules that would never have been detected by chest radiography. These nodules provide a particular challenge in general because although they have a high probability of being benign, it is difficult to predict the behavior of any particular nodule a priori. A second challenge is defining a nodule as it applies to screening, and it is clear that depending on the definition used, the reported prevalence of nodules will change. In recently reported studies, it is as low as 13 % for the I-ELCAP and as high as 27.3 % in the NLST [41, 66]. Combined with inherent difficulties in obtaining tissue from these small nodules, the typical approach is one of the watchful waiting to evaluate for changes in size and/or morphology that would warrant a more aggressive approach.

Solid Nodules

A nodule is considered solid if it obscures the underlying lung structure and the risk of malignancy is generally based on size, morphology, and risk factors. Assuming all screen-detected nodules are by definition in high-risk populations, the observations of size and morphology guide the initial management decisions, while growth is the key factor once a nodule is under periodic surveillance.

As has been previously noted, >95 % of nodules detected in the NLST turn out to be benign. This however accounts for all nodules or all sizes. Below the threshold of 1 cm, the risk of

Table 3.6 Fleischner Society recommendations for follow-up of small nodules

Nodule size	Low-risk patient	High-risk patient
Less than or equal to 4 mm	No follow-up	Follow-up in 12 months If no change in size—no follow-up
Greater than 4 mm up to and including 6 mm	Follow-up in 12 months If no change in size—no follow-up	Follow-up in 6–12 months If no change, follow-up in 18–14 months
Greater than 6 mm up to and including 8 mm	Follow-up in 6–12 months If no change, follow-up in 18–24 months	Follow-up in 3–6 months If no change, follow-up in 9–12 and 24 months
Greater than 8 mm	CT follow-up 3, 9, and 24 months. Also consider enhanced CT, PET, or biopsy	CT follow-up 3, 9, and 24 months. Also consider enhanced CT, PET, or biopsy

(From MacMahon H, Austin JH, Gamsu G, et al. Guidelines for management of small pulmonary nodules detected on CT scans: a statement from the Fleischner Society. Radiology 2005;237:395–400; with permission)

malignancy is <1 %, and for nodules ≤4 mm the risk of malignancy is approximately 0.2 % [67, 68]. Because of the low intrinsic risk of nodules in this size range, a guideline-based follow-up is generally appropriate. The guidelines as set out by the Fleischner Society (Table 3.6) prescribe periodic follow-up for a period of 2 years based on nodule size [69]. The absence of growth in a solid nodule after 2 years is said to indicate benignancy.

In a compliant screening population, some nodules regardless of size may safely be followed at 1-year time rather than intermediate time frame. In the NELSON study, nodules that were smooth, spherical, attached to the pleura or fissure or juxtavascular, and less than 500 mm^3 (8 mm diameter) were all nonmalignant at 1 year [70]. A common feature seen on CT is the intrapulmonary lymph node. The morphologic characteristics are similar to those nodules evaluated in the NELSON study, typically polygonal or oval, within 15 mm of the visceral pleura, often with linear attachment, and may be adjacent to a pulmonary vein [71, 72].

While seemingly straightforward, accurate measurement of size and growth is not always straightforward. The standard methodology in clinical practice uses electronic calipers on a PACS workstation. In a study of 54 nodules ranging from 3 to 18 mm in size, intra- and interobserver variability was ±1.7 mm [73]. As a practical matter, this suggests that manual changes less than 2 mm should be viewed with suspicion as indicators of growth nor should an apparent decrease of less than 2 mm be seen as regression. To overcome this inherent variability, a number of software programs have been created designed to segment and provide a volume measurement for small pulmonary nodules. The main advantage lies in the intrinsic reproducibility of the vendor-specific software measurement [74, 75]. For the most accurate depiction of volume, a thin slice collimation (preferably 1–1.25 mm or less) is required [76]. Because the segmentation parameters are not the same across software platforms, it is not clear that nodule volumes accurately translate across vendors. Another way to evaluate accuracy is to look at nodules using a "coffee break" design. In these studies the patient is scanned twice, the second time after getting off the scanner and back on. In these studies the volume variability approaches 10 % even for the most robust segmentation and may be up to 30 % for poorly segmented nodules, [77] and nodule volume is impacted by morphology [78], depth of inspiration [79], and cardiac cycle [80].

Coffee break designs provide a backdrop for assessing suspected growth, and knowing that volumes may vary by up to 30 % provides a reasonable window for defining rough stability. Volumetric analysis was specifically evaluated in a cohort of the NELSON trial and found that nodules <8 mm without apparent growth by volumetry at 3 months (2 months for incidence nodules) could be safely followed at 1-year intervals [81].

Table 3.7 Recommendations for follow-up of part-solid and ground-glass nodules

Nodule size	Nodule density	Follow-up
Less than or equal to 5 mm	Pure ground glass	None
Greater than 5 mm	Pure ground glass	Follow-up in 3 months for resolution
Greater than 5 mm	Pure ground glass Stable at 3 months	Annual follow-up for 3–5 years
Greater than 5 mm	Pure ground glass Growing or new solid component	Consider shorter interval follow-up (3–6 months) or surgical excision
Any size	Part solid	Follow-up in 3 months for resolution
Any size	Part solid Persistent	Consider shorter interval follow-up (3–6 months) or surgical excision
Any size	Part solid Persistent Solid core ≥10 mm	Consider PET/CT for staging prior to surgical excision
Any size; multiple	Pure ground glass or part solid	Follow-up in 3 months for resolution Base subsequent management on dominant lesion

(Adapted from Godoy MC, Naidich DP. Overview and strategic management of subsolid pulmonary nodules. Journal of thoracic imaging 2012;27:240–8, with permission)

Part-Solid Nodules

Nodules that either have a portion containing hazy, ground-glass opacity or are all ground-glass density are termed part-solid nodules (Table 3.7). As early as 2002 it was recognized that nodules with this density subtype had a higher rate of malignancy [82, 83]. It is now recognized that those that are malignant are frequently in the spectrum from preinvasive lesions (atypical adenomatous hyperplasia and adenocarcinoma in situ) to frankly invasive adenocarcinomas and that the relative solid component tends to predict histology [83]. In the screening or incidental detection setting, these need to be distinguished from benign etiologies such as acute inflammation and focal fibrosis.

Because the likelihood of malignancy for a pure ground-glass nodule less than 5 mm is sufficiently low, follow-up is generally not recommended. In cases where follow-up is desired or for lesions greater than 5 mm, the first follow-up is suggested in 3 months [84, 85]. This allows sufficient time for acute inflammatory nodules to resolve. Compared with persistent part-solid nodules, transient nodules are more likely to occur in younger subjects, males, and those that are smokers. Transient nodules may be multiple and tend to have ill-defined margins [85]. Unfortunately, there are no reliable findings to document benignity, necessitating short-term follow-up. As persistent nodules even when premalignant or malignant tend to grow quite slowly, further follow-ups are generally prescribed at 1-year intervals. At any point, increase in size or density should prompt more aggressive management. As percutaneous biopsy may not accurately reflect the correct diagnosis due to sampling error, surgical resection is favored [86]. It is difficult to know how long to follow nongrowing nodules. Volume doubling times for part-solid cancers may exceed 1,000 days [87]. Expert opinion suggests they should be followed at least 3 years [88].

In following part-solid nodules, both change in size and change in density must be considered. There is a continuum from preinvasive to minimally invasive to frankly invasive which seems to be reflected by nodule morphology. Pure ground-glass nodules are most often AAH or in situ carcinoma, and higher degrees of invasion are associated with solid components. In this manner a part solid may not change in diameter but rather fill in centrally. Paradoxically, lesions may decrease in size if the central invasive component and alveolar collapse retract the lesions margins [89]. Mass as defined as volume multiplied by mean attenuation +1,000 in early studies may be better able to predict future behavior than change in diameter [90]. In coffee break designs, the inter-scan variability in mean attenuation appears to be less than 10 % [91]. Finally, it should be noted that PET/CT is not reliable in the evaluation of part-solid nodules unless the solid component is greater than 1 cm as even malignant lesions may show little or no uptake [92, 93].

Conclusion

In a high-risk appropriately selected population, CT screening for lung cancer has the ability to reduce lung cancer mortality. An effective screening process needs to include adequate information for the participant, a clearly defined plan to deal with indeterminate nodules, and resources for current smokers to quit. Although not formally studied, tobacco cessation is at least as important if not more important than screening itself.

References

1. Aberle DR, Berg CD, Black WC, et al. The national lung screening trial: overview and study design. Radiology. 2011;258:243–53.
2. Tong L, Spitz MR, Fueger JJ, Amos CA. Lung carcinoma in former smokers. Cancer. 1996;78:1004–10.
3. Cancer Trends Progress Report—2005 Update. In: National Cancer Institute, NIH, DHHS, Bethesda, MD, December 2005.
4. Patz Jr E, Goodman P, Bepler G. Screening for lung cancer. N Engl J Med. 2000;343:1627–33.
5. Black W, Haggstrom D, Welch H. All-cause mortality in randomized trials of cancer screening. J Natl Cancer Inst. 2002;94:167–73.
6. Boucot KR, Weiss W. Is curable lung cancer detected by semiannual screening? JAMA. 1973;224:1361–5.
7. Brett GZ. Earlier diagnosis and survival in lung cancer. Br Med J. 1969;4:260–2.
8. Manser RL, Irving LB, Stone C, Byrnes G, Abramson M, Campbell D. Screening for lung cancer. Cochrane Database Syst Rev. 2001;3, CD001991.
9. Sobue T, Suzuki T, Naruke T. Efficacy of lung cancer screening; comparison of results from a case–control study and a survival analysis. The Japanese Lung Cancer Screening Research Group. Jpn J Cancer Res. 1992;83:424–30.
10. Tsukada H, Kurita Y, Yokoyama A, et al. An evaluation of screening for lung cancer in Niigata Prefecture, Japan: a population-based case–control study. Br J Cancer. 2001;85:1326–31.
11. Sagawa M, Tsubono Y, Saito Y, et al. A case–control study for evaluating the efficacy of mass screening program for lung cancer in Miyagi Prefecture, Japan. Cancer. 2001;92:588–94.
12. Nishii K, Ueoka H, Kiura K, et al. A case–control study of lung cancer screening in Okayama Prefecture, Japan. Lung Cancer. 2001;34:325–32.
13. Nakayama T, Baba T, Suzuki T, Sagawa M, Kaneko M. An evaluation of chest X-ray screening for lung cancer in Gunma Prefecture, Japan: a population-based case–control study. Eur J Cancer. 2002;38: 1380–7.
14. Sagawa M, Nakayama T, Tsukada H, et al. The efficacy of lung cancer screening conducted in 1990s: four case–control studies in Japan. Lung Cancer. 2003;41:29–36.
15. Dominioni L, Imperatori A, Rovera F, Ochetti A, Paolucci M, Dionigi G. Lung cancer screening in cigarette smokers in the province of Varese, Italy. Cancer. 2000;89:2345–8.
16. Salomaa ER. Does the early detection of lung carcinoma improve prognosis? The Turku study. Cancer. 2000;89:2387–91.
17. Wilde J. A 10 year follow-up of semi-annual screening for early detection of lung cancer in the Erfurt County, GDR. Eur Respir J. 1989;2:656–62.
18. Kubik A, Polak J. Lung cancer detection. Results of a randomized prospective study in Czechoslovakia. Cancer. 1986;57:2427–37.
19. Kubik A, Parkin D, Khlat M, Erban J, Polak J, Adamec M. Lack of benefit from semi-annual screening for cancer of the lung: follow-up report of a randomized controlled trial of population of high-risk males in Czechoslovakia. Int J Cancer. 1990;45: 26–33.
20. Kubik AK, Parkin DM, Zatloukal P. Czech study on lung cancer screening: post-trial follow-up of lung cancer deaths up to year 15 since enrollment. Cancer. 2000;89:2363–8.
21. Berlin NI, Buncher CR, Fontana RS, Frost JK, Melamed MR. The National Cancer Institute Cooperative Early Lung Cancer Detection Program. Results of the initial screen (prevalence). Early lung cancer detection: introduction. Am Rev Respir Dis. 1984;130:545–9.
22. Frost JK, Ball Jr WC, Levin ML, et al. Early lung cancer detection: results of the initial (prevalence) radiologic and cytologic screening in the Johns Hopkins study. Am Rev Respir Dis. 1984;130:549–54.
23. Flehinger BJ, Melamed MR, Zaman MB, Heelan RT, Perchick WB, Martini N. Early lung cancer detection: results of the initial (prevalence) radiologic and cytologic screening in the Memorial Sloan-Kettering study. Am Rev Respir Dis. 1984;130:555–60.

24. Melamed MR, Flehinger BJ, Zaman MB, Heelan RT, Perchick WA, Martini N. Screening for early lung cancer. Results of the Memorial Sloan-Kettering study in New York. Chest. 1984;86:44–53.
25. Melamed MR. Lung cancer screening results in the National Cancer Institute New York study. Cancer. 2000;89:2356–62.
26. Berlin NI. Overview of the NCI cooperative early lung cancer detection program. Cancer. 2000;89: 2349–51.
27. Fontana RS, Sanderson DR, Woolner LB, et al. Mayo lung cancer project: status report. Clin Notes Respir Dis. 1976;15:13–4.
28. Fontana R, Sanderson D, Taylor W, et al. Early lung cancer detection: results of the initial (prevalence) radiologic and cytologic screening in the Mayo Clinic Stu. Am Rev Respir Dis. 1984;130:561–5.
29. Fontana RS. The Mayo Lung Project: a perspective. Cancer. 2000;89:2352–5.
30. Fontana RS, Sanderson DR, Woolner LB, et al. Screening for lung cancer. A critique of the Mayo Lung Project. Cancer. 1991;67:1155–64.
31. Marcus P, Bergstralh E, Fagerstrom R, et al. Lung cancer mortality in Mayo Lung Project: impact of extended follow up. J Natl Cancer Inst. 2000;92: 1308–16.
32. Oken MM, Hocking WG, Kvale PA, et al. Screening by chest radiograph and lung cancer mortality: the prostate, lung, colorectal, and ovarian (PLCO) randomized trial. JAMA. 2011;306:1865–73.
33. Brenner DJ. Radiation risks potentially associated with low-dose CT screening of adult smokers for lung cancer. Radiology. 2004;231:440–5.
34. Mascalchi M, Belli G, Zappa M, et al. Risk-benefit analysis of X-ray exposure associated with lung cancer screening in the Italung-CT trial. AJR Am J Roentgenol. 2006;187:421–9.
35. Goodney PP, Lucas FL, Stukel TA, Birkmeyer JD. Surgeon specialty and operative mortality with lung resection. Ann Surg. 2005;241:179–84.
36. Little AG, Rusch VW, Bonner JA, et al. Patterns of surgical care of lung cancer patients. Ann Thorac Surg 2005;80:2051–6; discussion 6.
37. Crestanello JA, Allen MS, Jett JR, et al. Thoracic surgical operations in patients enrolled in a computed tomographic screening trial. J Thorac Cardiovasc Surg. 2004;128:254–9.
38. Sobue T, Moriyama N, Kaneko M, et al. Screening for lung cancer with low-dose helical computed tomography: anti-lung cancer association project. J Clin Oncol. 2002;20:911–20.
39. Nawa T, Nakagawa T, Kusano S, Kawasaki Y, Sugawara Y, Nakata H. Lung cancer screening using low-dose spiral CT: results of baseline and 1-year follow-up studies. Chest. 2002;122:15–20.
40. Sone S, Li F, Yang ZG, et al. Results of three-year mass screening programme for lung cancer using mobile low-dose spiral computed tomography scanner. Br J Cancer. 2001;84:25–32.
41. Sone S, Takashima S, Li F, et al. Mass screening for lung cancer with mobile spiral computed tomography scanner. Lancet. 1998;351:1242–5.
42. Henschke CI, Yankelevitz DF, Libby DM, Pasmantier MW, Smith JP, Miettinen OS. Survival of patients with stage I lung cancer detected on CT screening. N Engl J Med. 2006;355:1763–71.
43. Henschke CI, Yankelevitz DF, Miettinen OS. Computed tomographic screening for lung cancer: the relationship of disease stage to tumor size. Arch Intern Med. 2006;166:321–5.
44. Berg CD, Aberle DR. CT screening for lung cancer. N Engl J Med 2007;356:743–4; author reply 6–7.
45. Patz Jr EF, Swensen SJ, Herndon II JE. Estimate of lung cancer mortality from low-dose spiral computed tomography screening trials: implications for current mass screening recommendations. J Clin Oncol. 2004;22:2202–6.
46. Pedersen JH, Ashraf H, Dirksen A, et al. The Danish randomized lung cancer CT screening trial–overall design and results of the prevalence round. J Thorac Oncol. 2009;4:608–14.
47. Saghir Z, Dirksen A, Ashraf H, et al. CT screening for lung cancer brings forward early disease. The randomised Danish Lung Cancer Screening Trial: status after five annual screening rounds with low-dose CT. Thorax. 2012;67:296–301.
48. Infante M, Cavuto S, Lutman FR, et al. A randomized study of lung cancer screening with spiral computed tomography: three-year results from the DANTE trial. Am J Respir Crit Care Med. 2009;180:445–53.
49. van Iersel CA, de Koning HJ, Draisma G, et al. Risk-based selection from the general population in a screening trial: selection criteria, recruitment and power for the Dutch-Belgian randomised lung cancer multi-slice CT screening trial (NELSON). Int J Cancer. 2007;120:868–74.
50. Church TR. Chest radiography as the comparison for spiral CT in the national lung screening trial. Acad Radiol. 2003;10:713–5.
51. Aberle DR, Adams AM, Berg CD, et al. Baseline characteristics of participants in the randomized national lung screening trial. J Natl Cancer Inst. 2010;102:1771–9.
52. http://www.cancer.gov/newscenter/pressreleases/NLSTresultsRelease. Accessed 1 May 2011.
53. Field JK, Smith RA, Aberle DR, et al. International Association for the study of lung cancer computed tomography screening workshop 2011 report. J Thorac Oncol. 2012;7:10–9.
54. Jaklitsch MT, Jacobson FL, Austin JH, et al. The American Association for Thoracic Surgery guidelines for lung cancer screening using low-dose computed tomography scans for lung cancer survivors and other high-risk groups. J Thorac Cardiovasc Surg. 2012;144:33–8.
55. National Comprehensive Cancer Network. NCCN Clinical Practice Guidelines in Oncology: Lung Cancer Screening Version 1.2013. 2012.

56. Graham JD, Corso PS, Morris JM, Segui-Gomez M, Weinstein MC. Evaluating the cost-effectiveness of clinical and public health measures. Annu Rev Public Health. 1998;19:125–52.
57. Wisnivesky JP, Mushlin AI, Sicherman N, Henschke C. The cost-effectiveness of low-dose CT screening for lung cancer: preliminary results of baseline screening. Chest. 2003;124:614–21.
58. Mahadevia PJFL, Frick KD, Eng J, Goodman SN, Powe NR. Lung cancer screening with helical computed tomography in older adult smokers: a decision and cost-effectiveness analysis. JAMA. 2003;289:313–22.
59. Marshall D, Simpson KN, Earle CC, Chu C. Potential cost-effectiveness of one-time screening for lung cancer (LC) in a high risk cohort. Lung Cancer. 2001;32:227–36.
60. Marshall D, Simpson KN, Earle CC, Chu CW. Economic decision analysis model of screening for lung cancer. Eur J Cancer. 2001;37:1759–67.
61. Schwartz LM, Woloshin S, Fowler Jr FJ, Welch HG. Enthusiasm for cancer screening in the United States. JAMA. 2004;291:71–8.
62. Silvestri GA, Nietert PJ, Zoller J, Carter C, Bradford D. Attitudes towards screening for lung cancer among smokers and their non-smoking counterparts. Thorax. 2007;62:126–30.
63. Mazzone P. The rationale for, and design of, a lung cancer screening program. Cleve Clin J Med. 2012;79:337–45.
64. Rosen MP, Corey J, Siewert B. Establishing a computed tomography screening clinic. J Thorac Imaging. 2012;27:220–3.
65. McMahon PM, Kong CY, Johnson BE, et al. Chapter 9: the MGH-HMS lung cancer policy model: tobacco control versus screening. Risk Anal. 2012;32 Suppl 1:S117–24.
66. Aberle DR, Adams AM, Berg CD, et al. Reduced lung-cancer mortality with low-dose computed tomographic screening. N Engl J Med. 2011;365:395–409.
67. McWilliams AM, Mayo JR, Ahn MI, MacDonald SL, Lam SC. Lung cancer screening using multi-slice thin-section computed tomography and autofluorescence bronchoscopy. J Thorac Oncol. 2006;1:61–8.
68. Swensen SJ, Jett JR, Hartman TE, et al. CT screening for lung cancer: five-year prospective experience. Radiology. 2005;235:259–65.
69. MacMahon H, Austin JH, Gamsu G, et al. Guidelines for management of small pulmonary nodules detected on CT scans: a statement from the Fleischner Society. Radiology. 2005;237:395–400.
70. Xu DM, van der Zaag-Loonen HJ, Oudkerk M, et al. Smooth or attached solid indeterminate nodules detected at baseline CT screening in the NELSON study: cancer risk during 1 year of follow-up. Radiology. 2009;250:264–72.
71. Ishikawa H, Koizumi N, Morita T, Tsuchida M, Umezu H, Sasai K. Ultrasmall intrapulmonary lymph node: usual high-resolution computed tomographic findings with histopathologic correlation. J Comput Assist Tomogr. 2007;31:409–13.
72. Shaham D, Vazquez M, Bogot NR, Henschke CI, Yankelevitz DF. CT features of intrapulmonary lymph nodes confirmed by cytology. Clin Imaging. 2010;34:185–90.
73. Revel MP, Bissery A, Bienvenu M, Aycard L, Lefort C, Frija G. Are two-dimensional CT measurements of small noncalcified pulmonary nodules reliable? Radiology. 2004;231:453–8.
74. Gietema HA, Wang Y, Xu D, et al. Pulmonary nodules detected at lung cancer screening: interobserver variability of semiautomated volume measurements. Radiology. 2006;241:251–7.
75. Revel MP, Lefort C, Bissery A, et al. Pulmonary nodules: preliminary experience with three-dimensional evaluation. Radiology. 2004;231:459–66.
76. Ravenel JG, Leue WM, Nietert PJ, Miller JV, Taylor KK, Silvestri GA. Pulmonary nodule volume: effects of reconstruction parameters on automated measurements–a phantom study. Radiology. 2008;247:400–8.
77. Gietema HA, Schaefer-Prokop CM, Mali WP, Groenewegen G, Prokop M. Pulmonary nodules: interscan variability of semiautomated volume measurements with multisection CT—influence of inspiration level, nodule size, and segmentation performance. Radiology. 2007;245:888–94.
78. Petrou M, Quint LE, Nan B, Baker LH. Pulmonary nodule volumetric measurement variability as a function of CT slice thickness and nodule morphology. AJR Am J Roentgenol. 2007;188:306–12.
79. Goo JM, Kim KG, Gierada DS, Castro M, Bae KT. Volumetric measurements of lung nodules with multi-detector row CT: effect of changes in lung volume. Korean J Radiol. 2006;7:243–8.
80. Boll DT, Gilkeson RC, Fleiter TR, Blackham KA, Duerk JL, Lewin JS. Volumetric assessment of pulmonary nodules with ECG-gated MDCT. AJR Am J Roentgenol. 2004;183:1217–23.
81. van Klaveren RJ, Oudkerk M, Prokop M, et al. Management of lung nodules detected by volume CT scanning. N Engl J Med. 2009;361:2221–9.
82. Henschke CI, Yankelevitz DF, Mirtcheva R, McGuinness G, McCauley D, Miettinen OS. CT screening for lung cancer: frequency and significance of part-solid and nonsolid nodules. AJR Am J Roentgenol. 2002;178:1053–7.
83. Travis WD, Brambilla E, Noguchi M, et al. International association for the study of lung cancer/American thoracic society/European respiratory society international multidisciplinary classification of lung adenocarcinoma. J Thorac Oncol. 2011;6:244–85.
84. Godoy MC, Naidich DP. Overview and strategic management of subsolid pulmonary nodules. J Thorac Imaging. 2012;27:240–8.
85. Lee SM, Park CM, Goo JM, et al. Transient part-solid nodules detected at screening thin-section CT for lung cancer: comparison with persistent part-solid nodules. Radiology. 2010;255:242–51.
86. Franks TJ, Galvin JR, Jett JR, Naidich DP, Boiselle PM. Expert opinion: role of percutaneous biopsy of part-solid nodules in the IASLC/ATS/ERS international

multidisciplinary classification of lung adenocarcinoma. J Thorac Imaging. 2011;26:189.
87. Hasegawa M, Sone S, Takashima S, et al. Growth rate of small lung cancers detected on mass CT screening. Br J Radiol. 2000;73:1252–9.
88. Naidich DP, Bankier AA, Macmahon H, et al. Recommendations for the management of subsolid pulmonary nodules detected at CT: a statement from the Fleischner Society. Radiology. 2013;266(1):304–17.
89. Lindell RM, Hartman TE, Swensen SJ, Jett JR, Midthun DE, Mandrekar JN. 5-year lung cancer screening experience: growth curves of 18 lung cancers compared to histologic type, CT attenuation, stage, survival, and size. Chest. 2009;136:1586–95.
90. de Hoop B, Gietema H, van de Vorst S, Murphy K, van Klaveren RJ, Prokop M. Pulmonary ground-glass nodules: increase in mass as an early indicator of growth. Radiology. 2010;255:199–206.
91. Park CM, Goo JM, Lee HJ, Kim KG, Kang MJ, Shin YH. Persistent pure ground-glass nodules in the lung: interscan variability of semiautomated volume and attenuation measurements. AJR Am J Roentgenol. 2010;195:W408–14.
92. Kim TJ, Park CM, Goo JM, Lee KW. Is there a role for FDG PET in the management of lung cancer manifesting predominantly as ground-glass opacity? AJR Am J Roentgenol. 2012;198:83–8.
93. Okada M, Nakayama H, Okumura S, et al. Multicenter analysis of high-resolution computed tomography and positron emission tomography/computed tomography findings to choose therapeutic strategies for clinical stage IA lung adenocarcinoma. J Thorac Cardiovasc Surg. 2011;141:1384–91.

Assessment of the Solitary Pulmonary Nodule: An Overview

4

Aqeel A. Chowdhry and Tan-Lucien H. Mohammed

In this chapter, the evaluation of the nodules detected by chest radiograph is discussed. A solitary pulmonary nodule (SPN) is a single nodule that is defined as rounded with smooth margins, well-circumscribed lesion measuring less than 3 cm. It has been reported that SPNs are seen in up to 2 per 1,000 screening chest radiographs in the United States, with an estimated 130,000–150,000 single nodules detected annually [1]. These nodules may comprise both benign and malignant etiologies and are summarized in Table 4.1. Although the majority of detected SPNs are benign, often the sequel of granulomatous disease, it is of paramount importance to distinguish between benign and malignant causes. In particular, the chance of malignancy increases in patients over 50 and may be as high as 60 %. As the 5-year survival for resected early stage lung cancer approaches 70–80 % for chest X-ray detected nodules, proper identification and adequate follow-up is needed to ensure appropriate work-up of the SPN is performed resulting in adequate characterization of the nature of the lesion.

A.A. Chowdhry, M.D.
Department of Radiology, Radiology/South Pointe Hospital, Cleveland Clinic, Cleveland, OH, USA

T.-L.H. Mohammed, M.D., F.C.C.P. (✉)
Department of Radiology C5-XR, Virginia Mason Medical Center, Seattle, Washington 98101, USA
e-mail: mohammed10@gmail.com

Radiographic Evaluation

Chest Radiograph

An SPN is most commonly initially detected on a chest radiograph performed for some other reason. Common causes of an SPN are listed in Table 4.1. In order to be detected, a nodule must present sufficient size and density to create an opacity on the radiograph (Fig. 4.1). In general detected nodules under 7 mm are either calcified or "false-positive" findings such as a vessel on-end [2]. The first step in the evaluation should be reviewing prior radiographs that may show the nodule in question. This includes not only chest radiographs but also thoracic spine, shoulder radiographs, or any other study that may provide insight into the length of time that a nodule has been present. As a general rule, 2-year stability suggests benignity [3]. In patients with a low pretest probability of malignancy or when a "nodule" is suspected to be extrapulmonary, strategies such as repeat radiographs, additional oblique or apical lordotic views, or fluoroscopy may be sufficient to categorize a nodule as benign, extrapulmonary, or needing further evaluation.

After ascertaining whether the nodule is present on prior radiographs, the next step is the evaluation for the presence or absence of calcium. Calcification is suggested when the nodule is denser than an adjacent rib or may be suggested by differential density within the nodule itself [4] (Fig. 4.2). While this may seem straightforward,

J.G. Ravenel (ed.), *Lung Cancer Imaging*, Contemporary Medical Imaging,
DOI 10.1007/978-1-60761-620-7_4, © Springer Science+Business Media New York 2013

Table 4.1 Common cause of solitary pulmonary nodules

Benign nodules	Infectious (granuloma, lung abscess, round pneumonia, hydatid cyst)
	Inflammatory (sarcoidosis, Wegener granulomatosis, rheumatoid arthritis)
	Congenital (sequestration, arteriovenous malformation, cyst)
	Other (rounded atelectasis, mucoid impaction)
Malignant nodules	Primary lung cancer
	Metastasis
	Carcinoid tumor
	Lymphoma
	Sarcoma
	Neurofibroma

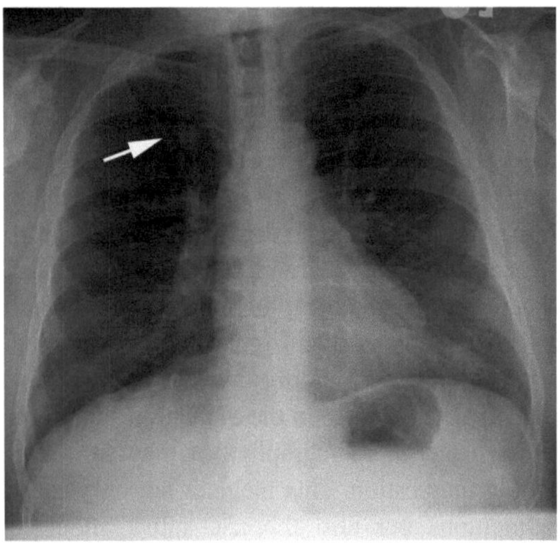

Fig. 4.1 Solitary pulmonary nodule. Frontal chest radiograph reveals a 1.8 cm lobulated opacity surrounded by air (*arrow*)

in clinical practice this can be difficult as it has been shown that up to 7 % of nodules considered "definitely calcified" may not have calcium present at CT [5]. Thus, a relatively low threshold for confirming the presence of calcium by other techniques is warranted. Dual-energy radiography can be used to produce individual soft tissue and bone-only images. This technique can also improve the detection of calcium within a nodule [6]. Similarly, low kV fluoroscopy can be efficacious at identifying calcium not clear on routine radiographs.

In regard to calcification, not only the detection but also the pattern of calcification is important. A completely calcified lesion or one with a large central nidus is typical for a benign lesion usually the sequelae of granulomatous inflammation. Nodules with chondroid- or "popcorn"-type calcifications are typical of hamartomas [7] (Fig. 4.3). Eccentric calcification should not be taken as evidence of benignity as malignant nodules may contain dystrophic calcification or envelop benign calcified nodules (Fig. 4.4).

Border characteristics can also be used to establish a probability of malignancy. Nodules with a smooth, regular edge are most often benign although up to 20 % may be malignant. As the contours become more lobular or irregular, the chance that a nodule is malignant increases. In particular, nodules with spiculated margins are found to be malignant in the majority of cases [7].

Ultimately, CT is the technique of choice when there is low likelihood that a nodule is calcified.

Computed Tomography

Chest CT is recommended in the majority of patients with a newly found SPN found on a routine chest radiograph. Intravenous contrast is not necessary as a rule [8]. CT allows better characterization of the nodule morphology, location, and density as well detects ancillary abnormalities that may provide clues to the diagnosis or establish the presence of multiple nodules. CT also can reveal the cause of "false-positive" nodules by localizing them to chest wall structures.

Calcification

The detection of calcium may be based on subjective visual data or objective attenuation values. An attenuation value above 185 HU is strongly predictive of calcification [9]. In either case, the use of thin sections through a nodule can be helpful for the detection of calcium (Fig. 4.5).

Morphology

Like chest radiography, morphology can play a role in establishing probability of malignancy.

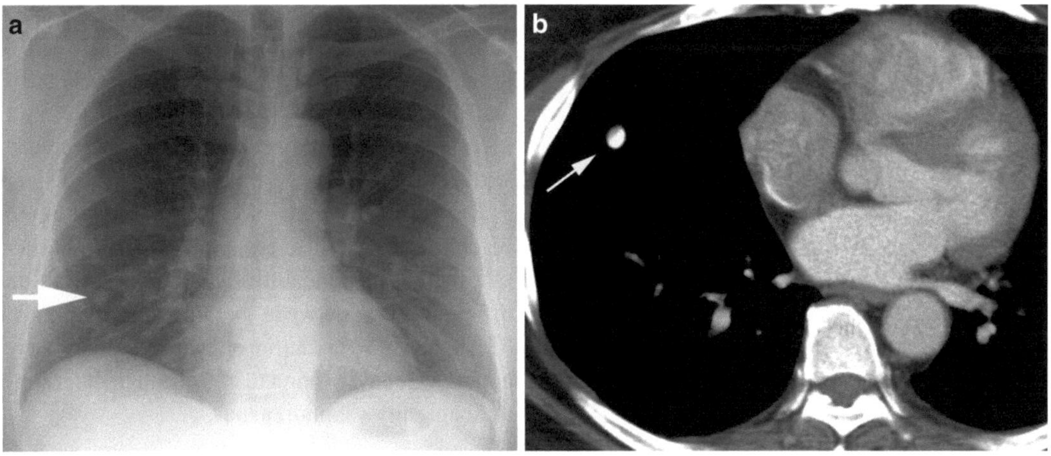

Fig. 4.2 Calcified pulmonary nodule. (**a**) Frontal chest radiograph reveals well-circumscribed 0.8 cm dense nodule (*arrow*). (**b**) Axial CT confirms nodule as densely calcified (*arrow*)

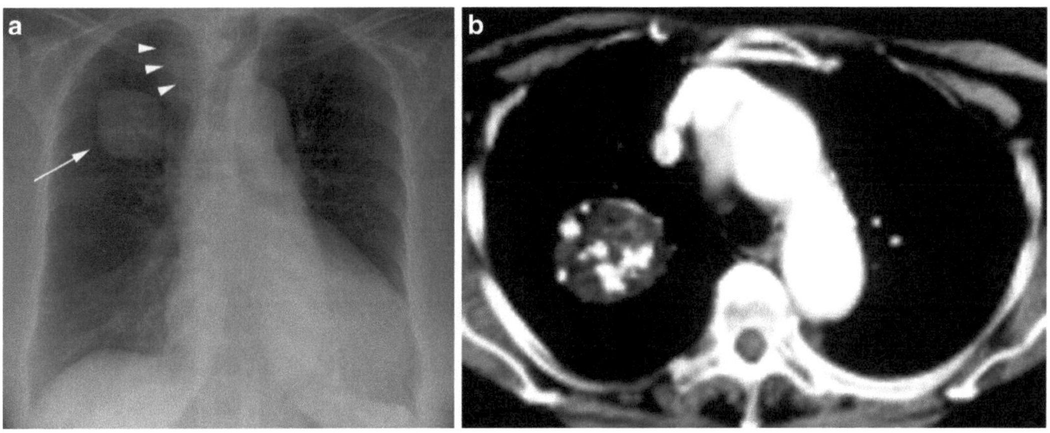

Fig. 4.3 Hamartoma. (**a**) Frontal chest radiograph reveals a 3 cm well-circumscribed right upper lobe nodule with internal chondroid calcifications (*arrow*). Note also right thyroid goiter (*arrowheads*). (**b**) Axial CT confirms nodule as heterogeneous with both internal fat and calcification diagnostic of hamartoma

Unfortunately, no single border characteristic can determine malignancy. Smooth borders are often benign while lobulated or spiculated borders are often malignant (Figs. 4.6–4.8) [10]. There is however significant overlap. Central cavitation may occur in both benign and malignant processes. An irregular inner wall and/or notches along the outer wall have been associated with malignancy [11].

Volumetry

Volume doubling time (VDT) is a useful albeit imperfect measure of malignant potential. As most malignant processes double in volume between 30 and 300 days [12], the calculation of VDT over time can aide management decisions. Simplistically, volume doubling has occurred when the original diameter has multiplied by 1.25 (e.g., a nodule that grows from 2 to 2.5 cm

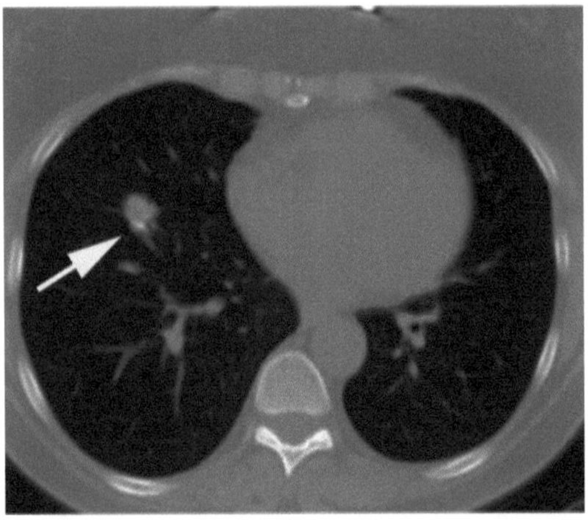

Fig. 4.4 Eccentric calcifications within nodule. Axial CT reveals spiculated nodule with coarse peripheral calcifications (*arrow*). Initial FNA non-diagnostic. Wedge resection revealed amyloidoma

has roughly doubled in volume). With transverse measurements, volumes can be estimated by the formula $4/3r^2$. Computer software programs have become widely available that allow nodule volume calculation. There is a wide variety of software algorithms currently on the market that all have the same basic features: that is, there is a computer-aided delineation of the nodule borders and segmentation from normal structures to produce a 3D rendering of the nodule (Fig. 4.9). Because of inherent differences in segmentation methodologies, different software algorithms will produce different volumes. Thus, it is important that nodules be measured using the same software each time. The inherent appeal, however, is the precision and reproducibility of measurements. Many studies have shown that computer-aided volumetry does not suffer from the variations that human measurements do [13, 14]. In addition, volumetry more accurately reflects the entire nodule which is not always best evaluated in the axial imaging plane. The ability to calculate volume does simplify the calculation of VDT, although this is more difficult to validate.

There are several caveats that need to be understood. Because the lung is a dynamic organ, differences in breath hold and cardiac activity influence nodule size on an individual study as well as effects of contrast administration [15–20]. Studies that have used a "coffee break" design (two scans with a short break in between) show that up to a 30 % variance in volume may occur [19]. Thus, small incremental volume growth must be viewed with caution.

3D volumetric data has also been reported to be helpful in the differential diagnosis. In particular the 3D shape features have can be helpful in differentiating between benign and malignant SPNs. Using attenuation, shape index, and curvedness value was found to be helpful in determining benignity vs. malignancy.

Enhancement

Contrast dynamics may help distinguish benign from malignant nodules. The patient is first scanned using unenhanced, thin-section CT followed by a weight based bolus of intravenous contrast and serial scans through the nodule at 1 min intervals for 4 min. In a multicenter study, nodules with a peak enhancement of <15 HU were very likely to be benign with a high sensitivity (98 %). Unfortunately specificity was relatively poor and enhancement characteristics could not be used to rule-in malignancy (Fig. 4.10) [21]. With the widespread availability of FDG PET, this technique is rarely used for diagnostic purposes.

Small Nodules

For nodules that are not clearly benign and less than one centimeter in size, periodic surveillance is generally the most appropriate strategy. In certain cases, particularly those with high pretest probability of malignancy, biopsy or 18F-fluorodeoxyglucose positron emission tomography (FDG PET) may be appropriate. As these nodules are not typically detected on chest radiographs, they are covered more fully in the chapter on lung cancer screening. Briefly, solid nodule management is outlined by Fleischner criteria [22] (see Table 3.6). Part-solid and ground glass nodules often represent a spectrum from preinvasive lesions such as atypical adenomatous hyperplasia (AAH) to low-grade adenocarcinomas [23]. Because these usually represent more indolent processes, periodic surveillance

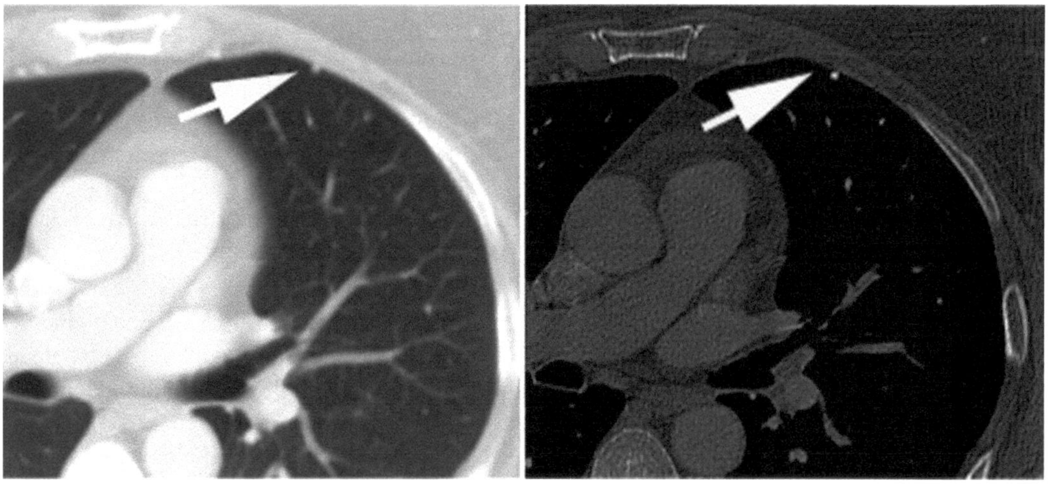

Fig. 4.5 Use of thin sections to detect calcium. Composite axial image at 5 mm (*left*) and 1 mm (*right*) reveals a 5 mm nodule in left upper lobe (*arrow*) that appears to be of soft tissue density at 5 mm slice thickness. Thin section image reveals nodule to be densely calcified and benign

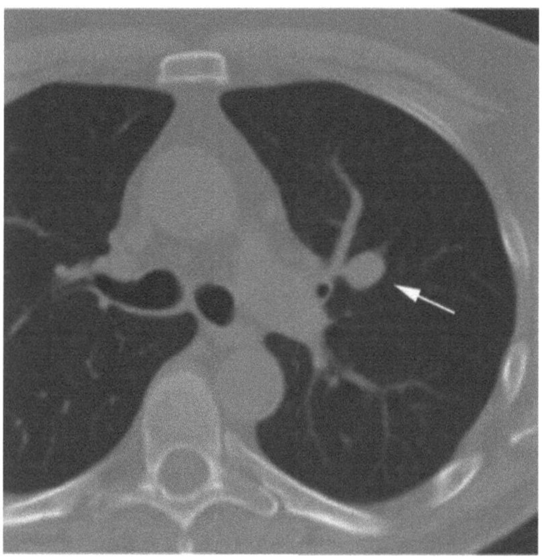

Fig. 4.6 Smooth pulmonary nodule (*arrow*). Found to be carcinoid at bronchoscopy

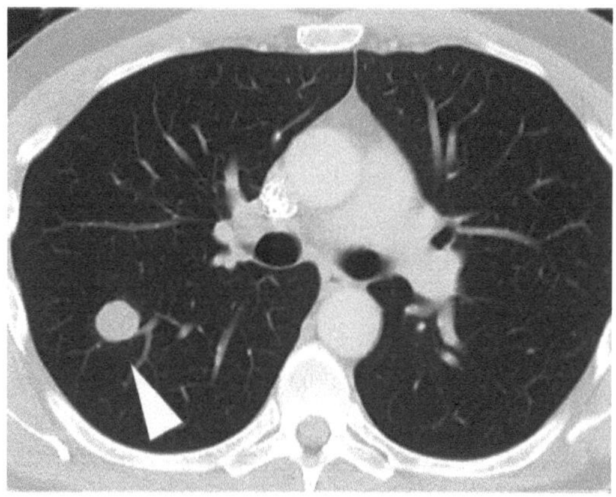

Fig. 4.7 Lobulated pulmonary nodule. Found to be adenocarcinoma at biopsy

and watchful waiting are appropriate [24] (see Table 3.7). The first follow-up can often be obtained at 3 months as many of these nodules will resolve. For those that persist, annual follow-up is appropriate. If tissue characterization is needed, the recommendation is for wedge resection as percutaneous biopsy may be subject to sampling error [25].

MRI

Although not typically used, MR may have an emerging role in delineation of benign and malignant nodules. The predominant techniques revolve around blood flow evaluation and diffusion-weighted imaging (DWI). Time-enhancement

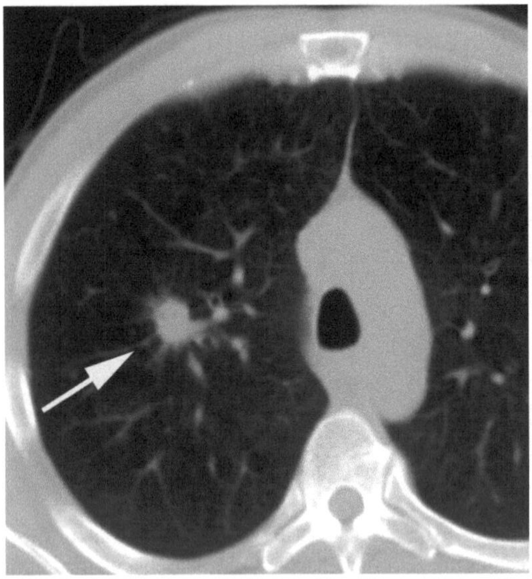

Fig. 4.8 Spiculated pulmonary nodule. Found to be adenocarcinoma at surgical resection

ratio curves can be calculated from MRI data. Observations have shown a correlation between enhancement and angiogenesis as well as collagen matrix and that this technique was particularly useful in evaluation microvessel density, a factor associated with vascular endothelial growth factor (VEGF) [26]. Certain enhancement patterns such as thin rim enhancement is suggestive of benignity often tuberculomas [12], a network enhancement pattern may be seen in hamartomas [27], while an angiogram sign may be seen with certain adenocarcinomas. In small studies, dynamic MR techniques have been shown to be an improvement compared with dynamic CT perfusion and FDG PET/CT [28].

DWI relies on the motion of water protons through tissues. As diffusion coefficients may differ between benign and malignant tissue, DWI has been proposed as an alternative or problem-solving tool. Mean diffusion has been shown to be higher in malignant pulmonary nodules [29]; however, there is overlap as small nodules and low-grade adenocarcinoma were found to have lower diffusion, while inflammatory lesions overlap with malignant nodules. Compared with FDG PET, DWI had a similar sensitivity and improved specificity [30]. In a recent meta-analysis of ten studies, DWI had a sensitivity and specificity of 84 % and was particularly helpful in ruling in malignancy with a high pretest probability and ruling out malignancy when pretest probability was low [31].

18F-FDG PET

PET imaging using 18-fluorine deoxyglucose (18-FDG) is a marker of glucose metabolism within a nodule. To that extent the amount of glucose metabolism (measured as a standard uptake value) predicts the likelihood of malignancy (Fig. 4.11). In interpreting activity, there are two basic approaches. The first is a quantitative approach to define a threshold over which malignancy is felt to be likely. The second is a qualitative approach that defines any activity above background as suspicious. For smaller and part-solid nodules the qualitative approach appears to result in fewer false negatives [32]. False-positive results for malignancy may occur in inflammatory nodules, active granulomatous disease, and other infections (Fig. 4.12), while false negatives may occur with small lesions, low-grade adenocarcinomas, and carcinoid tumors (Fig. 4.13). Inherent in either approach is the need to consider pretest probability of malignancy and nodule morphology which can in turn limit mischaracterization. Interpretation, therefore, must include correlation with CT preferably obtained at full-breath hold rather than for attenuation correction on an integrated PET/CT. In the seminal studies of FDG PET for pulmonary nodules, lesions had varying sizes in some cases up to 6 cm and the prevalence of malignancy ranged from 46 to 80 %. This resulted in a pooled sensitivity of 83 % and specificity of 87 % [12]. Thus, the quoted test characteristics for FDG PET are for intermediate to high pretest probability nodules, and masses do not necessarily reflect the performance of the test for low probability lesions.

From a probability perspective, patients with a nodule with a high pretest probability of malignancy may benefit from PET before biopsy. In this instance the PET serves as de facto staging

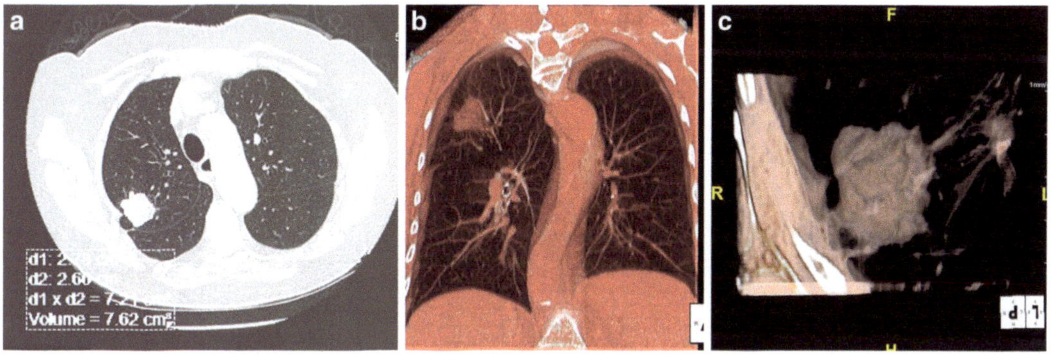

Fig. 4.9 Volumetric imaging. (**a**) Axial CT image shows automated nodule segmentation with calculation of nodule volume. (**b**) Thick slab volume rendered image of same nodule. (**c**) 3D volume rendered image

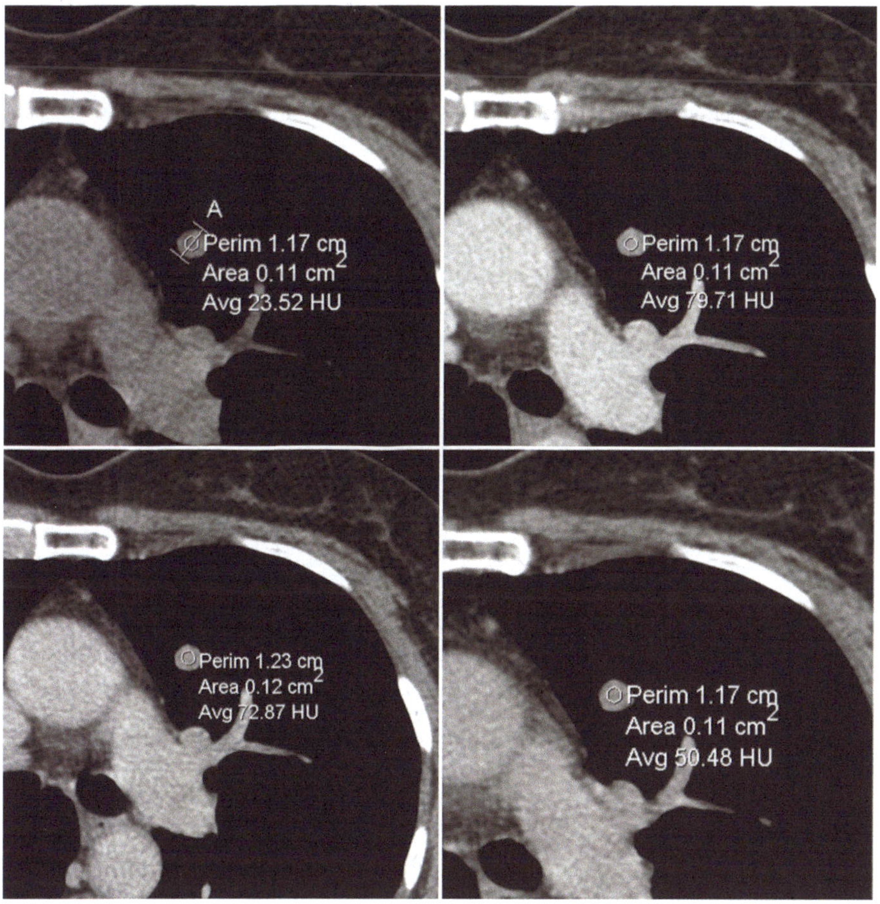

Fig. 4.10 Nodule enhancement. Axial CT images without contrast and at 1, 2, and 4 min following contrast injection show peak enhancement of 56 HU, an indeterminate result. Nodule considered benign after 2 years of no growth

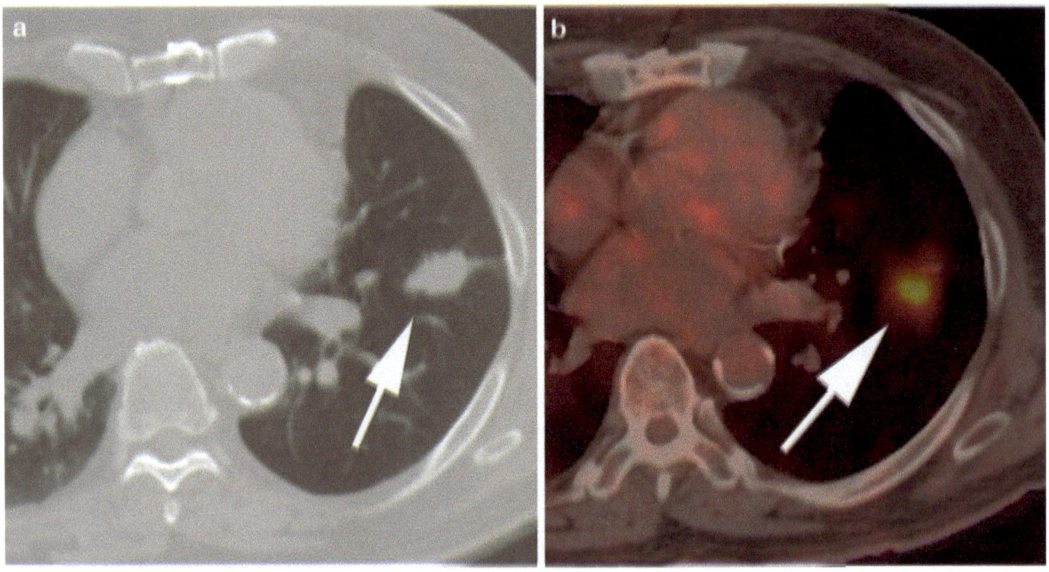

Fig. 4.11 True positive PET/CT. (**a**) Axial CT image reveals oblong lobulated left lower lobe nodule (*arrow*). (**b**) Fused PET/CT image shows elevated uptake within the nodule (*arrow*). Note slight misregistration of activity from anatomic site of disease. Biopsy revealed adenocarcinoma

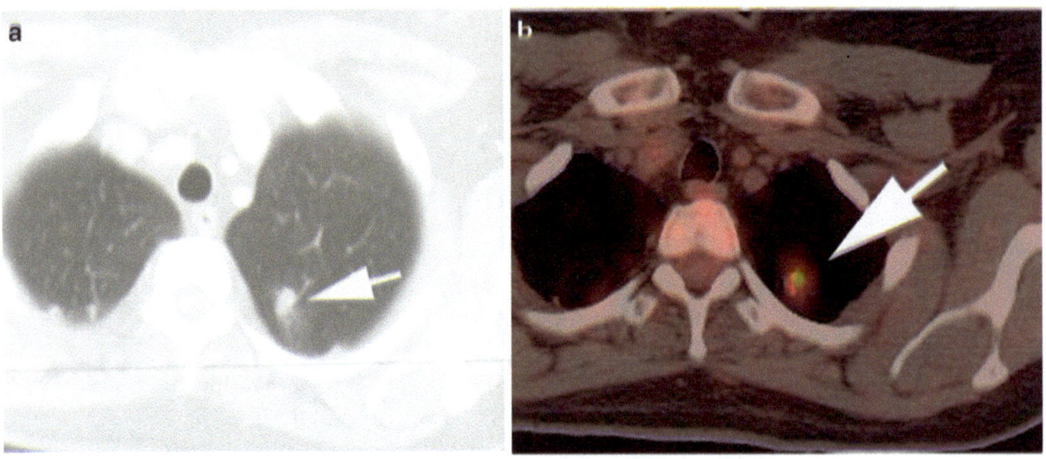

Fig. 4.12 False-positive PET/CT. (**a**) Axial CT image reveals spiculated left upper lobe nodule suspicious for malignancy. (**b**) Fused PET/CT image shows elevated uptake within nodule. Wedge resection revealed granulomatous inflammation and no evidence of malignancy

and may detect mediastinal or distant disease allowing for the diagnosis and final staging with one procedure. In cases where malignancy is suspected in a nodule that has characteristics known to result in false-negative findings such as a part-solid or small nodule, consideration should be given to biopsy or wedge resection and foregoing PET. For intermediate and low probability lesion, the choice of PET over watchful waiting is somewhat controversial [33, 34]. While the complete absence of metabolic activity may allow one to confidently exclude malignancy, low or moderate activity risks a more aggressive approach to ultimately arrive at a benign diagnosis. The impact

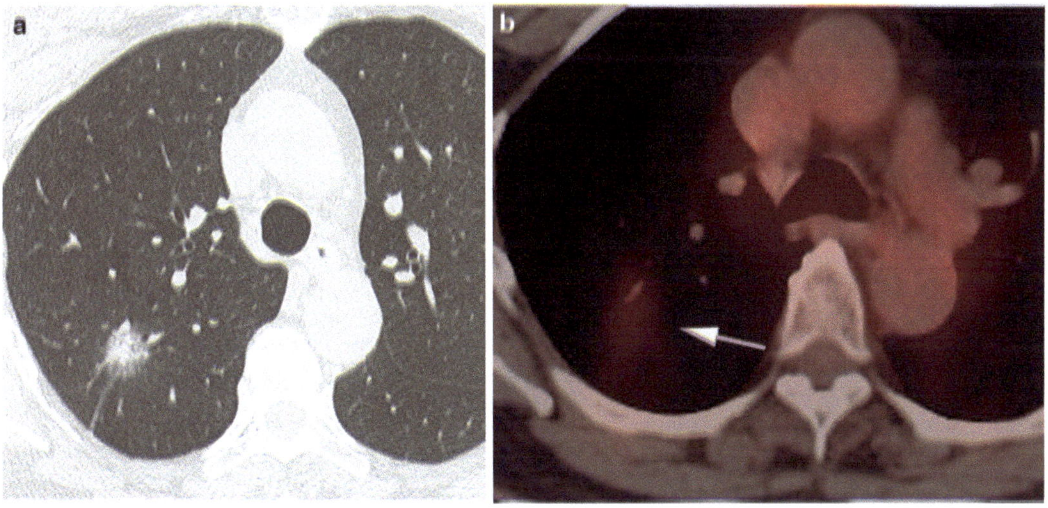

Fig. 4.13 False-negative PET/CT. (**a**) Axial CT image reveals part-solid nodule in right upper lobe. (**b**) Fused PET/CT reveals faint uptake slightly above background but below usual threshold for malignancy. Because of nodule morphology, wedge resection performed and confirmed low-grade adenocarcinoma

of PET on future management decisions must be considered in this regard prior to performing the test.

Summary

For the incidentally detected lung nodule, it is important to have a management pathway in mind. This should include an assessment of patient risk factors for malignancy, pretest probability based on morphologic characteristics, and patient expectations and safety. In general these pathways include the judicious use of CT at the outset to guide the pace and type of further evaluation.

References

1. Winer-Muram HT. The solitary pulmonary nodule. Radiology. 2006;239(1):34–49.
2. Ketai L, Malby M, Jordan K, Meholic A, Locken J. Small nodules detected on chest radiography: does size predict calcification? Chest. 2000;118(3):610–4.
3. Good CA, Wilson TW. The solitary circumscribed pulmonary nodule; study of seven hundred five cases encountered roentgenologically in a period of three and one-half years. J Am Med Assoc. 1958;166(3):210–5.
4. Erasmus JJ, McAdams HP, Connolly JE. Solitary pulmonary nodules: part II. Evaluation of the indeterminate nodule. Radiographics. 2000;20(1):59–66.
5. Berger WG, Erly WK, Krupinski EA, Standen JR, Stern RG. The solitary pulmonary nodule on chest radiography: can we really tell if the nodule is calcified? AJR Am J Roentgenol. 2001;176(1):201–4.
6. Kuhlman JE, Collins J, Brooks GN, Yandow DR, Broderick LS. Dual-energy subtraction chest radiography: what to look for beyond calcified nodules. Radiographics. 2006;26(1):79–92.
7. Erasmus JJ, Connolly JE, McAdams HP, Roggli VL. Solitary pulmonary nodules: part I. Morphologic evaluation for differentiation of benign and malignant lesions. Radiographics. 2000;20(1):43–58.
8. Ravenel JG, Mohammed TL, Movsas B, et al. ACR Appropriateness Criteria(R) noninvasive clinical staging of bronchogenic carcinoma. J Thorac Imaging. 2010;25(4):W107–11.
9. Siegelman SS, Khouri NF, Leo FP, Fishman EK, Braverman RM, Zerhouni EA. Solitary pulmonary nodules: CT assessment. Radiology. 1986;160(2): 307–12.
10. Brandman S, Ko JP. Pulmonary nodule detection, characterization, and management with multidetector computed tomography. J Thorac Imaging. 2011;26(2): 90–105.
11. Honda O, Tsubamoto M, Inoue A, et al. Pulmonary cavitary nodules on computed tomography: differentiation of malignancy and benignancy. J Comput Assist Tomogr. 2007;31(6):943–9.
12. Wahidi MM, Govert JA, Goudar RK, Gould MK, McCrory DC. Evidence for the treatment of patients with pulmonary nodules: when is it lung cancer?:

ACCP evidence-based clinical practice guidelines (2nd edition). Chest. 2007;132(3 Suppl):94S–107S.
13. Revel MP, Bissery A, Bienvenu M, Aycard L, Lefort C, Frija G. Are two-dimensional CT measurements of small noncalcified pulmonary nodules reliable? Radiology. 2004;231(2):453–8.
14. Revel MP, Lefort C, Bissery A, et al. Pulmonary nodules: preliminary experience with three-dimensional evaluation. Radiology. 2004;231(2):459–66.
15. Boll DT, Gilkeson RC, Fleiter TR, Blackham KA, Duerk JL, Lewin JS. Volumetric assessment of pulmonary nodules with ECG-gated MDCT. AJR Am J Roentgenol. 2004;183(5):1217–23.
16. de Hoop B, Gietema H, van Ginneken B, Zanen P, Groenewegen G, Prokop M. A comparison of six software packages for evaluation of solid lung nodules using semi-automated volumetry: what is the minimum increase in size to detect growth in repeated CT examinations. Eur Radiol. 2009;19(4):800–8.
17. Gietema HA, Schaefer-Prokop CM, Mali WP, Groenewegen G, Prokop M. Pulmonary nodules: Interscan variability of semiautomated volume measurements with multisection CT—influence of inspiration level, nodule size, and segmentation performance. Radiology. 2007;245(3):888–94.
18. Gietema HA, Wang Y, Xu D, et al. Pulmonary nodules detected at lung cancer screening: interobserver variability of semiautomated volume measurements. Radiology. 2006;241(1):251–7.
19. Rampinelli C, De Fiori E, Raimondi S, Veronesi G, Bellomi M. In vivo repeatability of automated volume calculations of small pulmonary nodules with CT. AJR Am J Roentgenol. 2009;192(6):1657–61.
20. Rampinelli C, Raimondi S, Padrenostro M, et al. Pulmonary nodules: contrast-enhanced volumetric variation at different CT scan delays. AJR Am J Roentgenol. 2010;195(1):149–54.
21. Swensen SJ, Viggiano RW, Midthun DE, et al. Lung nodule enhancement at CT: multicenter study. Radiology. 2000;214(1):73–80.
22. MacMahon H, Austin JH, Gamsu G, et al. Guidelines for management of small pulmonary nodules detected on CT scans: a statement from the Fleischner Society. Radiology. 2005;237(2):395–400.
23. Travis WD, Giroux DJ, Chansky K, et al. The IASLC Lung Cancer Staging Project: proposals for the inclusion of broncho-pulmonary carcinoid tumors in the forthcoming (seventh) edition of the TNM Classification for Lung Cancer. J Thorac Oncol. 2008;3(11):1213–23.
24. Godoy MC, Naidich DP. Subsolid pulmonary nodules and the spectrum of peripheral adenocarcinomas of the lung: recommended interim guidelines for assessment and management. Radiology. 2009;253(3):606–22.
25. Travis WD, Garg K, Franklin WA, et al. Bronchioloalveolar carcinoma and lung adenocarcinoma: the clinical importance and research relevance of the 2004 World Health Organization pathologic criteria. J Thorac Oncol. 2006;1(9 Suppl):S13–9.
26. Fujimoto K. Usefulness of contrast-enhanced magnetic resonance imaging for evaluating solitary pulmonary nodules. Cancer Imaging. 2008;8:36–44.
27. Kono R, Fujimoto K, Terasaki H, et al. Dynamic MRI of solitary pulmonary nodules: comparison of enhancement patterns of malignant and benign small peripheral lung lesions. AJR Am J Roentgenol. 2007;188(1):26–36.
28. Ohno Y, Koyama H, Nogami M, et al. Dynamic perfusion MRI: capability for evaluation of disease severity and progression of pulmonary arterial hypertension in patients with connective tissue disease. J Magn Reson Imaging. 2008;28(4):887–99.
29. Satoh S, Kitazume Y, Ohdama S, Kimula Y, Taura S, Endo Y. Can malignant and benign pulmonary nodules be differentiated with diffusion-weighted MRI? AJR Am J Roentgenol. 2008;191(2):464–70.
30. Mori T, Nomori H, Ikeda K, et al. Diffusion-weighted magnetic resonance imaging for diagnosing malignant pulmonary nodules/masses: comparison with positron emission tomography. J Thorac Oncol. 2008;3(4):358–64.
31. Wu LM, Xu JR, Hua J, et al. Can diffusion-weighted imaging be used as a reliable sequence in the detection of malignant pulmonary nodules and masses? Magn Reson Imaging. 2013;31(2):235–46.
32. Christensen JA, Nathan MA, Mullan BP, Hartman TE, Swensen SJ, Lowe VJ. Characterization of the solitary pulmonary nodule: 18F-FDG PET versus nodule-enhancement CT. AJR Am J Roentgenol. 2006; 187(5):1361–7.
33. Ost DE, Gould MK. Decision making in patients with pulmonary nodules. Am J Respir Crit Care Med. 2012;185(4):363–72.
34. Godoy MC, Naidich DP. Overview and strategic management of subsolid pulmonary nodules. J Thorac Imaging. 2012;27(4):240–8.

Imaging in Non-small Cell Lung Cancer

5

James G. Ravenel

Appropriate therapy is dependent on accurate staging to determine those amenable to surgery and define the appropriate role for chemotherapy and radiation therapy. In this chapter, the role of imaging in the staging and prognosis of lung cancer is discussed.

Chest Radiographs

Chest radiographs are typically the first studies performed in the evaluation of the patient with suspected lung cancer, although the paradigm may shift to a greater emphasis on CT as experience with screening CT increases. The typical radiographic finding is an irregular or spiculated nodule or mass, although border characteristics can vary and can be smooth or cavitary (Figs. 5.1–5.3). A second manifestation is collapse of a lobe owing to an endobronchial tumor (Fig. 5.4). The chest radiograph may also give evidence of mediastinal adenopathy or chest wall invasion. It is important to recognize that chest radiographs do not detect all lung tumors and that a negative radiograph in the setting of a high clinical suspicion should not necessarily end the radiographic evaluation. In addition, there are known "blind spots" on the radiographs particularly along mediastinal and hilar borders and beneath the rib and clavicular shadows (Fig. 5.5) [1].

CT, PET, and Histology

While on a practical basis for staging, the majority of primary lung cancers are grouped as either small cell or non-small cell lung carcinomas (NSCLC), the distinction of cell types in the NSCLC group is often of value in choosing certain treatment regimens. While this is truly the domain of pathology, certain imaging features may be present in the different histologic subtypes and may aid in diagnosis. While the classic teaching is that squamous cell carcinomas tend to be central and more likely to be cavitary than adenocarcinomas, there can certainly be overlap. One feature that appears to reliably predict adenocarcinoma as the histology is the presence of ground-glass opacity at CT [2] (Fig. 5.6). In the past, many of these tumors were grouped under the subtype bronchioloalveolar cell carcinoma (BAC), but owing to the confusion over terminology, these have been reclassified into in situ, minimally invasive and invasive adenocarcinoma to account for different biologic behavior and prognosis. Overall, the extent of ground-glass opacity appears to correlate with areas of hyperplasia, in situ carcinoma, or minimally invasive tumor which predicts slower growth and better overall prognosis [3–6]. Pure ground-glass nodules are typically atypical adenomatous

J.G. Ravenel, M.D. (✉)
Department of Radiology, Medical University of South Carolina, 96 Jonathan Lucas St, Room 211, P. O. Box 250322, Charleston, SC 29425, USA
e-mail: ravenejg@musc.edu

J.G. Ravenel (ed.), *Lung Cancer Imaging*, Contemporary Medical Imaging,
DOI 10.1007/978-1-60761-620-7_5, © Springer Science+Business Media New York 2013

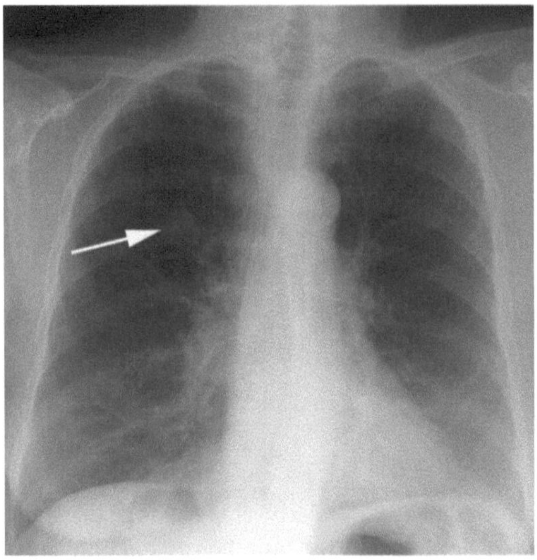

Fig. 5.1 Frontal chest radiograph reveals 2 cm right upper lobe solitary pulmonary nodule (*arrow*)

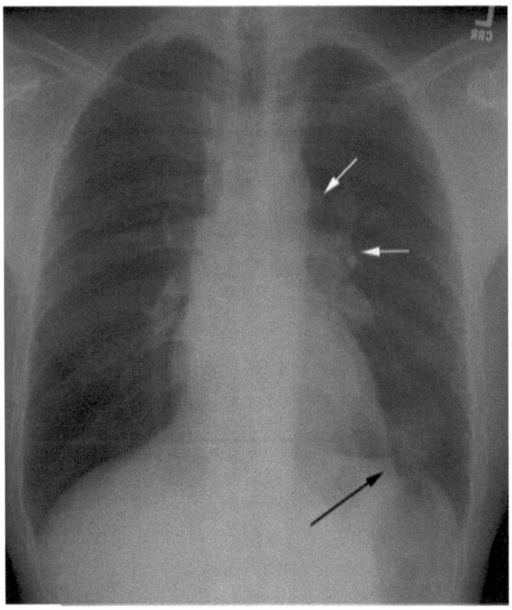

Fig. 5.2 Frontal chest radiograph reveals left lower lobe poorly defined nodule (*black arrow*) with associated left hilar and aortopulmonary window adenopathy (*white arrows*)

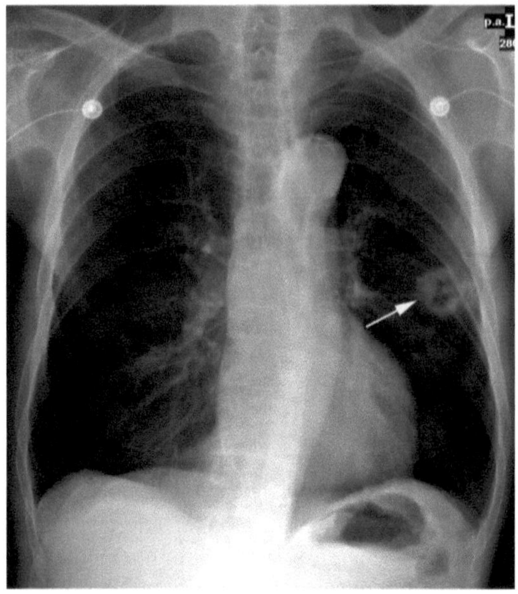

Fig. 5.3 Frontal chest radiograph reveals cavitary lung cancer in left upper lobe (*arrow*)

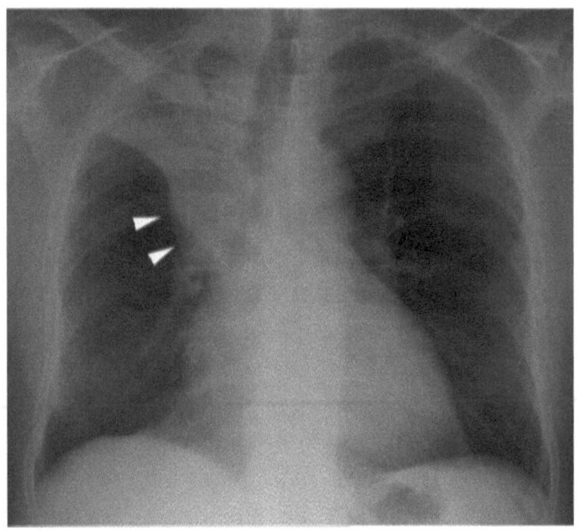

Fig. 5.4 Frontal chest radiograph reveals central right hilar mass (*arrowheads*) resulting in collapse of right upper lobe (also known as "S" sign of Golden)

hyperplasia or in situ adenocarcinomas but may on occasion contain an invasive component [7]. With FDG-PET, the standard uptake value tends to be higher with squamous and large cell histology [2], and similarly lung cancers that are not FDG avid are likely to be in the spectrum of low-grade adenocarcinoma [8–10].

The spectrum of low-grade adenocarcinoma is complex often requiring resection of the entire lesion to exclude an invasive component [11]. These tumors may present as a solitary pulmonary nodule or as diffuse confluent airspace

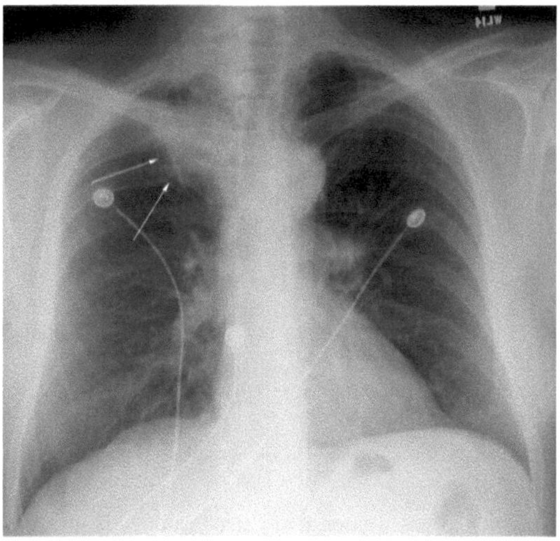

Fig. 5.5 Frontal chest radiograph reveals density differences between right (*arrows*) and left lung apices, although exact borders of mass are hard to define

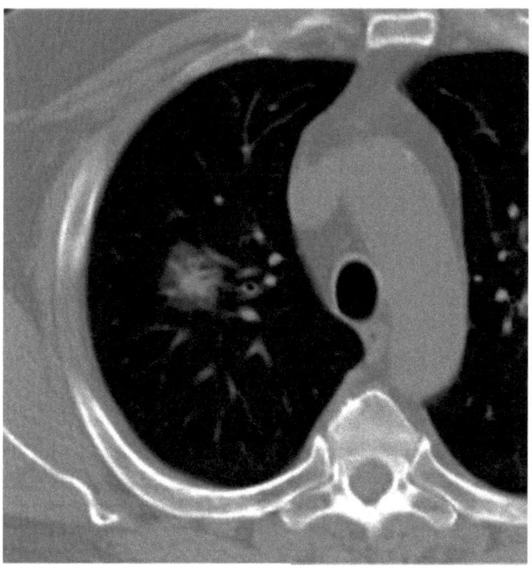

Fig. 5.6 Axial CT image reveals part-solid nodule with solid core and peripheral ground-glass opacity. Appearance is typical of invasive adenocarcinoma

disease. Nodules may have a variety of appearances including lobulated or spiculated borders, pleural tags, air bronchograms, and internal lucencies (pseudocavitation) [12] (Fig. 5.7). The ground-glass opacity histologically reflects the lepidic tumor growth with or without alveolar collapse [9], while the lucencies presumably

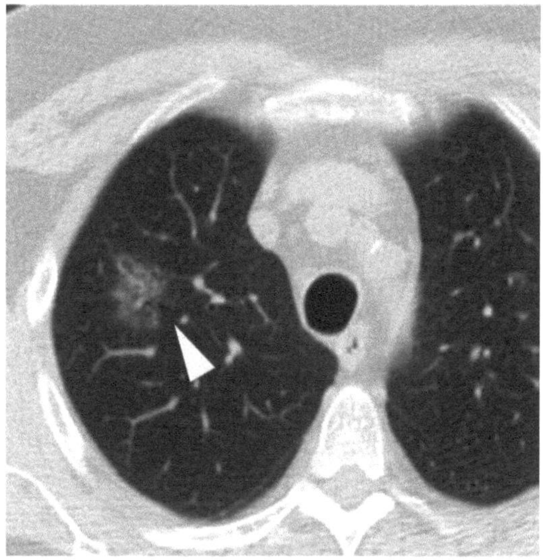

Fig. 5.7 Axial CT image reveals a pure ground-glass nodule with associated irregular borders air bronchograms and bubble-like lucencies (*arrowhead*) features often associate with preinvasive or minimally invasive histologies

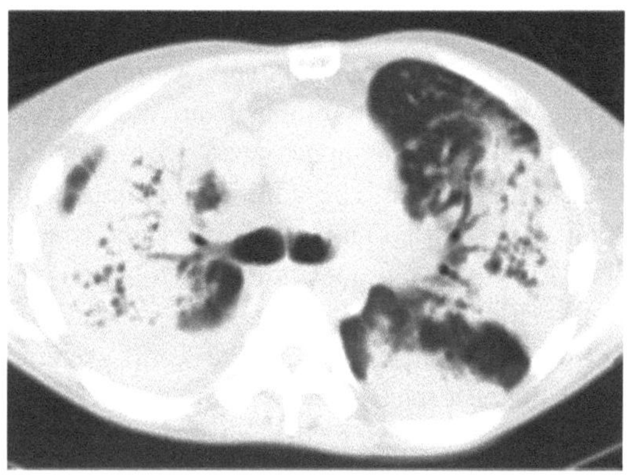

Fig. 5.8 Axial CT image reveals widespread parenchymal consolidation with pseudocavitation. Bronchoscopy revealed multifocal mucinous adenocarcinoma

reflect either uninvolved lobules or focal air trapping with bronchiolar obstruction [13, 14]. While a solid component may simply reflect alveolar collapse, it is more likely to represent areas of fibroblast proliferation or invasive adenocarcinoma [15].

A second radiographic appearance is the diffuse or multifocal form (Fig. 5.8). Findings range from multiple ground-glass opacities and nodules to lobar consolidation [12]. In many cases, the initial distinction from infection is impossible and the disease is not considered until the "pneumonia" does not resolve. The filling of airspaces is generally the result of mucin production, and with contrast-enhanced CT the underlying architecture of the lung is preserved. Sufficient mucin may eventually lead to attenuation of the pulmonary vessels and a bulging fissure [16]. The finding of discrete nodules in other lobes combined with non-resolving consolidation strongly supports the diagnosis [17]. The CT angiogram sign reflects normal pulmonary vasculature coursing through consolidated lung and can be seen in cases of infection, lipoid pneumonia, and obstructive pneumonitis [18].

NSCLC Staging

CT allows for anatomic staging of the primary lesion, mediastinal lymph nodes, and distant metastatic disease. The major limitations of anatomic imaging are the use of size criteria to define benign versus malignant lymph nodes, failure to distinguish tumor from atelectasis, and the nonspecific appearance of metastatic disease in general. The addition of metabolic imaging (FDG-PET) adds sensitivity and specificity to staging but does not replace histologic confirmation.

Staging is categorized by the TNM system, which is accepted by the American Joint Committee on Cancer (AJCC) [19]. This classification system takes into account the primary lesion (T), the presence or absence of mediastinal or supraclavicular lymph node involvement (N), and the presence or absence of distant metastasis (M) (Tables 5.1 and 5.2).

Table 5.1 Staging of lung cancer: AJCC TNM descriptors

Primary lesion
T0-no evidence of primary tumor
Tis-carcinoma in situ
T1-tumor <3 cm surrounded by lung or visceral pleura without invasion proximal to lobar bronchus
1a- ≤2 cm
1b- >2–3 cm
T2-tumors >3 cm, any tumor invading main bronchi but >2 cm from the carina, invasion of visceral pleura, obstructive pneumonitis extending to hila but does not involve entire lung
2a- >3–5 cm
2b- >5–7 cm
T3-tumor >7 cm. Tumor of any size that directly invades chest wall, diaphragm, mediastinal pleura, or parietal pericardium; or involves main bronchus within 2 cm of carina but does not involve carina; or results in obstructive atelectasis or pneumonitis of entire lung. Separate nodule(s) in same lobe
T4-tumor invades any of the following: mediastinum, heart great vessels, trachea, esophagus, vertebral body, or carina; malignant ipsilateral pleural or pericardial effusion; separate nodule(s) in a different ipsilateral lobe
Lymph nodes
N0-no regional lymph node metastases
N1-spread to ipsilateral peribronchial or hilar nodes
N2-spread to ipsilateral mediastinal or subcarinal nodes
N3-spread to contralateral mediastinal or hilar nodes, scalene nodes, supraclavicular nodes
Distant disease
M0-no distant metastases
M1-distant metastases present
M1a-separate tumor nodule in contralateral lung, pleural nodules, malignant pleural, or pericardial effusion
M1b-all other distant metastasis

T-Stage

The evaluation of T-stage is based upon size and location of the lesion, commonly using CT. The use of intravenous (IV) contrast while often specified in clinical trials is not mandatory as no clear superiority of contrast-enhanced CT scans has been established [20–22]. The use of IV contrast is therefore best left to the discretion of the interpreting physician.

T1 tumors are those that are less than 3 cm in greatest dimension and that do not invade the visceral pleura or mainstem bronchi. These can be further subdivided into T1a (<2 cm) and T1b (≥2 cm <3 cm) (Fig. 5.9). T2 tumors are greater

Table 5.2 Staging of NSCLC based on TNM classification

0-	Carcinoma in situ
1A-	T1N0M0
1B-	T2aN0M0
2A-	T2bN0M0 T1N1M0 T2aN1M0
2B-	T2bN1M0 T3N0M0
3A-	T3N1M0 T1-3N2M0 T4N0-1 M0
3B-	T4N2M0 Any N3
4-	Any M1

Used with the permission of the American Joint Committee on Cancer (AJCC), Chicago, Illinois. The original source for this material is the *AJCC Cancer Staging Manual*, Seventh Edition (2010) published by Springer Science and Business Media LLC. http://www.springer.com

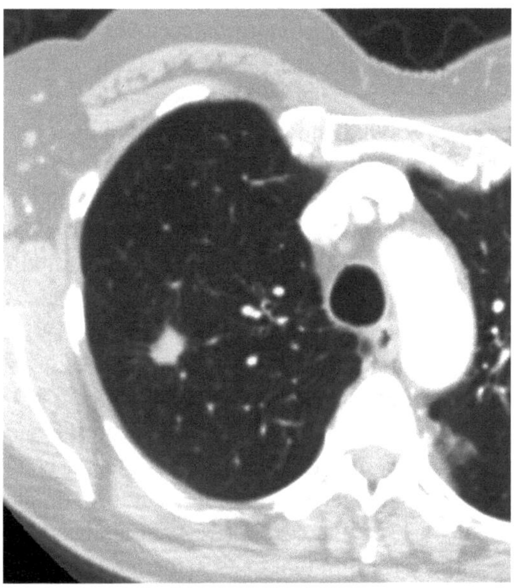

Fig. 5.9 T1 lesion. Axial CT image reveals a 1.4 cm spiculated right upper lobe nodule typical for lung neoplasm

than 3 cm and <7 cm in greatest dimension and/or involve the visceral pleura or mainstem bronchi, at least 2 cm from the carina (Fig. 5.10). T2 tumors can be subdivided into a and b categories based on whether tumor size is less than or

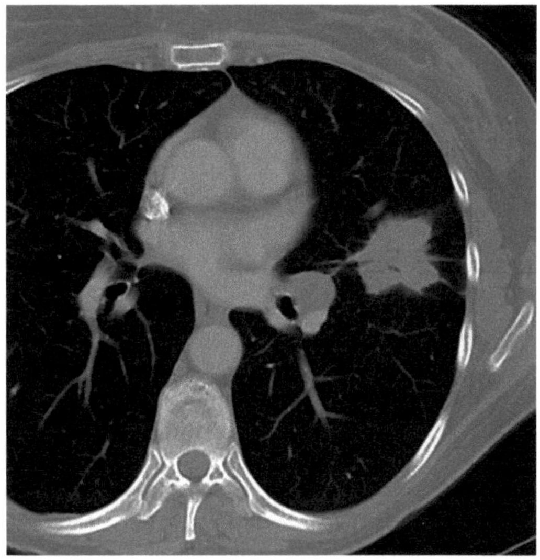

Fig. 5.10 T2 lesion. Axial CT image reveals a 4 cm spiculated mass in the left upper lobe

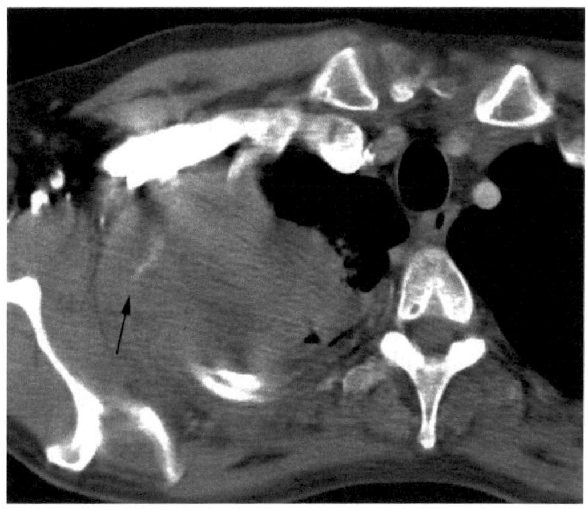

Fig. 5.11 T3 lesion. Axial CT reveals large right upper lobe mass with invasion into chest wall and destruction of right second rib (*arrow*)

greater than 5 cm. Regardless of size, it is important to note the relationship of the tumor to the pulmonary artery, lobar fissures, and incomplete fissures when applicable as this may alter the planned surgical approach [23]. T3 tumors include those ≥7 cm, are of any size that involve the chest wall, diaphragm, mediastinal pleura, parietal pericardium, or are within 2 cm of the carina but do not invade the carina (Fig. 5.11). Satellite nodules in the same tumor lobe are also

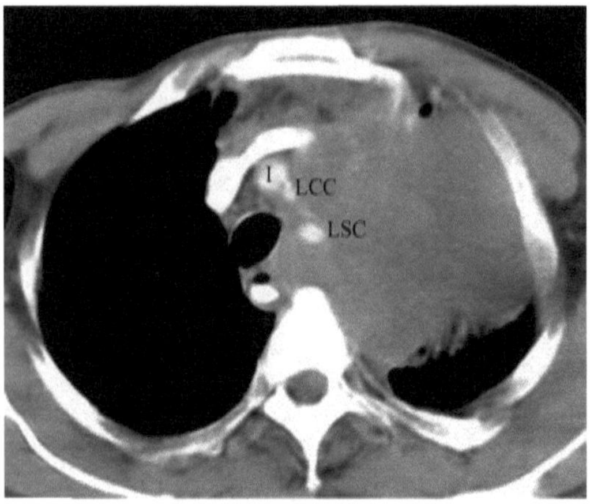

Fig. 5.12 T4 lesion. Axial CT reveals large left upper mass with invasion into the mediastinum and encasement of the innominate artery (I), left common carotid artery (LCC), and left subclavian artery (LSC)

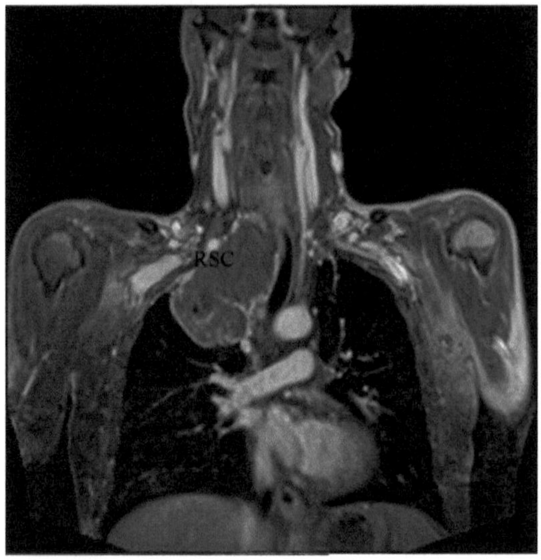

Fig. 5.13 Pancoast tumor. Coronal gadolinium-enhanced T1 sequence reveals cephalad extension of superior sulcus tumor, abutting the right subclavian artery (RSC)

considered T3 tumors regardless of the size of the dominant nodule/mass. T4 tumors invade vital structures including the heart, great vessels, esophagus, carina, or vertebral body or contain a satellite nodule in the ipsilateral lung non-tumor lobe (Fig. 5.12). While T4 tumors are generally considered unresectable, in certain circumstances, complete surgical resection may be feasible [23].

The distinction between T1 and T2 tumors is generally straightforward and does not usually impact initial treatment. Difficulty with T-staging may arise when there is need to determine chest wall (T3) or mediastinal (T4) invasion. Whereas primary signs such as bone destruction, rib erosion, or the presence of a tumor adjacent to mediastinal structures are reliable evidence of invasion, secondary signs such as absent fat planes, pleural thickening, and obtuse angle of tumor contact with the chest wall are not reliable [24–26]. Several CT features have been described to help determine chest wall invasion. These include greater than 3 cm of contact with the pleural surface, pleural thickening, absent fat planes, and obtuse angle of tumor with the chest wall [26]. Although sensitivity is relatively good with at least two features present (87 %), specificity remains relatively low (59 %), and localized chest pain remains a much more specific determinant [26]. Using thinner collimation with coronal and sagittal reformation improves accuracy for both chest wall and mediastinal invasion [27].

Magnetic resonance (MR) imaging can aid in problem solving and is clearly better at delineating extension of superior sulcus tumors [28]. In particular MR is superior to CT for the detection of involvement of the neural foramina, spinal canal, and brachial plexus. Surgery is contraindicated by local extension when the brachial plexus is involved above the level of T1, more than 50 % of a vertebral is invaded, or when there is invasion of the trachea or esophagus (Fig. 5.13). Invasion of the subclavian, common carotid, and vertebral arteries, less than 50 % vertebral body invasion and extension into the neural foramina, should be considered relative contraindications to surgery [28]. In other cases, the tumor should be considered a T3 lesion and treatment decisions should be based on the patient's medical condition as well as the presence or absence of metastatic disease.

MR can also be useful in excluding chest wall involvement. Using cine MR during free breathing, the finding of sliding between the tumor and mediastinum or chest wall has been shown to be diagnostic of lack of invasion. The converse however is not necessarily indicative of invasion as adhesion and local inflammatory changes may also restrict tumor motion [29–31].

In the appropriate hands, ultrasound also can be a useful adjunct in detecting chest wall invasion. In several studies, ultrasound has been shown to be superior to CT with sensitivity greater than 90 % [32, 33]. Sonographic features of chest wall invasion include direct invasion of the chest wall, interruption of the pleural reflection, and impairment of motion with respiration [32]. Ultrasound may be limited in certain circumstances, and false-negative and false-positive results may be obtained due to shadowing from osseous structures or fibrous adhesions of the tumor to pleura, respectively. Endoscopic ultrasound can also be utilized to assess mediastinal and aortic invasion [34, 35]. Because it is a relatively untested technique in this setting, the actual utility will depend on operator technique and experience.

PET/CT and T-Staging System

Due to the limited spatial resolution, 18F-FDG PET does not have a specific role in staging the primary tumor. While it has been suggested that fusion of CT and 18F-FDG PET images together may enhance T-stage determination (particularly for chest wall and mediastinal invasion) [36], care must be taken not to over- or under-stage tumors due to respiratory misregistration. By acquiring CT images at medium lung volumes rather than at deep inspiration, misregistration problems can be minimized. However, careful analysis of the CT images without 18F-FDG PET is still mandatory in order to avoid this pitfall. In rare circumstances, 18F-FDG PET may be helpful in detecting an occult primary tumor suspected based on detection of distant metastases.

Prognosis by PET/CT

As already seen, size and local invasion are predictors of survival at CT. FDG PET and PET/CT can also be used to evaluate long-term prognosis.

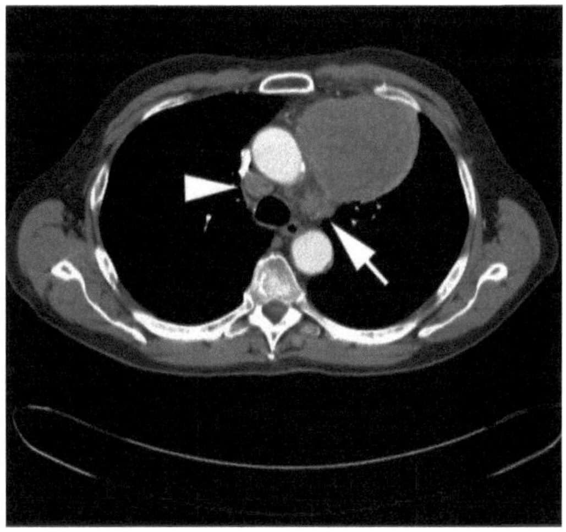

Fig. 5.14 Mediastinal adenopathy. Left upper lobe neoplasm with ipsilateral (N2) aortopulmonary adenopathy (*arrow*) and contralateral right paratracheal (N3) adenopathy (*arrowhead*)

In a retrospective study, 2-year survival was 96 % for surgically treated patients with an SUVmax <9 and 68 % if >9. The combination of tumor size >3 cm and SUVmax >9 resulted in only 47 % survival at 3 years [37]. However, when adjusting for surgical pathologic stage, SUVmax did not predict prognosis [38]. Other investigators have proposed a cutoff of SUVmax of 5–5.5 and found a survival advantage in the low SUV group [39–42]. This survival advantage was also supported by a recent meta-analysis showing that high SUV tumors were associated with reduced survival and a hazard ratio of 2.07 [43]. Unlike size, however, the use of SUV has not been included in the staging system and presumably reflects the variability in SUV across sites and scanners as well as the lack of an agreed upon measurement standard.

N-Stage

N-stage is defined by the presence or absence of lymphadenopathy and the relationship of the abnormal lymph nodes to the primary tumor (Fig. 5.14). Nodal location is defined by the IASLC lymph node map [44] (Fig. 5.15). N1 is defined as nodes which are ipsilateral intrapulmonary, peribronchial, and hilar. N2 nodes are ipsilateral mediastinal nodes, including the midline groups

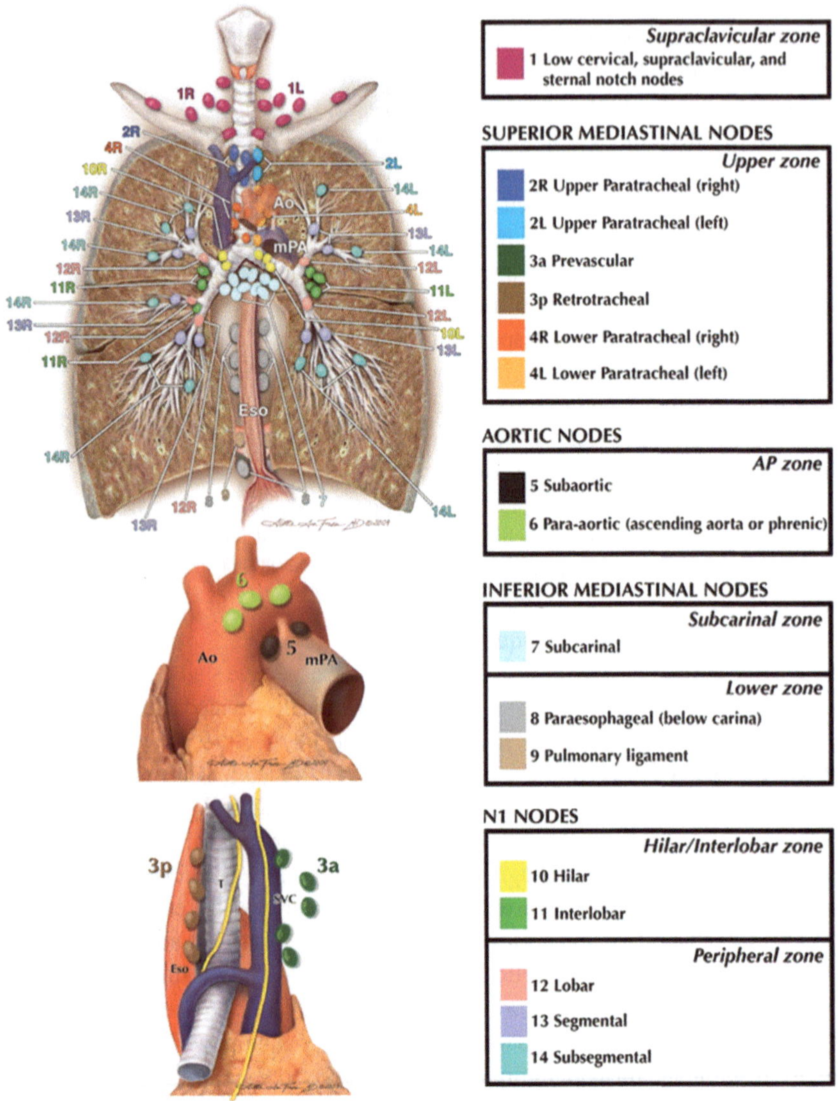

Fig. 5.15 IASLC lymph node map

(levels 3 and 7). Finally, N3 nodes are contralateral to the primary tumor or involve the scalene or supraclavicular nodes. The location of the primary tumor has a strong and relatively predictable influence on the likely location of metastatic nodes. Right upper lobe tumors most often drain to right paratracheal nodes (2R and 4R), while right middle and lower lobe tumors most frequently drain to lower right paratracheal and subcarinal nodes (4R and 7). On the left, the common sites for nodal metastases for the left upper lobe include AP window and prevascular nodes (5 and 6) and prevascular and subcarinal (6 and 7) for the left lower lobe [45]. For lower lobe tumors, the frequency of upper mediastinal lymph node involvement (levels 2, 4, 5, 6) is greater for tumors in the superior segment (64 %) versus basal segments (36 %) [46]. Because size is the main criteria for malignancy, CT is relatively inaccurate for staging the mediastinum. A lymph node measuring greater than 1 cm in short axis diameter is generally considered "positive" for clinical

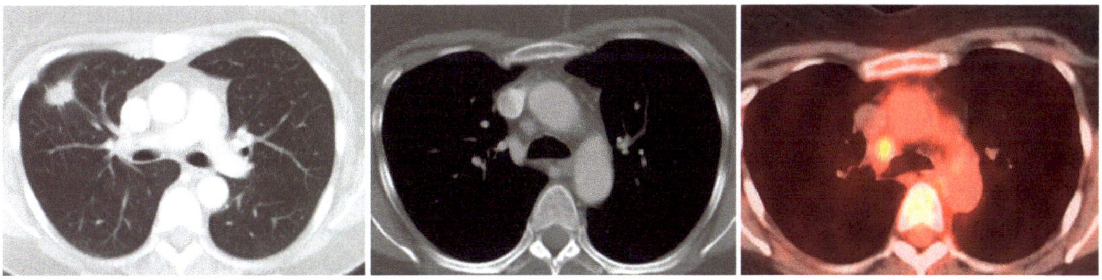

Fig. 5.16 T1N2 lung cancer. Composite of PET/CT reveals right upper lobe spiculated nodule with 1 cm borderline enlarged right paratracheal lymph node with FDG activity. Confirmed as lymph node metastasis by endobronchial ultrasound and biopsy

staging purposes [47]. While there is no lower limit of size that guarantees freedom from disease, the overall chance that a node is malignant is clearly influenced by size. For example, the prevalence of metastatic disease in lymph nodes is approximately 30 % for nodes 10–15 mm in size and 67 % for nodes >15 mm in size [48]. Among 43 studies conducted from 1991 to 2005, the sensitivities of CT for nodal disease ranged from 26 to 86 % and specificity ranged from 31 to 97 % with a pooled sensitivity and specificity from a total of 5,111 patients in whom prevalence of nodal disease was 28 % of 51/86 % [49]. CT, most importantly, provides anatomic relationships and landmarks critical for interpreting 18F-FDG PET studies and allows for selection of the most appropriate pathway for biopsy.

18F-FDG PET improves noninvasive staging but is not a substitute for tissue. Pooling all studies resulted in sensitivity/specificity of 74 %/85 % 2,865 patients with a prevalence of mediastinal disease of 29 % [49]. A prior meta-analysis showed a sensitivity and specificity of 85 %/90 % [50], suggesting that with more widespread acceptance and utilization, the true test characteristics are not as good as once thought. While 18F-FDG PET is not an endpoint in the staging work-up, 18F-FDG PET scans can decrease the number of futile thoracotomies by 20 % [51, 52]. The PLUS study [51] randomized stage I–III patients who were potentially operable to FDG PET or no PET and showed a reduction in the "futile" thoracotomy rate (thoracotomy performed in patients with unresectable disease) by 20 % (41 % without 18F-FDG PET vs. 21 % with 18F-FDG PET). However, for clinical 1A patients, the yield of 18F-FDG PET in preventing nontherapeutic pulmonary resection appears to be less than 10 % [53]. Thus, the ultimate success of 18F-FDG PET in the mediastinum may be to spare advanced-stage patients extensive surgery.

It is clear that 18F-FDG PET must be interpreted in the context of CT findings to maximize utility, and the value of 18F-FDG PET in staging the mediastinum is dependent on the CT findings [50, 54]. If a CT contains enlarged lymph nodes greater than 1 cm, sensitivity of 18F-FDG PET approaches 100 %, but specificity decreases (~78 %). In the setting of a negative CT scan, 18F-FDG PET shows lower sensitivity (82 %) but improved specificity (93 %) (Fig. 5.16) [50]. Modeling for size in combination with PET the likelihood of malignancy in a PET-negative node is 5 % when 10–15 mm in size and 21 % when greater than 15 mm in size. Conversely, the likelihood of malignancy in a PET-positive node is 62 % when 10–15 mm and 90 % when >15 mm [48].

The relationship of nodal SUV to malignancy is similar to that of size; the overall likelihood of malignancy increases with increasing SUV. Although a wide range of maximum SUV can be associated with benignity, accuracy improves with an SUV>5.3 [55]. Additionally, the true positive rate is higher in lymph nodes <1 cm with elevated SUV [56].

The ratio of SUV of the mediastinal lymph nodes to the primary tumor can also be helpful. A ratio of 0.56 predicted malignancy with a sensitivity of 94 % and specificity of 72 %, but like SUV alone, showed extensive overlap between benign and malignant lymph nodes [57]. The reality is that 18F-FDG PET should not replace histologic staging in the vast majority of cases. Most notably, a single positive finding should always be confirmed by histology before considering as stage 3 disease.

In regard to the 18F-FDG PET-negative mediastinum, there appear to be several caveats that can guide whether further mediastinal staging is necessary. A retrospective study of 18F-FDG false-negative results found that occult metastases were more likely to occur with increasing T-stage, central tumors, adenocarcinoma histology, and higher primary tumor SUV (>6), although the actual number of false-negative lymph nodes in this study was small ($n = 16$) [58]. Other groups have found that in addition to these features, upper lobe tumors and those with N1-positive disease also have a relatively high rate of occult disease in the mediastinum with histologic staging [59, 60]. The size of false-negative lymph nodes tends to be less than 1 cm; therefore, while the negative predictive value of the PET-negative mediastinum is quite high, the potential for a false-negative result is associated with decreasing node size. Tobacco use appears to lower maximum SUV and both smoking status and maximum pack years are independently associated with a decreased accuracy of 18F-FDG PET for mediastinal staging [61]. In summary, an 18F-FDG PET-negative mediastinum has an extremely high negative predictive value in small (T1), peripheral tumors with a low primary tumor SUV and no significant activity in the hilar lymph nodes. Under these conditions, it seems reasonable to proceed to surgery without prior pathological staging of the mediastinum.

Integrated 18F-FDG PET/CT imaging outperforms CT alone, 18F-FDG PET alone, and conventional visual correlation or superimposition of CT and 18F-FDG PET acquired individually [36, 62–64]. The diagnostic advantages touted in the literature include more precise demarcation of primary tumor (which can also be used to better define radiation ports), improved diagnosis of tumor invasion, demarcation of tumor within atelectasis or infection, more precise localization of mediastinal lymph nodes greater than 8 mm in size, as well as the precise localization of extrathoracic lesions [65]. Most notably, integrated systems allow more accurate staging impacting treatment decisions in up to 20 % of patients [62].

MR imaging is not typically used for mediastinal staging, although abnormal lymph nodes can be detected using this technique. A lack of standardization of protocols however makes comparison of results difficult. Most protocols utilize a short tau inversion recovery (STIR) sequence which allows for whole-body staging with a total exam time of 60 min [66]. Using this approach, MR imaging approaches the accuracy of PET/CT for detecting nodal metastases at 1.5 T [67]. A slightly shorter imaging time is feasible with 3.0 T MR and likewise has relatively similar, albeit slightly less accurate [68]. In one study STIR images using quantitative analysis using a lymph node-saline ratio were found to be more sensitive and specific compared to PET/CT [69].

Owing to the increased cellularity, larger nuclear size, and decreased extracellular space, the motion of water molecules is restricted. One attempt to improve evaluation with MR is the addition of diffusion-weighted imaging (DWI) to evaluate the apparent diffusion coefficient (ADC). The results, however, have been mixed. Ohno et al. evaluated 250 consecutive patients with T1 or T2 NSCLC using a STIR sequence, DWI, and FDG PET/CT and found STIR images to be slightly more accurate than either DWI or FDG PET/CT [70]. In a smaller study of 63 subjects, Usada et al. found DWI to be superior in detecting both primary tumor and lymph node metastasis [71]. Pauls et al. were unable to demonstrate an advantage of DWI over FDG-PET and noted that MR had a greater tendency to understage patients [72]. DWI may improve delineation of central tumors from post-obstructive pneumonitis [73]. It is clear that MR imaging can be used to stage lung cancer with similar test characteristics to standard techniques but requires agreement on the optimal technique and validation in a multicenter trial.

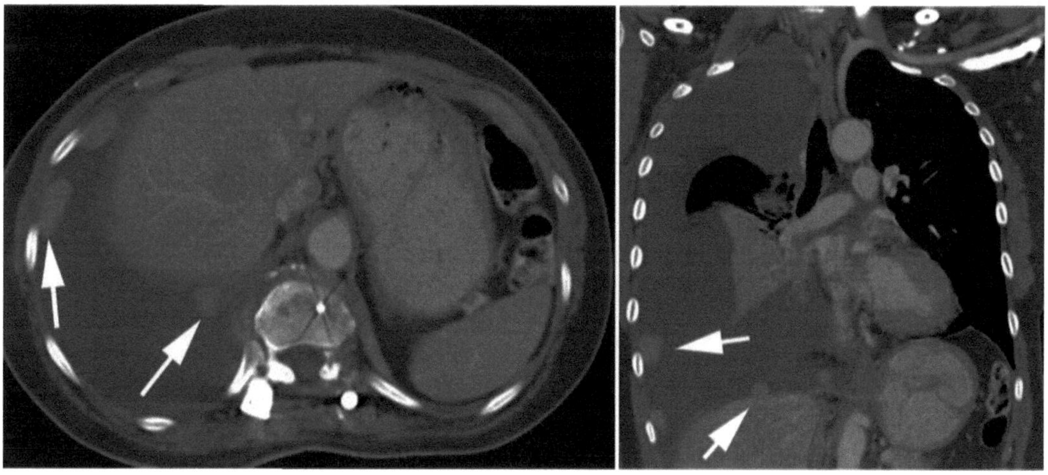

Fig. 5.17 Pleural metastases. Axial and coronal CT images reveal large right pleural effusion with enhancing pleural nodules (*arrows*)

M-Stage

M-stage is defined by the absence (M0) or presence (M1) of distant metastasis. The M-category is further subdivided into M1a-malignant pleural effusion and M1b-other distant metastases. Lung cancer most commonly metastasizes to bone, brain, liver, and adrenal glands. CT and whole-body 18F-FDG PET imaging are usually used for the evaluation of distant metastases. In the absence of symptoms, the negative predictive value is usually 95 % for liver, brain, and adrenal and 90 % for bone [74, 75]. Whole-body MR imaging as discussed previously also has the capability of providing accurate staging in a single exam. In limited studies, whole-body MR is as accurate as 18F-FDG PET in detecting distant metastases and seems to have a particular advantage in detecting brain and liver lesions [68]. The addition of diffusion-weighted images may ultimately increase yield [76].

Pleural Metastasis

Ipsilateral malignant pleural effusions are considered to be M1a by staging criteria and are most frequently associated with adenocarcinoma histology. However, pleural effusions are not uncommon in patients with lung cancer and are not necessarily due to the presence of malignant disease in the pleural space. Malignant pleural effusions by definition have tumor cells in the pleural space and almost always exudates (3–10 % will be transudates) [77]. In some cases the effusions are paramalignant due to central venous or lymphatic obstruction or effusions due to post-obstructive atelectasis/pneumonitis [78]. Effusions in lung cancer patients may also result unrelated to the tumor itself (cardiac, hepatic, renal disease, etc.), thus sampling of the fluid is mandatory prior to labeling a patient unresectable. CT findings suggesting a malignant effusion include parietal pleural thickness >1 cm, circumferential thickening, and nodules and mediastinal pleural involvement (Fig. 5.17) [77]. 18F-FDG PET has been shown to be quite accurate (>90 %) in the confirmation of metastatic pleural disease in two series [79, 80].

Adrenal Metastasis

Adrenal nodules are a common incidental finding in the general population and in patients with lung cancer (Fig. 5.17). The majority of these lesions represent benign adenomas. In this case, unenhanced CT holds an advantage over contrast-enhanced CT, as a density measurement of <10 HU virtually assures the diagnosis of benign adenoma [81]. The low attenuation is due to intracellular lipid accumulation within benign lesions. However, a number of adrenal lesions have a density >10 HU and are considered indeterminate.

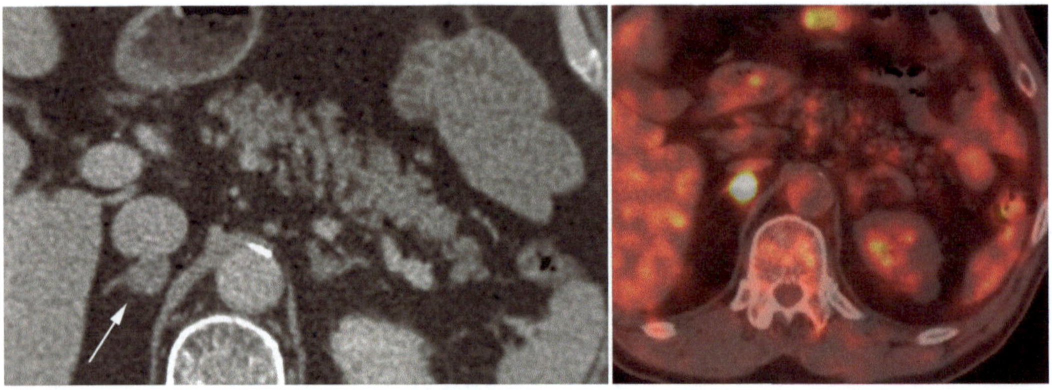

Fig. 5.18 Indeterminate adrenal lesion (*arrow*). Axial CT and fused PET/CT images reveal a metabolically active right adrenal nodule. Because this was only potential site of metastatic disease, biopsy was performed and revealed nonfunctioning pheochromocytoma

Similarly, on contrast-enhanced CT, both benign and malignant lesions invariably exceed the threshold of 10 HU. If an adrenal lesion is recognized after contrast administration, but prior to leaving the scanner, a delayed washout technique can be employed to distinguish benign and malignant lesions. If greater than 50 % of the attenuation "washes out" after 15 min, the lesion is an adenoma [82, 83]. For indeterminate lesion on unenhanced CT, histogram analysis can also improve sensitivity. If the lesion has >10 % pixels with a negative HU value, it is invariably a benign adenoma. This technique appears to be able to characterize indeterminate adrenal lesions as benign lipid-poor adenomas in approximately ½ of cases [84–86]. This technique can also help characterize lesions that remain indeterminate after washout studies [87].

MR imaging with in-phase and out-of-phase sequences is an alternative to CT. Signal dropout can be used to reliably confirm the benign nature of an incidental adrenal lesion [88]. While it has been suggested that MR is of limited utility when CT attenuation values are >10 [89, 90], it can be a useful strategy for following up lesions detected on contrast-enhanced scan without using additional contrast media, and in one study signal intensity dropout of >20 % performed better than histogram analysis at CT [85].

18F-FDG PET has been shown to differentiate benign and malignant adrenal lesions, even those indeterminate at CT and MR, with a sensitivity and specificity of 94–100 % and 74–91 % in a total of four studies [91–94]. The most important observation is that benign nodules can be FDG avid, and therefore PET activity in the adrenal gland should not necessarily confirm a patient as stage IV disease (Fig. 5.18).

Liver Metastasis

The most common hepatic lesions detected by CT in the evaluation of lung cancer are benign cysts or hemangiomas. Given the frequency of indeterminate findings, it is reassuring that the liver is rarely the sole site of metastatic disease at time of diagnosis, occurring in approximately 3 % of cases [95]. As most chest CT scans will cover the majority of the liver, dedicated hepatic imaging is generally not indicated. While this suggests a benefit to enhanced CT for staging, careful evaluation of the unenhanced CT with narrow window settings will allow for visualization of most hepatic metastases. In cases where differentiation of benign and malignant lesion is necessary, MR can often be definitive in distinguishing the two (Fig. 5.19). 18F-FDG PET has not been formally evaluated for imaging of liver metastasis related to lung cancer; however, experience in other malignancies suggests that 18F-FDG PET can accurately detect liver metastases by focal uptake greater than the background of the liver [96].

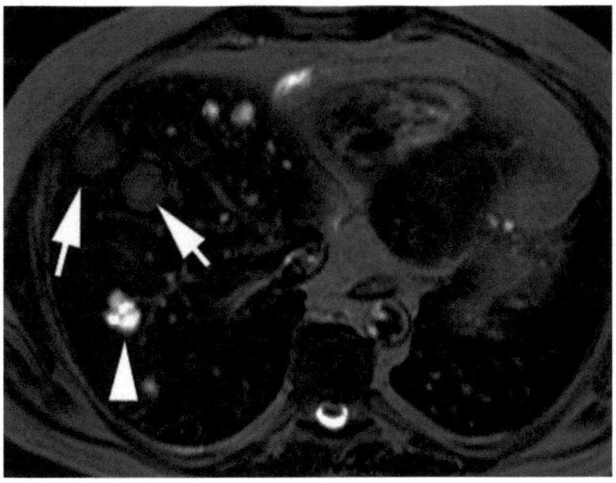

Fig. 5.19 Liver metastases and cysts. T2-weighted axial MR in patients noted to have multiple hypointense lesions on CT. MR clearly distinguishes the marked high signal in cysts (*arrowhead*) and differentiates them from metastatic lesions (*arrows*)

Bone Metastasis

Most patients with bone metastases are symptomatic or have an elevated alkaline phosphatase. While bone scintigraphy is quite sensitive for the detection of osseous metastases, the false-positive rate approaches 40 %. Since fewer than 5 % of lung cancer patients have occult bone metastases at presentation [97], routine bone scintigraphy is probably not warranted. Bone scintigraphy, the current standard for osseous metastases, suffers from a relatively low specificity.

Routine CT allows for evaluation of the thoracic spine, upper lumbar spine, scapula, and ribs. While CT is not thought of as a modality for the detection of bone metastases, careful evaluation of osseous structures, with an appropriate window and level setting, frequently allows for the detection of metastases, particularly when correlated with either bone scintigraphy or 18F-FDG PET. In particular, using CT in this manner may limit false-positive studies by confirming degenerative changes as a cause of increased uptake on bone scintigraphy. Bone metastases may appear as lytic or destructive lesions or as regional areas of sclerosis (Fig. 5.12). In some cases, CT may in fact be the first clue to the presence of osseous metastasis.

Several studies have shown 18F-FDG PET to have a similar sensitivity and accuracy, with improved specificity and negative predictive value [98–100]. Thus, if whole-body 18F-FDG PET has already been performed, bone scintigraphy is usually superfluous (Fig. 5.20).

Brain Metastasis

CT with contrast is accurate for the detection of cerebral metastasis, although MR performance characteristics are slightly better (Fig. 5.21) [101]. Not surprisingly, the incidence of brain metastasis also increases with increasing size of the primary lesion and nodal stage [102]. However, in the absence of neurological symptoms, cerebral metastases are unusual and the routine staging of subjects with a normal clinical exam yields positive findings in less than 10 % [103–105]. Of the various histologic subtypes, adenocarcinoma and large cell carcinoma are most frequently associated with asymptomatic cerebral metastases [106]. Cerebral imaging is therefore most efficaciously utilized in patients with neurologic symptoms or prior to resection of T2 tumors or planned resection of IIIA disease. 18F-FDG PET has relatively low sensitivity and is not a suitable modality for the evaluation of metastatic disease, due to the brain's high metabolic activity and glucose consumption [107].

New Frontiers/Novel Imaging Techniques

Although clinical practice standards are generally guided by the concepts previously outlined, newer techniques for imaging are emerging and in a relative infancy of use. Whether any of these techniques improve on current staging and treatment algorithms, remain niche techniques for specific clinical questions or fall by the wayside remain to be seen. Several potential approaches are briefly discussed below.

Perfusion CT

CT perfusion is based on the theory that iodine maps are a surrogate for tumor vascularity. The evaluation of lung tumors with perfusion CT is

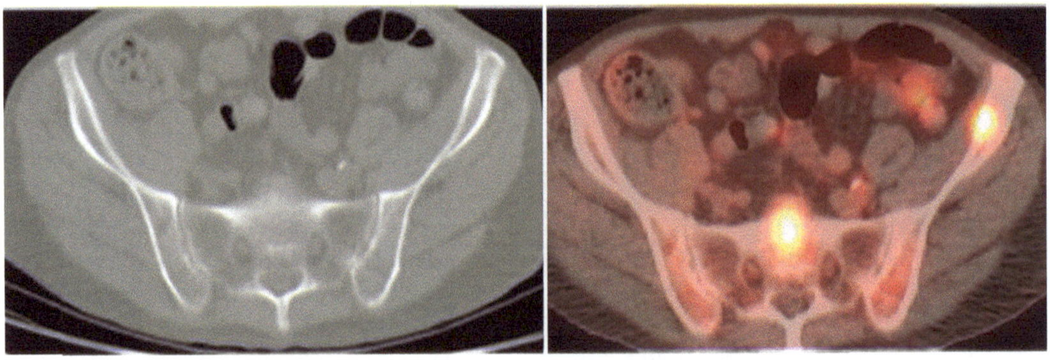

Fig. 5.20 Bone marrow metastases. Axial CT and fused PET/CT image show foci of FDG uptake in sacrum and left ilium with evidence of bone erosion or destruction. Such lesions can be occult on bone scintigraphy due to lack of bone remodeling

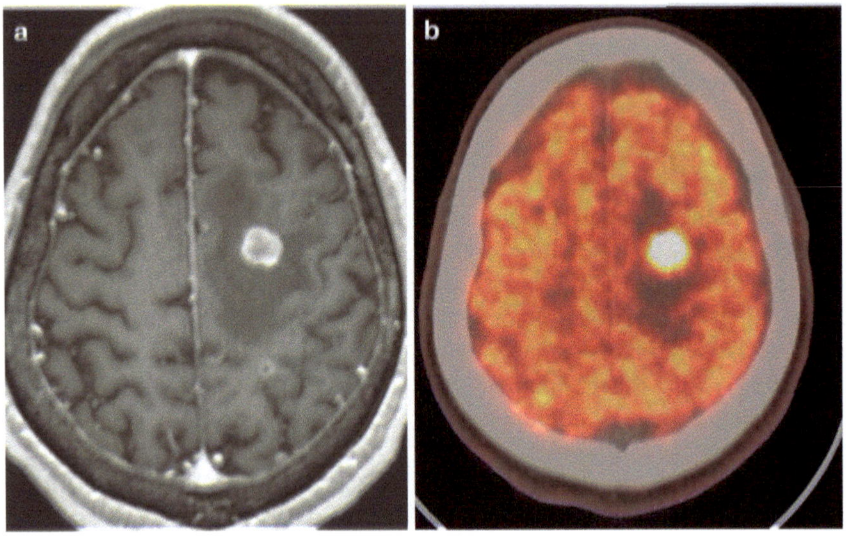

Fig. 5.21 Brain metastasis. (**a**) Axial gadolinium-enhanced MR reveals enhancing left parietal metastasis with surrounding vasogenic edema. (**b**) Axial 4-h delayed time point fused FDG PET/CT reveals metabolic activity above background. The activity is often masked at the time of the whole-body PET acquisition

challenging owing to a long imaging time and therefore long breathhold compared with static regions such as rectal and head and neck tumors where perfusion CT has been more widely studied. A recent small study in lung tumors has suggested that an increase in tumor blood volume is associated with better prognosis and that changes in permeability during therapy (decrease in permeability correlates with improved survival) can also predict outcome [108]. Another potential use is detecting a response to anti-angiogenic therapy where perfusion changes may be more predictive than size [109].

Positron Agents

Imaging Tumor Proliferation-18F-Fluorothymidime (FLT-PET)

Alternative imaging approaches to response may be evaluated by assessment of cellular proliferation. In theory the use of proliferation may lead to a better prediction of tumor behavior than metabolism. Proof of concept for FLT-PET has been shown similar to FDG-PET in subjects treated with gefitinib where time to progression was longer for responders compared to nonresponders [110]. A similar proof of concept showed that

FLT-PET can be used in tracking response to radiation therapy, although the significance of response was not evaluated [111]. However, in small studies FLT-PET does not appear superior to FDG-PET. In a study of 18 subjects with NSCLC, FLT had and lower mean SUV and a lower sensitivity than FDG, nor was it superior to FDG with regard to correlation with Ki-67 proliferation index [112]. FLT also has a tendency to understage patients owing to its relatively lower SUV compared with FDG [113]. A major limitation of these studies is that they do not address whole-body staging. Because of uptake in the liver, FLT is unreliable for the detection of liver metastases due to high physiologic activity and limits its potential as a staging agent [114].

Imaging Tumor Hypoxia-18F-Fluoromisonidazole (F-MISO)

Another approach is to assess tissue hypoxia. F-MISO is the most widely studied PET agent for tissue hypoxia [115]. Higher levels of hypoxia are predictive of poor local and distant control, and F-MISO appears to be a better predictor of outcome compared with FDG-PET in head and neck cancers [116] and perhaps for lung cancer.

Conclusion

Imaging plays a critical role in staging patients with non-small cell lung cancer. While mediastinoscopy is still considered the gold standard in mediastinal staging, imaging is beneficial in that it is noninvasive and highly accurate, especially when anatomic and physiologic information is acquired simultaneously through integrated 18F-FDG PET/CT systems.

References

1. Woodring JH. Pitfalls in the radiologic diagnosis of lung cancer. AJR Am J Roentgenol. 1990;154(6):1165–75.
2. Aquino SL, Halpern EF, Kuester LB, Fischman AJ. FDG-PET and CT features of non-small cell lung cancer based on tumor type. Int J Mol Med. 2007;19(3):495–9.
3. Aoki T, Nakata H, Watanabe H, et al. Evolution of peripheral lung adenocarcinomas: CT findings correlated with histology and tumor doubling time. AJR Am J Roentgenol. 2000;174(3):763–8.
4. Aoki T, Tomoda Y, Watanabe H, et al. Peripheral lung adenocarcinoma: correlation of thin-section CT findings with histologic prognostic factors and survival. Radiology. 2001;220(3):803–9.
5. Kim EA, Johkoh T, Lee KS, et al. Quantification of ground-glass opacity on high-resolution CT of small peripheral adenocarcinoma of the lung: pathologic and prognostic implications. AJR Am J Roentgenol. 2001;177(6):1417–22.
6. Kuriyama K, Seto M, Kasugai T, et al. Ground-glass opacity on thin-section CT: value in differentiating subtypes of adenocarcinoma of the lung. AJR Am J Roentgenol. 1999;173(2):465–9.
7. Nakata M, Saeki H, Takata I, et al. Focal ground-glass opacity detected by low-dose helical CT. Chest. 2002;121(5):1464–7.
8. Cheran SK, Nielsen ND, Patz Jr EF. False-negative findings for primary lung tumors on FDG positron emission tomography: staging and prognostic implications. AJR Am J Roentgenol. 2004;182(5):1129–32.
9. Lee KS, Jeong YJ, Han J, Kim BT, Kim H, Kwon OJ. T1 non-small cell lung cancer: imaging and histopathologic findings and their prognostic implications. Radiographics. 2004;24(6):1617–36; discussion 1632–6.
10. Lindell RM, Hartman TE, Swensen SJ, et al. Lung cancer screening experience: a retrospective review of PET in 22 non-small cell lung carcinomas detected on screening chest CT in a high-risk population. AJR Am J Roentgenol. 2005;185(1):126–31.
11. Travis WD, Garg K, Franklin WA, et al. Evolving concepts in the pathology and computed tomography imaging of lung adenocarcinoma and bronchioloalveolar carcinoma. J Clin Oncol. 2005;23(14):3279–87.
12. Patsios D, Roberts HC, Paul NS, et al. Pictorial review of the many faces of bronchioloalveolar cell carcinoma. Br J Radiol. 2007;80(960):1015–23.
13. Gaeta M, Caruso R, Blandino A, Bartiromo G, Scribano E, Pandolfo I. Radiolucencies and cavitation in bronchioloalveolar carcinoma: CT-pathologic correlation. Eur Radiol. 1999;9(1):55–9.
14. Weisbrod GL, Towers MJ, Chamberlain DW, Herman SJ, Matzinger FR. Thin-walled cystic lesions in bronchioalveolar carcinoma. Radiology. 1992;185(2):401–5.
15. Gandara DR, Aberle D, Lau D, et al. Radiographic imaging of bronchioloalveolar carcinoma: screening, patterns of presentation and response assessment. J Thorac Oncol. 2006;1(9 Suppl):S20–6.
16. Jung JI, Kim H, Park SH, et al. CT differentiation of pneumonic-type bronchioloalveolar cell carcinoma and infectious pneumonia. Br J Radiol. 2001;74(882):490–4.

17. Aquino SL, Chiles C, Halford P. Distinction of consolidative bronchioloalveolar carcinoma from pneumonia: do CT criteria work? AJR Am J Roentgenol. 1998;171(2):359–63.
18. Shah RM, Friedman AC. CT angiogram sign: incidence and significance in lobar consolidations evaluated by contrast-enhanced CT. AJR Am J Roentgenol. 1998;170(3):719–21.
19. Mountain CF. Revisions in the International System for Staging Lung Cancer. Chest. 1997;111(6):1710–7.
20. Cascade PN, Gross BH, Kazerooni EA, et al. Variability in the detection of enlarged mediastinal lymph nodes in staging lung cancer: a comparison of contrast-enhanced and unenhanced CT. AJR Am J Roentgenol. 1998;170(4):927–31.
21. Haramati LB, Cartagena AM, Austin JH. CT evaluation of mediastinal lymphadenopathy: noncontrast 5 mm vs postcontrast 10 mm sections. J Comput Assist Tomogr. 1995;19(3):375–8.
22. Patz EJ, Erasmus J, McAdams H, et al. Lung cancer staging and management: comparison of contrast-enhanced and nonenhanced helical CT of the thorax. Radiology. 1999;212(1):56–60.
23. Munden RF, Swisher SS, Stevens CW, Stewart DJ. Imaging of the patient with non-small cell lung cancer. Radiology. 2005;237(3):803–18.
24. Pearlberg JL, Sandler MA, Beute GH, Lewis Jr JW, Madrazo BL. Limitations of CT in evaluation of neoplasms involving chest wall. J Comput Assist Tomogr. 1987;11(2):290–3.
25. Pennes DR, Glazer GM, Wimbish KJ, Gross BH, Long RW, Orringer MB. Chest wall invasion by lung cancer: limitations of CT evaluation. AJR Am J Roentgenol. 1985;144(3):507–11.
26. Glazer HS, Duncan-Meyer J, Aronberg DJ, Moran JF, Levitt RG, Sagel SS. Pleural and chest wall invasion in bronchogenic carcinoma: CT evaluation. Radiology. 1985;157(1):191–4.
27. Higashino T, Ohno Y, Takenaka D, et al. Thin-section multiplanar reformats from multidetector-row CT data: utility for assessment of regional tumor extent in non-small cell lung cancer. Eur J Radiol. 2005;56(1):48–55.
28. Bruzzi JF, Komaki R, Walsh GL, et al. Imaging of non-small cell lung cancer of the superior sulcus: part 2: initial staging and assessment of resectability and therapeutic response. Radiographics. 2008;28(2):561–72.
29. Akata S, Kajiwara N, Park J, et al. Evaluation of chest wall invasion by lung cancer using respiratory dynamic MRI. J Med Imaging Radiat Oncol. 2008;52(1):36–9.
30. Sakai S, Murayama S, Murakami J, Hashiguchi N, Masuda K. Bronchogenic carcinoma invasion of the chest wall: evaluation with dynamic cine MRI during breathing. J Comput Assist Tomogr. 1997;21(4):595–600.
31. Seo JS, Kim YJ, Choi BW, Choe KO. Usefulness of magnetic resonance imaging for evaluation of cardiovascular invasion: evaluation of sliding motion between thoracic mass and adjacent structures on cine MR images. J Magn Reson Imaging. 2005;22(2):234–41.
32. Bandi V, Lunn W, Ernst A, Eberhardt R, Hoffmann H, Herth FJ. Ultrasound vs. CT in detecting chest wall invasion by tumor: a prospective study. Chest. 2008;133(4):881–6.
33. Suzuki N, Saitoh T, Kitamura S. Tumor invasion of the chest wall in lung cancer: diagnosis with US. Radiology. 1993;187(1):39–42.
34. Schroder C, Schonhofer B, Vogel B. Transesophageal echographic determination of aortic invasion by lung cancer. Chest. 2005;127(2):438–42.
35. Varadarajulu S, Schmulewitz N, Wildi SM, et al. Accuracy of EUS in staging of T4 lung cancer. Gastrointest Endosc. 2004;59(3):345–8.
36. Lardinois D, Weder W, Hany TF, et al. Staging of non-small-cell lung cancer with integrated positron-emission tomography and computed tomography. N Engl J Med. 2003;348(25):2500–7.
37. Downey RJ, Akhurst T, Gonen M, et al. Preoperative F-18 fluorodeoxyglucose-positron emission tomography maximal standardized uptake value predicts survival after lung cancer resection. J Clin Oncol. 2004;22(16):3255–60.
38. Downey RJ, Akhurst T, Gonen M, Park B, Rusch V. Fluorine-18 fluorodeoxyglucose positron emission tomographic maximal standardized uptake value predicts survival independent of clinical but not pathologic TNM staging of resected non-small cell lung cancer. J Thorac Cardiovasc Surg. 2007;133(6):1419–27.
39. Goodgame B, Pillot GA, Yang Z, et al. Prognostic value of preoperative positron emission tomography in resected stage I non-small cell lung cancer. J Thorac Oncol. 2008;3(2):130–4.
40. Higashi K, Ueda Y, Arisaka Y, et al. 18F-FDG uptake as a biologic prognostic factor for recurrence in patients with surgically resected non-small cell lung cancer. J Nucl Med. 2002;43(1):39–45.
41. Sasaki R, Komaki R, Macapinlac H, et al. [18F]fluorodeoxyglucose uptake by positron emission tomography predicts outcome of non-small-cell lung cancer. J Clin Oncol. 2005;23(6):1136–43.
42. Vansteenkiste JF, Stroobants SG, Dupont PJ, et al. Prognostic importance of the standardized uptake value on (18)F-fluoro-2-deoxy-glucose-positron emission tomography scan in non-small-cell lung cancer: an analysis of 125 cases. Leuven Lung Cancer Group. J Clin Oncol. 1999;17(10):3201–6.
43. Berghmans T, Dusart M, Paesmans M, et al. Primary tumor standardized uptake value (SUVmax) measured on fluorodeoxyglucose positron emission tomography (FDG-PET) is of prognostic value for survival in non-small cell lung cancer (NSCLC): a systematic review and meta-analysis (MA) by the European Lung Cancer Working Party for the IASLC Lung Cancer Staging Project. J Thorac Oncol. 2008;3(1):6–12.

44. Rusch VW, Asamura H, Watanabe H, et al. The IASLC lung cancer staging project: a proposal for a new international lymph node map in the forthcoming seventh edition of the TNM classification for lung cancer. J Thorac Oncol. 2009;4(5):568–77.
45. Cerfolio RJ, Bryant AS. Distribution and likelihood of lymph node metastasis based on the lobar location of nonsmall-cell lung cancer. Ann Thorac Surg. 2006;81(6):1969–73; discussion 1973.
46. Watanabe S, Suzuki K, Asamura H. Superior and basal segment lung cancers in the lower lobe have different lymph node metastatic pathways and prognosis. Ann Thorac Surg. 2008;85(3):1026–31.
47. Glazer GM, Gross BH, Quint LE, Francis IR, Bookstein FL, Orringer MB. Normal mediastinal lymph nodes: number and size according to American Thoracic Society mapping. AJR Am J Roentgenol. 1985;144(2):261–5.
48. de Langen AJ, Raijmakers P, Riphagen I, Paul MA, Hoekstra OS. The size of mediastinal lymph nodes and its relation with metastatic involvement: a meta-analysis. Eur J Cardiothorac Surg. 2006;29(1):26–9.
49. Silvestri GA, Gould MK, Margolis ML, et al. Noninvasive staging of non-small cell lung cancer: ACCP evidenced-based clinical practice guidelines (2nd edition). Chest. 2007;132(3 Suppl):178S–201.
50. Gould MK, Kuschner WG, Rydzak CE, et al. Test performance of positron emission tomography and computed tomography for mediastinal staging in patients with non-small-cell lung cancer: a meta-analysis. Ann Intern Med. 2003;139(11):879–92.
51. van Tinteren H, Hoekstra O, Smit E, et al. Effectiveness of positron emission tomography in the preoperative assessment of patients with suspected non-small cell lung cancer: the PLUS multicentre randomised trial. Lancet. 2002;359(9315):1388–93.
52. Reed CE, Harpole DH, Posther KE, et al. Results of the American College of Surgeons Oncology Group Z0050 trial: the utility of positron emission tomography in staging potentially operable non-small cell lung cancer. J Thorac Cardiovasc Surg. 2003;126(6):1943–51.
53. Kozower BD, Meyers BF, Reed CE, Jones DR, Decker PA, Putnam JB Jr. Does positron emission tomography prevent nontherapeutic pulmonary resections for clinical stage IA lung cancer? Ann Thorac Surg. 2008;85(4):1166–9; discussion 1169–70.
54. Kelly RF, Tran T, Holmstrom A, Murar J, Segurola Jr RJ. Accuracy and cost-effectiveness of [18F]-2-fluoro-deoxy-D-glucose-positron emission tomography scan in potentially resectable non-small cell lung cancer. Chest. 2004;125(4):1413–23.
55. Bryant AS, Cerfolio RJ, Klemm KM, Ojha B. Maximum standard uptake value of mediastinal lymph nodes on integrated FDG-PET-CT predicts pathology in patients with non-small cell lung cancer. Ann Thorac Surg. 2006;82(2):417–22; discussion 422–3.
56. Nomori H, Watanabe K, Ohtsuka T, Naruke T, Suemasu K, Uno K. The size of metastatic foci and lymph nodes yielding false-negative and false-positive lymph node staging with positron emission tomography in patients with lung cancer. J Thorac Cardiovasc Surg. 2004;127(4):1087–92.
57. Cerfolio RJ, Bryant AS. Ratio of the maximum standardized uptake value on FDG-PET of the mediastinal (N2) lymph nodes to the primary tumor may be a universal predictor of nodal malignancy in patients with nonsmall-cell lung cancer. Ann Thorac Surg. 2007;83(5):1826–9; discussion 1829–30.
58. Lee PC, Port JL, Korst RJ, Liss Y, Meherally DN, Altorki NK. Risk factors for occult mediastinal metastases in clinical stage I non-small cell lung cancer. Ann Thorac Surg. 2007;84(1):177–81.
59. Cerfolio RJ, Bryant AS, Eloubeidi MA. Routine mediastinoscopy and esophageal ultrasound fine-needle aspiration in patients with non-small cell lung cancer who are clinically N2 negative: a prospective study. Chest. 2006;130(6):1791–5.
60. Hishida T, Yoshida J, Nishimura M, Nishiwaki Y, Nagai K. Problems in the current diagnostic standards of clinical N1 non-small cell lung cancer. Thorax. 2008;63(6):526–31.
61. Bryant AS, Cerfolio RJ. The clinical stage of non-small cell lung cancer as assessed by means of fluorodeoxyglucose-positron emission tomographic/computed tomographic scanning is less accurate in cigarette smokers. J Thorac Cardiovasc Surg. 2006;132(6):1363–8.
62. Antoch G, Stattaus J, Nemat AT, et al. Non-small cell lung cancer: dual-modality PET/CT in preoperative staging. Radiology. 2003;229(2):526–33.
63. Aquino SL, Asmuth JC, Alpert NM, Halpern EF, Fischman AJ. Improved radiologic staging of lung cancer with 2-[18F]-fluoro-2-deoxy-D-glucose-positron emission tomography and computed tomography registration. J Comput Assist Tomogr. 2003;27(4):479–84.
64. Cerfolio RJ, Ojha B, Bryant AS, Raghuveer V, Mountz JM, Bartolucci AA. The accuracy of integrated PET-CT compared with dedicated PET alone for the staging of patients with nonsmall cell lung cancer. Ann Thorac Surg. 2004;78(3):1017–23; discussion 1017–23.
65. Goerres GW, Kamel E, Seifert B, et al. Accuracy of image coregistration of pulmonary lesions in patients with non-small cell lung cancer using an integrated PET/CT system. J Nucl Med. 2002;43(11):1469–75.
66. Schlemmer HP, Schafer J, Pfannenberg C, et al. Fast whole-body assessment of metastatic disease using a novel magnetic resonance imaging system: initial experiences. Invest Radiol. 2005;40(2):64–71.
67. Plathow C, Aschoff P, Lichy MP, et al. Positron emission tomography/computed tomography and whole-body magnetic resonance imaging in staging of advanced nonsmall cell lung cancer–initial results. Invest Radiol. 2008;43(5):290–7.

68. Yi CA, Shin KM, Lee KS, et al. Non-small cell lung cancer staging: efficacy comparison of integrated PET/CT versus 3.0-T whole-body MR imaging. Radiology. 2008;248(2):632–42.
69. Ohno Y, Koyama H, Nogami M, et al. Whole-body MR imaging vs. FDG-PET: comparison of accuracy of M-stage diagnosis for lung cancer patients. J Magn Reson Imaging. 2007;26(3):498–509.
70. Ohno Y, Koyama H, Yoshikawa T, et al. N stage disease in patients with non-small cell lung cancer: efficacy of quantitative and qualitative assessment with STIR turbo spin-echo imaging, diffusion-weighted MR imaging, and fluorodeoxyglucose PET/CT. Radiology. 2011;261(2):605–15.
71. Usuda K, Zhao XT, Sagawa M, et al. Diffusion-weighted imaging is superior to positron emission tomography in the detection and nodal assessment of lung cancers. Ann Thorac Surg. 2011;91(6):1689–95.
72. Pauls S, Schmidt SA, Juchems MS, et al. Diffusion-weighted MR imaging in comparison to integrated [(18)F]-FDG PET/CT for N-staging in patients with lung cancer. Eur J Radiol. 2012;81(1):178–82.
73. Baysal T, Mutlu DY, Yologlu S. Diffusion-weighted magnetic resonance imaging in differentiation of postobstructive consolidation from central lung carcinoma. Magn Reson Imaging. 2009;27(10):1447–54.
74. Silvestri G, Littenberg B, Colice G. The clinical evaluation for detecting metastatic lung cancer: a meta-analysis. Am J Respir Crit Care Med. 1995;152(1):225–30.
75. Silvestri GA, Tanoue LT, Margolis ML, Barker J, Detterbeck F, American College of Chest Physicians. The noninvasive staging of non-small cell lung cancer: the guidelines. Chest. 2003;123(1 Suppl):147S–56.
76. Ohno Y, Koyama H, Onishi Y, et al. Non-small cell lung cancer: whole-body MR examination for M-stage assessment–utility for whole-body diffusion-weighted imaging compared with integrated FDG PET/CT. Radiology. 2008;248(2):643–54.
77. Heffner JE, Klein JS. Recent advances in the diagnosis and management of malignant pleural effusions. Mayo Clin Proc. 2008;83(2):235–50.
78. American Thoracic Society. Management of malignant pleural effusions. Am J Respir Crit Care Med. 2000;162(5):1987–2001.
79. Erasmus JJ, McAdams HP, Rossi SE, Goodman PC, Coleman RE, Patz EF. FDG PET of pleural effusions in patients with non-small cell lung cancer. AJR Am J Roentgenol. 2000;175(1):245–9.
80. Gupta NC, Rogers JS, Graeber GM, et al. Clinical role of F-18 fluorodeoxyglucose positron emission tomography imaging in patients with lung cancer and suspected malignant pleural effusion. Chest. 2002;122(6):1918–24.
81. Boland GW, Lee MJ, Gazelle GS, Halpern EF, McNicholas MM, Mueller PR. Characterization of adrenal masses using unenhanced CT: an analysis of the CT literature. AJR Am J Roentgenol. 1998;171(1):201–4.
82. Boland GW, Hahn PF, Pena C, Mueller PR. Adrenal masses: characterization with delayed contrast-enhanced CT. Radiology. 1997;202(3):693–6.
83. Pena CS, Boland GW, Hahn PF, Lee MJ, Mueller PR. Characterization of indeterminate (lipid-poor) adrenal masses: use of washout characteristics at contrast-enhanced CT. Radiology. 2000;217(3):798–802.
84. Ho LM, Paulson EK, Brady MJ, Wong TZ, Schindera ST. Lipid-poor adenomas on unenhanced CT: does histogram analysis increase sensitivity compared with a mean attenuation threshold? AJR Am J Roentgenol. 2008;191(1):234–8.
85. Jhaveri KS, Wong F, Ghai S, Haider MA. Comparison of CT histogram analysis and chemical shift MRI in the characterization of indeterminate adrenal nodules. AJR Am J Roentgenol. 2006;187(5):1303–8.
86. Remer EM, Motta-Ramirez GA, Shepardson LB, Hamrahian AH, Herts BR. CT histogram analysis in pathologically proven adrenal masses. AJR Am J Roentgenol. 2006;187(1):191–6.
87. Jhaveri KS, Lad SV, Haider MA. Computed tomographic histogram analysis in the diagnosis of lipid-poor adenomas: comparison to adrenal washout computed tomography. J Comput Assist Tomogr. 2007;31(4):513–8.
88. Heinz-Peer G, Honigschnabi S, Schneider B, Niederle B, Kaserer K, Lechner G. Characterization of adrenal masses using MR imaging with histopathologic correlation. AJR Am J Roentgenol. 1999;173(1):15–22.
89. Korobkin M, Giordano TJ, Brodeur FJ, et al. Adrenal adenomas: relationship between histologic lipid and CT and MR findings. Radiology. 1996;200(3):743–7.
90. Outwater EK, Siegelman ES, Huang AB, Birnbaum BA. Adrenal masses: correlation between CT attenuation value and chemical shift ratio at MR imaging with in-phase and opposed-phase sequences. Radiology. 1996;200(3):749–52.
91. Erasmus J, Patz Jr E, McAdams H, et al. Evaluation of adrenal masses in patients with bronchogenic carcinoma using 18F-fluorodeoxyglucose positron emission tomography. AJR Am J Roentgenol. 1997;168(5):1357–60.
92. Gupta NC, Graeber GM, Tamim WJ, Rogers JS, Irisari L, Bishop HA. Clinical utility of PET-FDG imaging in differentiation of benign from malignant adrenal masses in lung cancer. Clin Lung Cancer. 2001;3(1):59–64.
93. Vikram R, Yeung HD, Macapinlac HA, Iyer RB. Utility of PET/CT in differentiating benign from malignant adrenal nodules in patients with cancer. AJR Am J Roentgenol. 2008;191(5):1545–51.
94. Yun M, Kim W, Alnafisi N, Lacorte L, Jang S, Alavi A. 18F-FDG PET in characterizing adrenal lesions detected on CT or MRI. J Nucl Med. 2001;42(12):1795–9.

95. Kagohashi K, Satoh H, Ishikawa H, Ohtsuka M, Sekizawa K. Liver metastasis at the time of initial diagnosis of lung cancer. Med Oncol. 2003;20(1):25–8.
96. Delbeke D, Martin WH, Sandler MP, Chapman WC, Wright JK Jr, Pinson CW. Evaluation of benign vs malignant hepatic lesions with positron emission tomography. Arch Surg. 1998;133(5):510–5; discussion 515–6.
97. Little AG, Stitik FP. Clinical staging of patients with non-small cell lung cancer. Chest. 1990;97(6):1431–8.
98. Cheran SK, Herndon 2nd JE, Patz Jr EF. Comparison of whole-body FDG-PET to bone scan for detection of bone metastases in patients with a new diagnosis of lung cancer. Lung Cancer. 2004;44(3):317–25.
99. Gayed I, Vu T, Johnson M, Macapinlac H, Podoloff D. Comparison of bone and 2-deoxy-2-[18F]fluoro-D-glucose positron emission tomography in the evaluation of bony metastases in lung cancer. Mol Imaging Biol. 2003;5(1):26–31.
100. Hsia TC, Shen YY, Yen RF, Kao CH, Changlai SP. Comparing whole body 18F-2-deoxyglucose positron emission tomography and technetium-99m methylene diophosphate bone scan to detect bone metastases in patients with non-small cell lung cancer. Neoplasma. 2002;49(4):267–71.
101. Davis PC, Hudgins PA, Peterman SB, Hoffman Jr JC. Diagnosis of cerebral metastases: double-dose delayed CT vs contrast-enhanced MR imaging. AJNR Am J Neuroradiol. 1991;12(2):293–300.
102. Mujoomdar A, Austin JH, Malhotra R, et al. Clinical predictors of metastatic disease to the brain from non-small cell lung carcinoma: primary tumor size, cell type, and lymph node metastases. Radiology. 2007;242(3):882–8.
103. Cole JFH, Thomas JE, Wilcox AB, Halford 3rd HH. Cerebral imaging in the asymptomatic preoperative bronchogenic carcinoma patient: is it worthwhile? Ann Thorac Surg. 1994;57(4):838–40.
104. Colice G, Birkmeyer J, Black W, Littenberg B, Silvestri G. Cost-effectiveness of head CT in patients with lung cancer without clinical evidence of metastases. Chest. 1995;108(5):1264–71.
105. Ferrigno D, Buccheri G. Cranial computed tomography as a part of the initial staging procedures for patients with non-small cell lung cancer. Chest. 1994;106(4):1025–9.
106. Mintz BJ, Turhim S, Alexander S, Yang WC, Shanzer S. Intracranial metastases in the initial staging of bronchogenic carcinoma. Chest. 1984;86:850–3.
107. Rohren EM, Provenzale JM, Barboriak DP, Coleman RE. Screening for cerebral metastases with FDG PET in patients undergoing whole-body staging of non-central nervous system malignancy. Radiology. 2003;226(1):181–7.
108. Wang J, Wu N, Cham MD, Song Y. Tumor response in patients with advanced non-small cell lung cancer: perfusion CT evaluation of chemotherapy and radiation therapy. AJR Am J Roentgenol. 2009;193(4):1090–6.
109. Fraioli F, Anzidei M, Zaccagna F, et al. Whole-tumor perfusion CT in patients with advanced lung adenocarcinoma treated with conventional and anti-angiogenetic chemotherapy: initial experience. Radiology. 2011;259(2):574–82.
110. Sohn HJ, Yang YJ, Ryu JS, et al. [18F] Fluorothymidine positron emission tomography before and 7 days after gefitinib treatment predicts response in patients with advanced adenocarcinoma of the lung. Clin Cancer Res. 2008;14(22):7423–9.
111. Everitt S, Hicks RJ, Ball D, et al. Imaging cellular proliferation during chemo-radiotherapy: a pilot study of serial 18F-FLT positron emission tomography/computed tomography imaging for non-small-cell lung cancer. Int J Radiat Oncol Biol Phys. 2009;75(4):1098–104.
112. Yamamoto Y, Nishiyama Y, Ishikawa S, et al. Correlation of 18F-FLT and 18F-FDG uptake on PET with Ki-67 immunohistochemistry in non-small cell lung cancer. Eur J Nucl Med Mol Imaging. 2007;34(10):1610–6.
113. Yang W, Zhang Y, Fu Z, et al. Imaging of proliferation with 18F-FLT PET/CT versus 18F-FDG PET/CT in non-small-cell lung cancer. Eur J Nucl Med Mol Imaging. 2010;37(7):1291–9.
114. Dittmann H, Dohmen BM, Paulsen F, et al. [18F] FLT PET for diagnosis and staging of thoracic tumours. Eur J Nucl Med Mol Imaging. 2003;30(10):1407–12.
115. Krohn KA, Link JM, Mason RP. Molecular imaging of hypoxia. J Nucl Med. 2008;49 Suppl 2:129S–48.
116. Rajendran JG, Schwartz DL, O'Sullivan J, et al. Tumor hypoxia imaging with [F-18] fluoromisonidazole positron emission tomography in head and neck cancer. Clin Cancer Res. 2006;12(18):5435–41.

Preoperative Evaluation for Lung Cancer Resection

6

Mario Gomez, Clayton J. Shamblin, and Gerard A. Silvestri

Age

Age is considered an independent predictor of complications from lung resection. In patients >70 years old, the mortality rate is between 4 and 7 % for lobectomy and 14 % for pneumonectomy [1–3] as compared to a mortality rate of 1–4 % for lobectomy and 5–9 % for pneumonectomy in those <70. Furthermore, previous studies [4, 5] have reported substantial perioperative morbidity and mortality in patients >80 years and proposed that either nonsurgical treatment or a less than anatomic resection is more appropriate for this age group. A large national survey in the United States from 1994 to 2003 [6] demonstrated that perioperative mortality in 24,804 patients >80 years who underwent lung cancer resection was 6.7 % and 3.7 % in 70,416 patients aged 65–69 years. Additionally, 5-year survival rates were 31 % in octogenarians vs. 47 % in patients aged 65–69 years, although stage at diagnosis was not reported in this study. These data correlate with a series from Johns Hopkins [7] in which 68 patients in their 80s that underwent surgical resection for stage I non-small cell lung cancer (NSCLC) had a 30-day mortality rate of 8.8 % and a 5-year survival of 34 %. Another series of 61 octogenarians with stage I NSCLC from Cornell University [8] had a 1.6 % perioperative mortality and a 5-year survival of 38 %. In contrast, a more recent study by Palma et al. showed similar percent survival at 5 years between patients less than 75 and those greater than 75 years old (65 % and 69 %, respectively) who underwent surgical resection for stage I NSCLC [9]. Alternatively, in the National Chest Hospital Study Group for Lung Cancer in Japan [10], 799 patients who were treated nonoperatively had a 5-year survival rate of 16.6 %. In the United States [11], 49 patients with stage I or IIa lung cancer who did not receive treatment had a median survival time of 14.2 ± 2.4 months. This value was significantly worse compared to the median survival time of 46.2 ± 3.2 months for 43 patients who underwent lobectomy. In summary, it seems that postoperative morbidity is higher and operative mortality may be greater in the elderly. However, long-term survival after surgery is much higher in those who can undergo surgery. Evidence suggests that age alone should not be a reason to deny a potentially curative surgical resection but rather a careful assessment of comorbidities and patient preferences should take priority in this patient population.

M. Gomez, M.D.
Pulmonary and Sleep Center of the Valley,
1604 East 8th Street, Suite A, Weslaco,
TX 78596, USA

C.J. Shamblin, M.D. • G.A. Silvestri, M.D., M.S. (✉)
Department of Internal Medicine, Division of Pulmonary and Critical Care, Allergy and Sleep Medicine,
Medical University of South Carolina, 96 Jonathan Lucas Street, Suite 812-CSB, MSC 630, Charleston,
SC 29425-6300, USA
e-mail: silvestr@musc.edu

J.G. Ravenel (ed.), *Lung Cancer Imaging*, Contemporary Medical Imaging,
DOI 10.1007/978-1-60761-620-7_6, © Springer Science+Business Media New York 2013

Pulmonary Function Testing

Different pulmonary function tests have been studied as predictors of risk for lung resection. In addition, several techniques have been used to predict postoperative values based on preoperative tests and the type of surgery to be undertaken.

Forced Expiratory Volume in 1 s

The forced expiratory volume in 1 s (FEV1) obtained by spirometry is the most common test used to assess the eligibility of patients with lung cancer for surgery. Data from more than 2,000 patients in three large series in the 1970s have shown that a mortality rate of <5 % should be expected if the preoperative FEV1 is >1.5 L for a lobectomy and >2 L for a pneumonectomy [12–14]. It is recognized that these values represent a range of lung function based on an individual's age, sex, and height and may create a bias against older patients, people of small stature, and women who might be able to tolerate lower levels of lung function [15]. Although it is not possible to recalculate percent predicted values from published data, an FEV1 of >80 % predicted has been accepted as an indicator that patients could undergo pneumonectomy without further evaluation [16].

Diffusing Capacity for Carbon Monoxide

The diffusing capacity for carbon monoxide (DLCO) has been shown to be a strong independent predictor of postoperative complications and death [17–19]. Individuals with a preoperative DLCO <60 % predicted were found to have more frequent pulmonary complications, hospitalizations for respiratory compromise, and worse median dyspnea scores than individuals with preoperative DLCO >60 % predicted [20]. Furthermore, spirometry and DLCO should be seen as complementary tests. If there is evidence of diffuse parenchymal lung disease on chest radiographs or exertional dyspnea that is clinically out of proportion to the FEV1, DLCO should be measured. In a prospective study of 137 patients with resectable lung cancer, those with an FEV1 of >80 % predicted and DLCO of >80 % predicted without a cardiac history who underwent pneumonectomy survived the operation [16].

Predicted Postoperative Lung Function

In patients with a preoperative FEV1 or DLCO of <80 % predicted, the predicted postoperative (PPO) lung function may be calculated by estimating the amount of functioning lung tissue that will be lost after surgical resection. Several methods are used to calculate the PPO lung function including the anatomic estimation based on counting the number of segments to be removed, ventilation scans, perfusion scans, and quantitative CT scans [15]. The radionuclide perfusion scan method is preferred to estimate the PPO FEV1 and DLCO after pneumonectomy because the anatomic method tends to underestimate actual postoperative FEV1 values [21]. The anatomic method is preferred to estimate lung function after a lobectomy [1, 15].

Segment Method

This method involves calculating the portion of all bronchopulmonary segments that will remain after resection. The PPO FEV1 is calculated based on the number of lung segments resected: $\text{PPOFEV1} = \text{preoperativeFEV1} \times (1 - 0.0526 \times S)$, where S = number of segments resected. Each segment is considered to represent 1/19 of the lung function (1/19 = 0.0526) [22]. The lower lobes are considered to have five pulmonary segments each, the right upper lobe to have three segments, the right middle lobe to have two segments, and the left upper lobe to have four segments. For example, in a patient with an FEV1 of 2.0 L undergoing a right upper lobe, PPO FEV1 $= 2.0 \times (1 - 0.0526 \times 3) = 1.68$ L.

Using this, the PPO lung function was found to correlate well with actual function for those undergoing lobectomy ($r = 0.867$) and has a fair correlation for pneumonectomy ($r = 0.677$) [22].

However, the actual lung function was consistently underestimated using this technique, particularly in those patients with baseline impairment of their lung function (by 250 cc for lobectomy and 500 cc for pneumonectomy) [23].

Radionuclide Scanning Techniques

This technique has the same principle of the segment methods, and the relative function of the portion of lung to be resected is estimated by quantifying the perfusion to that area. Postoperative lung function is then estimated by the product of the preoperative function and the portion of lung function that will remain after resection as estimated by the scan. The accuracy of this technique has been questioned; a study using technetium scanning calculated values of imprecision from 18 to 21 % despite showing reasonable correlation [24]. Additionally, the FEV1 was consistently underestimated, particularly if the starting value was lower.

Quantitative Computed Tomography

Quantitative computed tomography scanning has also been described as a technique to estimate postresection lung function. The volume of lung with attenuation between 500 and 910 HU is used to estimate functional lung volume. The portion of lung remaining postresection was predicted by calculating lung volume in the area to be resected as a portion of total lung volume and using the principles stated prior. Using this method the PPO function correlated as well or better than that calculated using radionuclide quantitative perfusion imaging [25]. Potential advantages of this technique include that its routine use for staging purposes may eliminate the need for additional testing such as perfusion scans and that it may also be a more sensitive indicator of diffuse parenchymal lung disease than the FEV1 and DLCO combined [26].

A threshold PPO FEV1 of 0.7–0.8 L has been described as the lower limit to allow patients to undergo surgical resection [27, 28]. However, using absolute values for PPO lung function have the same limitations as using an absolute value of preoperative FEV1, as it may prevent people who may be able to tolerate lower values, such as older patients, people of small stature, and women, from a potentially curative intervention. For the aforementioned reasons, the percent PPO (%PPO) values for FEV1 and DLCO should be used instead of absolute values.

The %PPO FEV1 after pneumonectomy is calculated using the perfusion method with the following formula:

$$\text{PPO FEV1 postpneumonectomy} = \text{preoperative FEV1} \times (1 - \text{fraction of total perfusion of resected lung})$$

The PPO FEV1 can be converted into the %PPO FEV1 using standard equations. The PPO and %PPO DLCO postpneumonectomy can be determined using the same formula. The %PPO values estimated by perfusion scan may be up to 10 % less than the actual measured values 3 months after the patient have undergone resection [15]. For example, a 60-year-old male with a tumor located in the right lung is evaluated for pneumonectomy. His FEV1 is 1.5 L and the perfusion scan demonstrates that the right lung perfusion is 30 %. The PPO FEV1 = 1.5 × (1 − 0.3) = 1.05 L, and the %PPO FEV1 is 70 %. This means that following resection of the right lung, 1.05 L of the left lung will remain. The minimum acceptable PPO FEV1 is 0.8 L. In this case the patient will be an acceptable candidate for pneumonectomy.

The %PPO FEV1 after lobectomy is calculated using the anatomic method with the following formula:

$$\text{PPO FEV1 postlobectomy} = \text{preoperative FEV1} \times (1 - y / z)$$

where y is the number of functional or unobstructed lung segments to be removed and z is the total number of functional segments. The PPO FEV1 can be converted into %PPO FEV1 using standard equations. The PPO and %PPO DLCO postlobectomy can be determined using the same formula. The %PPO FEV1 using the anatomic method correlates strongly with the actual postoperative FEV1. This method can also be applied in patients undergoing segmentectomies [15]. For example, in a patient with an FEV1 of 1.8 L undergoing a right lower lobectomy, the PPO FEV1 = $2.0\times(1-5/19)=1.48$ L, and the %PPO FEV1 = 82 %.

The perioperative risk increases when the FEV1 or DLCO are <40 % PPO. Several series have reported perioperative mortality rates from 16 to 50 % in such patients [18, 29–32]. While a PPO FEV1 and DLCO <40 % is likely to eliminate patients from surgical consideration, successful surgical resections have been reported in patients with poor lung function reserve. For this reason, it is prudent to more thoroughly evaluate these patients to further assess risk.

A combined value, the PPO product (PPP), was found to be the best predictor of surgical mortality in one study [31]. The PPP is the product of the PPO FEV1 and PPO DLCO. A PPP <1,650 was found in 75 % of those who died and 11 % of those who survived surgery.

Cardiopulmonary Exercise Testing

Previous guidelines [1, 33] have recommended the use of cardiopulmonary exercise testing (CPET) as the next step in the preoperative risk assessment process in those patients with either FEV1 or DLCO <40 % PPO. The risk for perioperative complications has been reported to be higher in patients with a lower measured VO_2 max. Patients with preoperative VO_2 max of 15–20 mL/kg/min can undergo curative-intent lung cancer surgery with an acceptable low mortality rate [15]. A meta-analysis of four studies [15] demonstrated that patients with VO_2 max of <10 mL/kg/min had a very high risk for postoperative death. In three of these studies [30, 34, 35], the mortality rate ranged from 27 to 50 %, and in one small series [18], there were no deaths among the five patients with very low VO_2 max. In addition, a VO_2 max of 10–15 mL/kg/min indicates an increased risk of perioperative death [15]. Recently, Brunelli et al. found that all deaths after lung resection occurred in patients with a VO_2 max <20 mL/kg/min [36]. In summary, in patients with both an FEV1 and a DLCO of <40 % PPO, a VO_2 max of <15 mL/kg/min indicates a very high surgical risk [39] and alternative treatment strategies should be considered.

Stair Climbing

If CPET were unavailable, another type of exercise test should be considered. Stair climbing has been used as a surrogate of CPET. Climbing three flights of stairs indicates an FEV1 of >1.7 L and climbing five flights of stairs indicates an FEV1 of >2 L [37]. Patients who can climb five flights of stairs will have a VO_2 max of >20 mL/kg/min, and patients who cannot climb one flight of stairs will have a VO_2 max of <10 mL/kg/min [38]. Several groups have shown that the ability to climb >12–14 m of stairs, which correlates with three flights of stairs, identifies patients who are at low risk for postoperative complications following lobectomy, even if they might have had an FEV1 or DLCO of <40 % PPO [15]. A recent study including 640 patients showed that climbing <12 m had a twofold rate of complications and 13-fold rate of mortality with major lung resection as compared to those climbing >22 m. It was also demonstrated that in those patients with FEV1 and/or DLCO <40 % PPO, the mortality rate in those who could climb >22 m was 0 % [39]. Limitations to this test include that it has not been standardized, and the duration of stair climbing, the speed of ascent, the number of steps per flight, the height of each step, and the criteria for stopping the test have varied from study to study.

Shuttle Walking

The distance traveled while performing a shuttle walk test, during which an individual walks back and forth over a defined distance at an incremental and progressive rate, has correlated well with VO_2 max obtained on a treadmill. Walking 25 shuttles (10 m each) approximated a VO_2 max in excess of 10 mL/kg/min [40].

Oxygen Desaturation

Oxygen desaturation during standardized exercise has been studied as a predictor of risk from lung resection. A 4 % or greater desaturation performed better than measures of FEV1 and DLCO in predicting respiratory failure, major morbidity, intensive care unit admission, length of stay, and home oxygen requirements. If desaturation was not noted, there was a 1–9 % chance of complications [41].

Methods to Reduce Perioperative Risks and Long-Term Pulmonary Disability

Lung Volume Reduction Surgery

Lung volume reduction surgery (LVRS) has been shown to improve survival in patients with severe heterogeneous emphysema with upper lobe predominance and low exercise capacity [42]. Patients with an FEV1 of <20 % predicted and either homogeneous emphysema or a DLCO <20 % predicted do poorly with LVRS [43]. Published data suggests that patients with extremely poor lung function can tolerate combined LVRS and resection of the lung cancer with acceptable mortality rates and good postoperative outcomes. Although indications for combined LVRS and lung cancer resection are still under development, it is believed that patients with lung cancer in the upper lobe that is also affected by emphysema and who have a DLCO and FEV1 of >20 % predicted may benefit from this procedure the most [15].

Smoking Cessation

The benefit of smoking cessation just prior to surgery in preventing postoperative pulmonary complications has not been proven. Some early studies suggested that stopping smoking only a few weeks prior to surgery may actually have led to an unexpected or paradoxical increase in the rate of pulmonary complications [44, 45]. A recent meta-analysis of nine studies found this not to be true, however. Quitting smoking within 8 weeks before surgery was not associated with an increase or decrease in overall postoperative complications for all available studies (relative risk 0.78; 95 % confidence interval [CI], 0.57–1.07) [46]. A retrospective study [47] of 300 patients undergoing lung cancer surgical resection found that postoperative pulmonary complication rates for patients who had quit smoking >2 months prior to undergoing surgery were similar to those who had quit within 2 months of the procedure (19 % vs. 23 %, respectively; $p>0.05$). A study conducted in Japan [48] examined the relationship between the duration of the preoperative smoke-free period and the development of postoperative pulmonary complications in 288 patients who underwent pulmonary surgery to define the optimal timing of smoking cessation. They found that the incidence of postoperative pulmonary complications among current smokers and recent smokers was 43.6 % and 53.8 %, respectively, and each was higher than that in the never-smokers (23.9 %; $p<0.05$). In addition, they found that the moving average of the incidence of complications gradually decreased in patients whose smoke-free period was 5–8 weeks or longer. In general, patients should be advised to stop smoking as early as possible prior to surgery.

Pulmonary Rehabilitation

There are no data to support the routine use of preoperative pulmonary rehabilitation for patients with lung cancer. However, it may be helpful in preparing patients with COPD for LVRS, as it was found to improve dyspnea, quality of life, and exercise ability in such patients [49].

Quality of Life Before and After Surgery

The long-term goal of surgical therapy in lung cancer includes not only improvement in survival but also quality of life. Handy et al. [50] reported that the preoperative functional health status in patients who undergo lung cancer surgery is significantly impaired. In addition, pain and impairment of the functional status persisted for 6 months after resection. Other factors such as preoperative chemoradiation, extent of lung resection, postoperative complications, or adjuvant therapy did not adversely affect functional health status or quality of life 6 months after surgery. A low preoperative DLCO, not FEV1, was a predictor of postoperative quality of life.

Current Guidelines

The British Thoracic Society and Society of Cardiothoracic Surgeons of Great Britain and Ireland Working Party in 2001 [1] and the American College of Chest Physicians (ACCP) in 2007 [15] have developed guidelines for the preoperative evaluation for lung cancer resection. In 2009, the European Respiratory Society and European Society of Thoracic Surgeons (ERS/ESTS) published guidelines on fitness for radical therapy in lung cancer patients as well [51]. Although their suggestions have slight differences, most recommendations are similar. All guidelines recommend initial spirometry with the ERS/ESTS also recommending routine DLCO measurements on all patients. ACCP indicates measuring DLCO in those patients with normal spirometry but who have unexplained dyspnea or diffuse parenchymal disease on imaging. A major difference between the guidelines is the timing of calculation of PPO lung function and performing CPET. BTS and ACCP favor FEV1 and DLCO PPO values if spirometry is abnormal, followed by exercise testing in those patients with PPO values >30 % but less than 40 %. ERS/ESTS guidelines recommend exercise testing much earlier in their algorithm, followed by calculation of PPO values if VO_2 max values are between 10 and 20 mL/kg/min. These differences highlight the lack of consensus in this area and emphasize the importance of individualizing cases based on the best optimal treatment for each patient. (See Figs. 6.1 and 6.2 for the proposed algorithms for preoperative physiologic assessment of perioperative risk from the ACCP and ERS/ESTS, respectively.)

A summary of the current ACCP recommendations include:

- Patients with lung cancer should be assessed by a multidisciplinary team, which includes a thoracic surgeon, a medical oncologist, and a pulmonologist, to determine their suitability for lung resection.
- Patients with lung cancer should not be denied lung resection surgery on the basis of age alone.
- Patients with lung cancer who have major factors for increased perioperative cardiovascular risk should have a preoperative cardiologic evaluation.
- Patients with an FEV1 >2 L or >80 % predicted normal are suitable for pneumonectomy without further evaluation unless there is evidence of undue dyspnea on exertion or interstitial lung disease. In that case, the DLCO should be measured.
- Patients with an FEV1 >1.5 L are suitable for lobectomy without further evaluation unless there is evidence of undue dyspnea on exertion or interstitial lung disease. In that case, the DLCO should be measured.
- If a patient is not clearly operable after initial testing (FEV1 or DLCO <80 % predicted normal), PPO lung function should be estimated.
- If the PPO FEV1 or PPO DLCO is <40 % predicted normal, exercise testing should be considered.
- If the PPO FEV1 <30 % predicted normal or the product of the PPO FEV1 and PPO DLCO <1,650, there is a very high risk of perioperative death and cardiopulmonary complications. Other options should be considered.
- Patients with a VO_2 max of < 10 mL/kg/min regardless of other values, or <15 mL/kg/min with both PPO FEV1 and PPO DLCO <40 % predicted, are at high risk for perioperative death and cardiopulmonary complications. Other options should be considered.

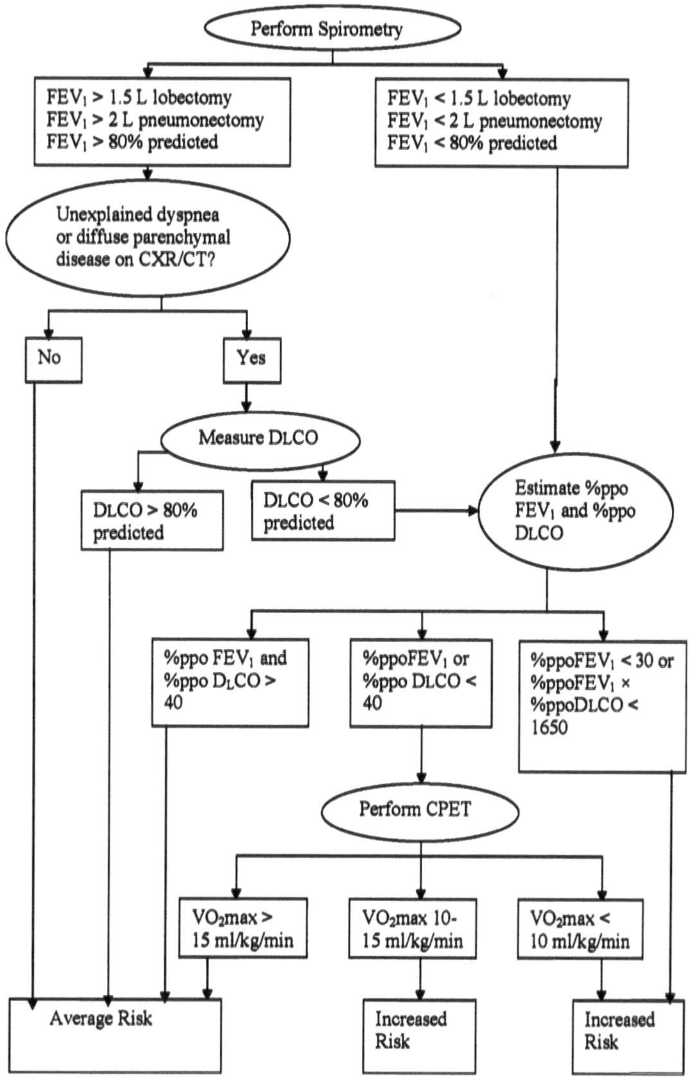

Fig. 6.1 Preoperative physiologic assessment of perioperative risk. *CXR* chest radiograph (from Colice GL, et al.: Physiologic evaluation of the patient with lung cancer being considered for resectional surgery: ACCP evidenced-based clinical practice guidelines (2nd edition). Chest 2007; 132; 161–177 [15]; with permission)

- Patients who walk <25 shuttles (250 m) on two shuttle walks, climb <1 flight of stairs, or desaturate >4 % during testing are at high risk of perioperative death and cardiopulmonary complications. Other options should be considered.
- Patients with very poor lung function and a lung cancer in an area of upper emphysema may be considered for combined LVRS and lung cancer resection if both the FEV1 and DLCO are >20 % predicted.
- All patients with lung cancer should be counseled regarding smoking cessation.

Summary

The objective of preoperative evaluation for lung cancer resection is to identify those patients who have an acceptable chance of tolerating resection and those that are at increased risk of perioperative complications, including death and long-term disability. Risk assessment is based on a combination of patient comorbidities, exercise tolerance, and objective physiologic data. A multidisciplinary approach including cardiothoracic surgeons, medical oncologists, radiation

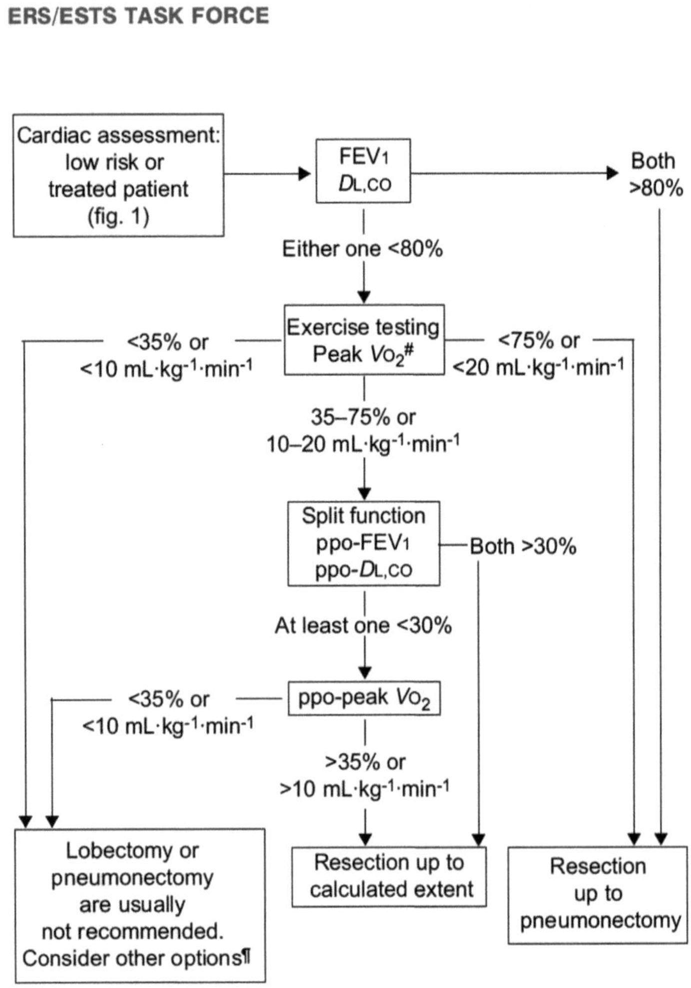

Fig. 6.2 Algorithm for assessment of cardiopulmonary reserve before lung resection in lung cancer patients. *FEV1* forced expiratory volume in 1 s, *DLCO* diffusing capacity of the lung for carbon monoxide, *VO_2* oxygen consumption, *PPO* predicted postoperative; #: if peak VO_2 is not available, cardiopulmonary exercise testing (CPET) can be replaced by stair climbing; however, if altitude reaching during stair climbing is <22 m, CPET with peak VO_2 measurement is highly recommended (from Brunelli A, Charloux A, Bolliger CT, Rocco G, et al. ERS/ESTS clinical guidelines on fitness for radical therapy in lung cancer patients (surgery and chemo-radiotherapy). Eur Respir J. 2009; 34(1):17–41 [51]; with permission)

oncologists, and pulmonologists is essential when evaluating the preoperative risk assessment of a patient for a curative-intent surgery. This is especially true for those patients who may be inoperable or marginal surgical candidates as emerging noninvasive treatment strategies may be reasonable alternatives to consider. For example, an elderly patient with marginal lung function who is a surgical candidate may choose an alternative therapeutic approach if given the option. Preoperative evaluation algorithms are available, but assessments must be individualized to facilitate patient preference-based decision making in regards to treatment of lung cancer.

References

1. British Thoracic Society, Society of Cardiothoracic Surgeons of Great Britain and Ireland Working Party. Guidelines on the selection of patients with lung cancer for surgery. Thorax. 2001;56:89–108.
2. Damhuis RA, Schutte PR. Resection rates and postoperative mortality in 7,899 patients with lung cancer. Eur Respir J. 1996;9:7–10.
3. Yellin A, Hill LR, Lieberman Y. Pulmonary resections in patients over 70 years of age. Isr J Med Sci. 1985;21:833–40.
4. Harvey JC, Erdman C, Pisch J, Beattie EJ. Surgical treatment of non-small cell lung cancer in patients older than seventy years. J Surg Oncol. 1995;60: 247–9.

5. Pagni S, Federico JA, Ponn RB. Pulmonary resection for lung cancer in octogenarians. Ann Thorac Surg. 1997;63:785–9.
6. Finlayson E, Fan Z, Birkmeyer J. Outcomes in octogenarians undergoing high-risk cancer operation: a national study. J Am Coll Surg. 2007;205:729–34.
7. Brock MV, Kim MP, Hooker CM, et al. Pulmonary resection in octogenarians with stage I nonsmall cell lung cancer. Ann Thorac Surg. 2004;77:271–7.
8. Port JL, Kent M, Korst RJ, et al. Surgical resection for lung cancer in the octogenarian. Chest. 2004;126: 733–8.
9. Palma DA, Tyldesley S, Sheehan F, et al. Stage I non-small cell lung cancer (NSCLC) in patients aged 75 years and older: does age determine survival after radical treatment? J Thorac Oncol. 2010;5(6): 818–24.
10. Motohiro A, Ueda H, Komatsu H, Yanai N, Mori T, National Chest Hospital Study Group for Lung Cancer. Prognosis of non-surgically treated, clinical stage I lung cancer patients in Japan. Lung Cancer. 2002;36:65–9.
11. McGarry RC, Song G, des Rosiers P, Timmerman R. Observation-only management of early stage, medically inoperable lung cancer: poor outcome. Chest. 2002;121(4):1155–8.
12. Boushy SF, Billig DM, North LB, Helgason AH. Clinical course related to preoperative and postoperative pulmonary function in patients with bronchogenic carcinoma. Chest. 1971;59(4):383–91.
13. Miller JI Jr. Physiologic evaluation of pulmonary function in the candidate for lung resection. J Thorac Cardiovasc Surg. 1993;105(2):347–51; discussion 351–2.
14. Wernly JA, DeMeester TR, Kirchner PT, Myerowitz PD, Oxford DE, Golomb HM. Clinical value of quantitative ventilation-perfusion lung scans in the surgical management of bronchogenic carcinoma. J Thorac Cardiovasc Surg. 1980;80(4):535–43.
15. Colice GL, Shafazand S, Griffin JP, Keenan R, Bolliger CT, American College of Chest Physicians. Physiologic evaluation of the patient with lung cancer being considered for resectional surgery: ACCP evidenced-based clinical practice guidelines (2nd edition). Chest. 2007;132(3 Suppl):161S–77S.
16. Wyser C, Stulz P, Soler M, et al. Prospective evaluation of an algorithm for the functional assessment of lung resection candidates. Am J Respir Crit Care Med. 1999;159(5 Pt 1):1450–6.
17. Ferguson MK, Little L, Rizzo L, et al. Diffusing capacity predicts morbidity and mortality after pulmonary resection. J Thorac Cardiovasc Surg. 1988;96(6):894–900.
18. Markos J, Mullan BP, Hillman DR, et al. Preoperative assessment as a predictor of mortality and morbidity after lung resection. Am Rev Respir Dis. 1989;139(4): 902–10.
19. Liptay MJ, Basu S, Hoaglin MC, et al. Diffusion lung capacity for carbon monoxide (DLCO) is an independent prognostic factor for long-term survival after curative lung resection for cancer. J Surg Oncol. 2009;100(8):703–7.
20. Bousamra M 2nd, Presberg KW, Chammas JH, et al. Early and late morbidity in patients undergoing pulmonary resection with low diffusion capacity. Ann Thorac Surg. 1996;62(4):968–74; discussion 974–5.
21. Smulders SA, Smeenk FW, Janssen-Heijnen ML, Postmus PE. Actual and predicted postoperative changes in lung function after pneumonectomy: a retrospective analysis. Chest. 2004;125(5):1735–41.
22. Zeiher BG, Gross TJ, Kern JA, Lanza LA, Peterson MW. Predicting postoperative pulmonary function in patients undergoing lung resection. Chest. 1995; 108(1):68–72.
23. Mazzone PJ, Arroliga AC. Lung cancer: preoperative pulmonary evaluation of the lung resection candidate. Am J Med. 2005;118(6):578–83.
24. Giordano A, Calcagni ML, Meduri G, Valente S, Galli G. Perfusion lung scintigraphy for the prediction of postlobectomy residual pulmonary function. Chest. 1997;111(6):1542–7.
25. Wu MT, Pan HB, Chiang AA, et al. Prediction of postoperative lung function in patients with lung cancer: comparison of quantitative CT with perfusion scintigraphy. AJR Am J Roentgenol. 2002;178(3): 667–72.
26. Ueda K, Kaneda Y, Sudoh M, et al. Role of quantitative CT in predicting hypoxemia and complications after lung lobectomy for cancer, with special reference to area of emphysema. Chest. 2005;128(5): 3500–6.
27. Olsen GN, Block AJ, Tobias JA. Prediction of post-pneumonectomy pulmonary function using quantitative macroaggregate lung scanning. Chest. 1974;66(1):13–6.
28. Pate P, Tenholder MF, Griffin JP, Eastridge CE, Weiman DS. Preoperative assessment of the high-risk patient for lung resection. Ann Thorac Surg. 1996;61(5):1494–500.
29. Bolliger CT, Jordan P, Soler M, et al. Exercise capacity as a predictor of postoperative complications in lung resection candidates. Am J Respir Crit Care Med. 1995;151(5):1472–80.
30. Holden DA, Rice TW, Stelmach K, Meeker DP. Exercise testing, 6-min walk, and stair climb in the evaluation of patients at high risk for pulmonary resection. Chest. 1992;102(6):1774–9.
31. Pierce RJ, Copland JM, Sharpe K, Barter CE. Preoperative risk evaluation for lung cancer resection: predicted postoperative product as a predictor of surgical mortality. Am J Respir Crit Care Med. 1994; 150(4):947–55.
32. Wahi R, McMurtrey MJ, DeCaro LF, et al. Determinants of perioperative morbidity and mortality after pneumonectomy. Ann Thorac Surg. 1989; 48(1):33–7.
33. Beckles MA, Spiro SG, Colice GL, Rudd RM, American College of Chest Physicians. The physio-

logic evaluation of patients with lung cancer being considered for resectional surgery. Chest. 2003;123(1 Suppl):105S–14S.
34. Bechard D, Wetstein L. Assessment of exercise oxygen consumption as preoperative criterion for lung resection. Ann Thorac Surg. 1987;44(4):344–9.
35. Olsen GN, Weiman DS, Bolton JW, et al. Submaximal invasive exercise testing and quantitative lung scanning in the evaluation for tolerance of lung resection. Chest. 1989;95(2):267–73.
36. Brunelli A, Belardinelli R, Refai M, et al. Peak oxygen consumption during cardiopulmonary exercise test improves risk stratification in candidates to major lung resection. Chest. 2009;135(5):1260–7.
37. Bolton JW, Weiman DS, Haynes JL, Hornung CA, Olsen GN, Almond CH. Stair climbing as an indicator of pulmonary function. Chest. 1987;92(5):783–8.
38. Pollock M, Roa J, Benditt J, Celli B. Estimation of ventilatory reserve by stair climbing. A study in patients with chronic airflow obstruction. Chest. 1993;104(5):1378–83.
39. Brunelli A, Refai M, Xiumé F, et al. Performance at symptom-limited stair-climbing test is associated with increased cardiopulmonary complications, mortality, and costs after major lung resection. Ann Thorac Surg. 2008;86(1):240–47; discussion 247–8.
40. Singh SJ, Morgan MD, Hardman AE, Rowe C, Bardsley PA. Comparison of oxygen uptake during a conventional treadmill test and the shuttle walking test in chronic airflow limitation. Eur Respir J. 1994;7(11):2016–20.
41. Rao V, Todd TR, Kuus A, Buth KJ, Pearson FG. Exercise oximetry versus spirometry in the assessment of risk prior to lung resection. Ann Thorac Surg. 1995;60(3):603–8.
42. Fishman A, Martinez F, Naunheim K, et al. A randomized trial comparing lung-volume-reduction surgery with medical therapy for severe emphysema. N Engl J Med. 2003;348(21):2059–73.
43. National Emphysema Treatment Trial Research Group. Patients at high risk of death after lung-volume-reduction surgery. N Engl J Med. 2001; 345(15):1075–83.
44. Bluman LG, Mosca L, Newman N, Simon DG. Preoperative smoking habits and postoperative pulmonary complications. Chest. 1998;113(4):883–9.
45. Warner MA, Offord KP, Warner ME, et al. Role of preoperative cessation of smoking and other factors in postoperative pulmonary complications: a blinded prospective study of coronary artery bypass patients. Mayo Clin Proc. 1989;64(6):609–16.
46. Myers K, Hajek P, Hinds C, McRobbie H. Stopping smoking shortly before surgery and postoperative complications: a systematic review and meta-analysis. Arch Intern Med. 2011;171(11):983–9.
47. Barrera R, Shi W, Amar D, et al. Smoking and timing of cessation: impact on pulmonary complications after thoracotomy. Chest. 2005;127(6):1977–83.
48. Nakagawa M, Tanaka H, Tsukuma H, Kishi Y. Relationship between the duration of the preoperative smoke-free period and the incidence of postoperative pulmonary complications after pulmonary surgery. Chest. 2001;120(3):705–10.
49. Ries AL, Make BJ, Lee SM, et al. The effects of pulmonary rehabilitation in the national emphysema treatment trial. Chest. 2005;128(6):3799–809.
50. Handy Jr JR, Asaph JW, Skokan L, et al. What happens to patients undergoing lung cancer surgery? Outcomes and quality of life before and after surgery. Chest. 2002;122(1):21–30.
51. Brunelli A, Charloux A, Bolliger CT, et al. ERS/ESTS clinical guidelines on fitness for radical therapy in lung cancer patients (surgery and chemo-radiotherapy). Eur Respir J. 2009;34(1):17–41.

7 Small Cell Carcinoma

James G. Ravenel

Small cell lung carcinoma (SCLC) is an aggressive neoplasm of neuroendocrine cell origin with a distinct biologic behavior and is therefore grouped separately from other primary lung neoplasms. SCLC represents about 15–25 % of all lung cancers and tends to occur in younger patients than those with the other lung cancers. SCLC mostly originates in the submucosa of proximal airways such as the lobar bronchi or main bronchi while a small percentage (<5 %) originates in the peripheral areas of the lung. The tumor itself is highly cellular and has a limited fibrotic or inflammatory response. Consequently, the tumor spreads rapidly through the lymphatics and blood vessels at an early stage, resulting in early nodal and distant metastatic deposits [1, 2]. From a practical standpoint, SCLC may be thought of as a "systemic" disease at the time of diagnosis.

Extrathoracic non-metastatic manifestations, or the paraneoplastic syndromes (PNS), are more common in SCLC than in NSCLC. These may be in the form of endocrinopathy, neurologic dysfunction, or skin disease. While the primary tumor is in general easily visualized by conventional imaging, FDG-PET may be helpful in documenting the tumor location when there are nonspecific conventional imaging findings [3]. The most common PNS is hyponatremia of malignancy which occurs in up to 15 % of cases and may be caused by inappropriate secretion of arginine vasopressin (antidiuretic hormone) or atrial natriuretic peptide [4, 5]. Production of ectopic corticotrophin is relatively common in SCLC but results in clinical disease, Cushing syndrome, in only 2–5 % of cases [6, 7]. Hypertrophic pulmonary osteoarthropathy is distinctly uncommon in SCLC, unlike NSCLC.

Neuromuscular PNS include Eaton–Lambert myasthenic syndrome, encephalomyelitis, and cerebellar degeneration. Eaton–Lambert myasthenic syndrome results from autoantibodies against P/Q voltage-gated calcium channels resulting in proximal muscle weakness and/or autonomic symptoms including dry mouth and constipation and occurs in approximately 3 % of SCLC cases [8]. Paraneoplastic limbic encephalitis is usually associated with anti-Hu antibody. Symptoms include psychiatric manifestations such as hallucinations, agitation, anxiety, or depression as well as memory loss, confusion, or seizures. Cerebellar degeneration has also been associated with SCLC and is manifest by ataxia, nystagmus, and dysarthria [9]. Still, the most common cause of neurological symptoms in a patient with SCLC is brain metastasis. The imaging features of PNS will be discussed later.

J.G. Ravenel, M.D. (✉)
Department of Radiology, Medical University of South Carolina, 96 Jonathan Lucas St, Room 211, P.O. Box 250322, Charleston, SC 29425, USA
e-mail: ravenejg@musc.edu

J.G. Ravenel (ed.), *Lung Cancer Imaging*, Contemporary Medical Imaging,
DOI 10.1007/978-1-60761-620-7_7, © Springer Science+Business Media New York 2013

Staging

Historically, SCLC was stratified by a two-stage system developed by the Veterans Administration Lung Cancer Study Group [10]. Limited-stage disease included disease confined to the chest and supraclavicular nodes that can be contained within a single, tolerable radiation port. The definition of limited disease was further refined by the International Association of the Study of Lung Cancer (IASLC) to state that the classification of limited SCLC should include patients with the disease restricted to one hemithorax with regional lymph node metastases, including ipsilateral hilar, ipsilateral and contralateral mediastinal, ipsilateral and contralateral supraclavicular, and ipsilateral pleural effusion independent of cytology [11].

As a practical rule, SCLC that would encompass stages I–IIIB under the current TNM system can be characterized as limited disease. Extensive stage disease included all lesions not characterized as limited stage and those with distant metastases analogous to stage IV. About 70 % of patients with SCLC present with extensive disease, and only 30 % have disease limited to the thorax. One group reported 2-year survival rates of about 10 % for limited disease and about 3 % for extensive disease. Extensive disease with only brain metastasis may have a survival rate similar to that of limited disease.

A relatively large retrospective series suggested that 5-year survival was enhanced (37.1 %) with surgery (the majority diagnosed prior to surgery) for pathologic stages IA–IIB, and survival was further improved with the addition of at least four cycles of chemotherapy to surgery [12]. Based on further analysis of resected SCLCs, the IASLC has found sufficient prognostic variability using the TNM system to warrant replacing the previous staging system [13]. For surgically resected SCLC ($n=349$), there is a marked survival enhancement (>2 years) for both stage T1a and N0 cases compared with other surgically resected SCLCs [13]. Moreover, 5-year survival for resected stage I tumors is 57 %. Unfortunately, comparisons with standard chemoradiotherapy are difficult since complete TNM pathologic staging is unavailable for nonsurgical cases and nonsurgical cases are traditionally labeled as limited disease and also biased toward higher TNM stages. Given these limitations, the overall 5-year survival for all surgically resected "limited disease" is 34.5 % and favorable compared to the 12–25 % for traditional chemoradiotherapy [1]. It should be noted that surgically resected cases account for only 3 % of all SCLC cases. The survival differences across pathologically staged SCLC are considered sufficient to warrant using the TNM system to stratify patients for treatment trials rather than the prior limited/extensive classification, although for clinical purposes outside of therapeutic trials the relatively simple limited/extensive classification probably is sufficient to guide treatment.

Imaging of Small Cell Lung Cancer

Imaging Chest and Abdomen

Because of the predilection for early metastatic spread, the primary site is often not visible by conventional radiography or CT. The typical primary site is radiographically occult submucosal endobronchial lesion that subsequently metastasizes to the mediastinal and hilar lymph nodes resulting in detection and the usual radiographic presentation of a large hilar and/or mediastinal mass (Fig. 7.1) [1]. Approximately 4 % of lung cancers presenting as a solitary pulmonary nodule (SPN) turn out to be SCLC (Fig. 7.2) and approximately 4 % of small cell cancers of the lung will present as an SPN [14]. There are no imaging features that otherwise distinguish SCLC and NSCLC when presenting as an SPN.

The mediastinum is by far the most common site of detected disease and varies in series from 66 to 92 % of cases [1, 15]. The mediastinal mass may grow so large that it obstructs the superior vena cava (SVC) (Fig. 7.3). SVC syndrome is a clinical diagnosis based on generalized swelling of the upper limbs, neck, and face associated with a mediastinal or paramediastinal lesion. Tumor growth in the mediastinum may also be associated

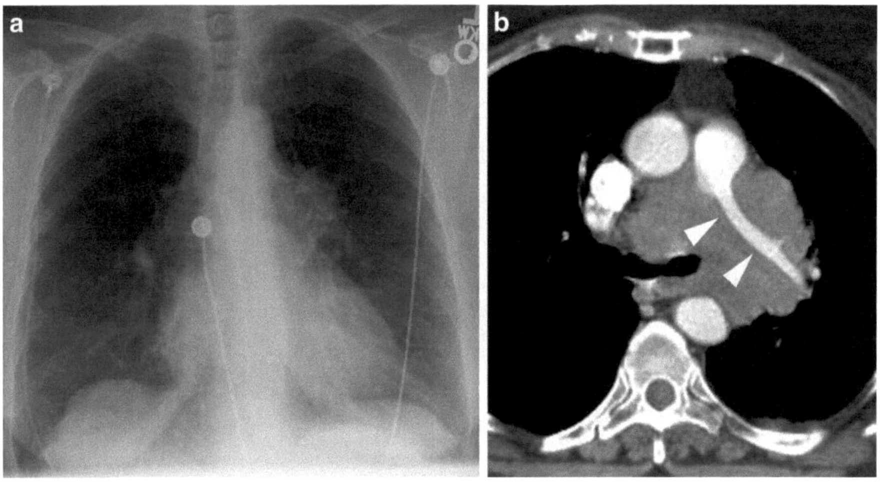

Fig. 7.1 Typical radiographic appearance of small cell lung cancer. (**a**) Frontal radiograph reveals mass involving the left hilum and aorto-pulmonary window without discrete parenchymal lesion. (**b**) Contrast-enhanced CT confirms mass as well as shows attenuation and narrowing of the left pulmonary artery (*arrowheads*)

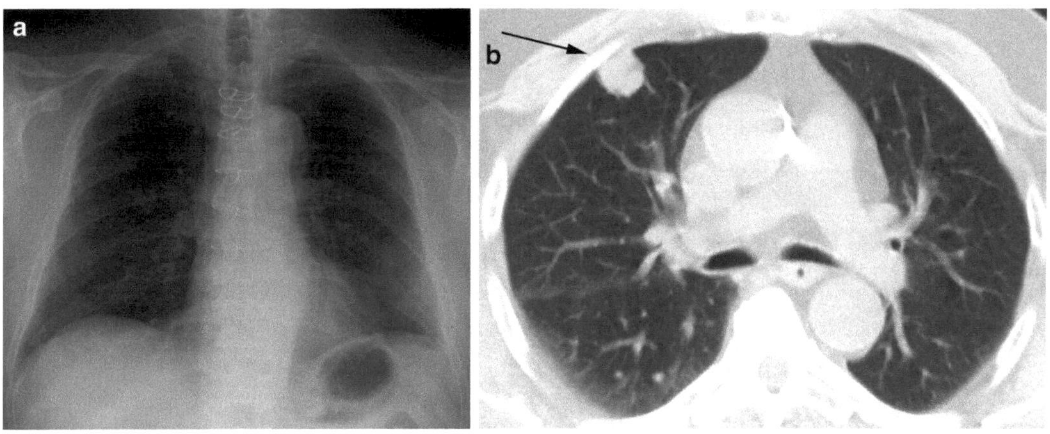

Fig. 7.2 (**a**, **b**) Small cell carcinoma (SCLC) presenting as a solitary pulmonary nodule (SPN). CT reveals slightly lobulated right upper lobe nodule (*arrow*). There are no radiographic features by which to differentiate from non-small cell lung cancers

with dyspnea, hoarseness, and dysphagia. In up to12 % of cases of SCLC, SVC syndrome is present at the time of initial diagnosis [4]. Invasion of the pericardium (38 %) and narrowing of central bronchi (68 %) can also occur and be detected with CT (Fig. 7.4) [3].

Once the tumor has access to the mediastinum, there are pathways of spread into the abdomen via the aortic and esophageal hiatus and into the neck. This can result in intra-abdominal lymphadenopathy primarily along the celiac vessels resulting in celiac, periportal (Fig. 7.5), and peripancreatic adenopathy. Previous studies show the incidence of disease in the peripancreatic and retroperitoneal lymph nodes to be 6 % [6]. Disease may also reach the gastrohepatic ligament either by spread along vascular planes or through the esophageal hiatus. Spread into the

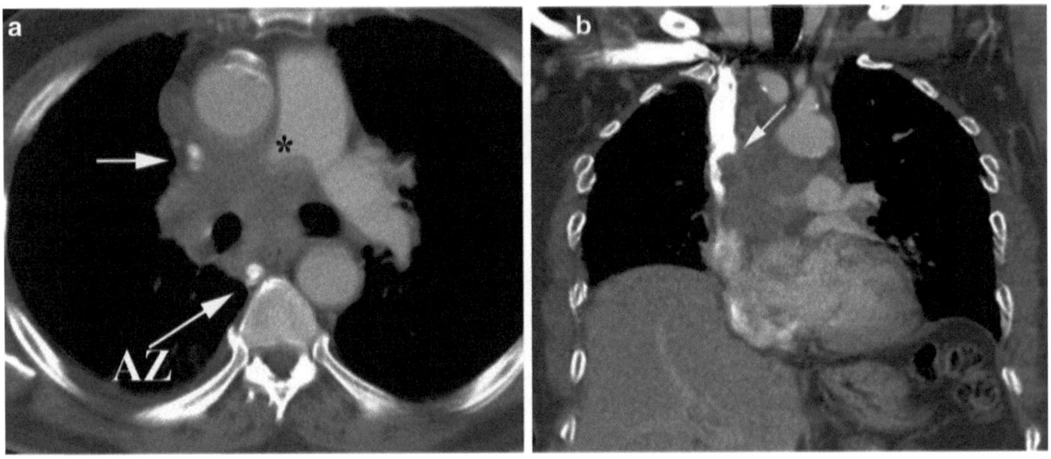

Fig. 7.3 Superior vena cava (SVC) obstruction. (**a**) Axial CT image reveals large mass surrounding and narrowing the SVC (*arrow*) as well as obstructing the right pulmonary artery (*asterisk*). Note collateral retrograde venous flow through the azygous vein (*AZ*). (**b**) Coronal reformation shows the mass invading the medial wall of the SVC (*arrow*)

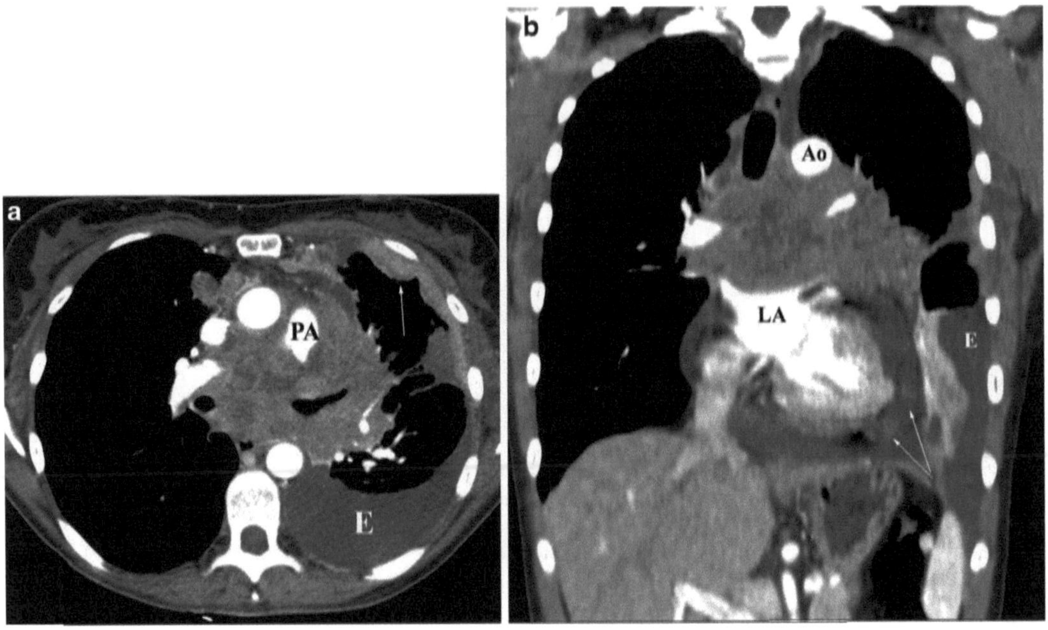

Fig. 7.4 SCLC with pleural and pericardial metastases. (**a**) Axial CT image reveals large mass infiltrating the mediastinum and markedly narrowing the origin of the left pulmonary artery (*PA*). There is associated left pleural effusion (*E*) with metastatic pleural implants anteriorly (*arrow*). (**b**) Coronal reformation reveals mass effect on the transverse aorta (*Ao*) and left atrium (*LA*) as well as a pericardial effusion with two discrete pericardial nodules (*arrow*) and left pleural effusion (*E*)

neck via the cervicothoracic continuum can result in ipsilateral supraclavicular adenopathy.

A majority of patients will have distant metastatic disease at presentation with up to 60 % having metastatic disease in the abdomen at the time of diagnosis. The adrenal gland and liver are the most frequent sites of disease (Figs. 7.6 and 7.7), although any abdominal organ can be affected

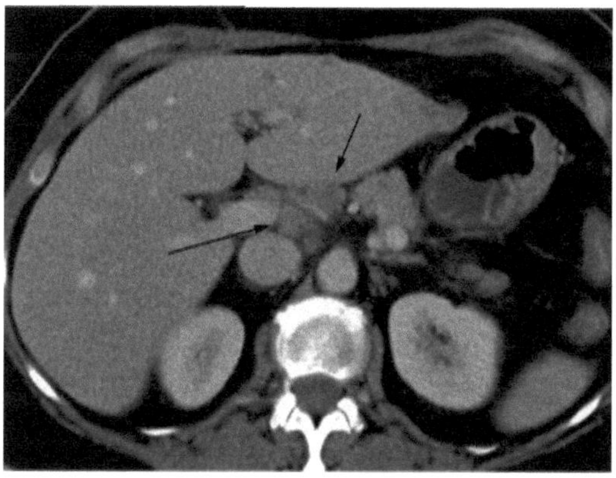

Fig. 7.5 Periportal adenopathy. Axial CT image reveals enlarged lymph nodes in the porta hepatis (*arrows*) surrounding common hepatic artery from SCLC

Table 7.1 Sites of metastatic disease

Site	% Involved at presentation	% Involved at autopsy
Mediastinal nodes	66–92	73–87
Bone	27–41	54
Liver	21–27	69
Adrenal	5–31	35–65
CNS	10–14	28–50
Retroperitoneal nodes	3–13	29–52
Supraclavicular nodes	17	42
Pleural effusion	16–20	30
Contralateral lung	1–12	8–27
Soft tissue	5	19

Adapted from Jackman DM, Johnson BE. Small-cell lung cancer. Lancet 2005;366(9494):1385–96

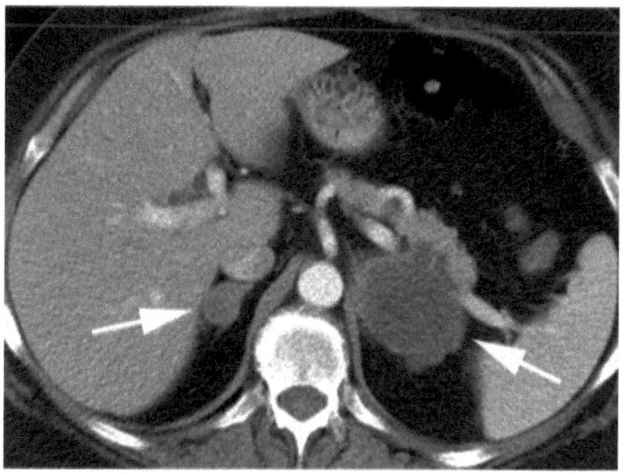

Fig. 7.6 Adrenal metastases. Axial CT image reveals necrotic low attenuation adrenal metastases (*arrows*)

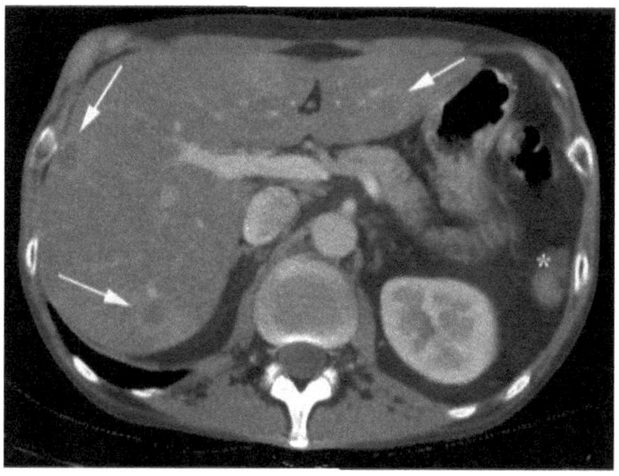

Fig. 7.7 Hepatic metastases. Axial CT image reveals multiple low attenuation nodules within the hepatic parenchyma

[16, 17] (Table 7.1). Because of this high frequency, a CT of the abdomen with contrast is considered indicated as part of routine staging [18].

Imaging of CNS in SCLC

Due to the high incidence of brain metastases, routine imaging of the central nervous system (CNS) is warranted. Cerebral metastases have been said to be present in up to 10 % of individuals at the time of diagnosis [19, 20]. The use of routine MR of the brain has resulted in a higher incidence and number of detected brain metastases, particularly in the neurologically asymptomatic patients [21]. PET/CT is generally not helpful for detection of cerebral metastases in SCLC regardless of the level of activity in the primary tumor [22]. While important for staging and treatment planning, it is unclear that early detection of asymptomatic cerebral metastases results in improved survival [18, 23]. The typical imaging appearance of a brain metastasis is a single or multiple rim-enhancing lesions (Fig. 7.8). If small the entire lesion may show homogeneous contrast enhancement. These lesions are, in general, easily distinguished for paraneoplastic lesions. For example, PLE will show high signal in the medial temporal lobe on FLAIR or T2-weighted images (Fig. 7.9), while cerebellar degeneration may be manifest early by transient

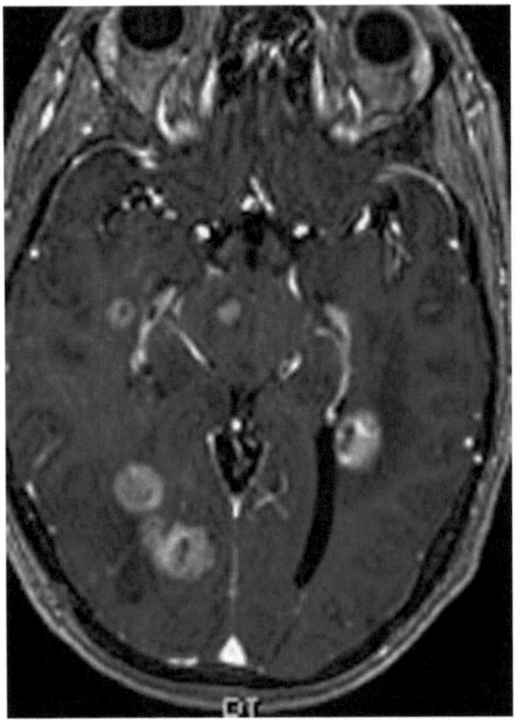

Fig. 7.8 Cerebral metastases. Axial gadolinium-enhanced T1-weighted image reveals multiple enhancing brain lesions with surrounding low signal vasogenic edema in the cerebrum and pons

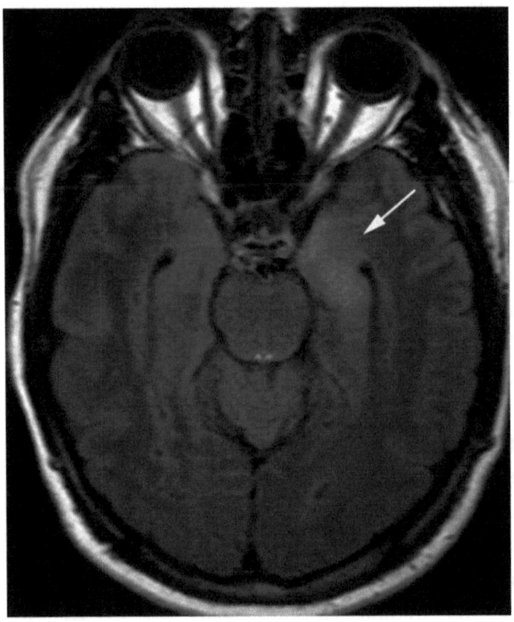

Fig. 7.9 Paraneoplastic limbic encephalitis. Axial FLAIR image reveals faintly increased signal in the left temporal lobe (*arrow*)

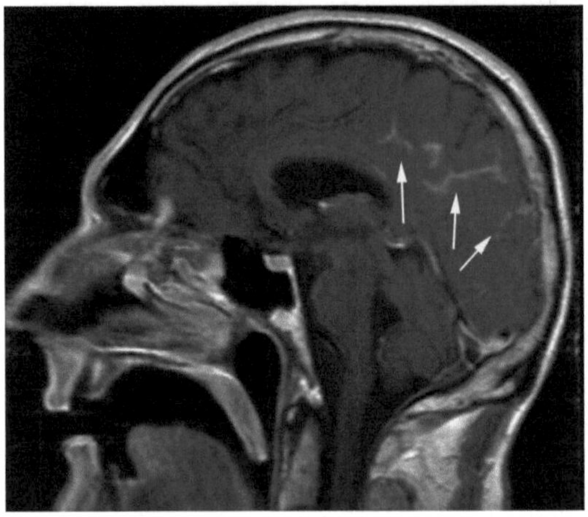

Fig. 7.10 Leptomeningeal carcinomatosis. Sagittal gadolinium-enhanced T1-weighted image reveals meningeal enhancement along the sulci of the posterior cerebral cortex (*arrows*)

enlargement of the cerebellum and meningeal enhancement and late by cerebellar atrophy [24]. Leptomeningeal disease is rare occurring in <2 % of cases (Fig. 7.10) [25].

Imaging of Osseous Metastases

Bone is considered to be the most common site of metastatic disease overall (35 % of cases), and therefore bone scintigraphy is generally part of the initial staging evaluation [26]. A whole body technique, bone scintigraphy detects signs of osseous repair, thus uptake is nonspecific and can be seen in healing fractures, degenerative joint, or spine disease as well as metastatic lesions. For the indeterminate lesion on bone scintigraphy, MR is useful to determine the etiology of the increased uptake. As data accumulates in other malignancies as well as SCLC, it is likely that bone scintigraphy will be replaced in the imaging algorithm by whole body PET/CT. Historically, bilateral bone marrow biopsies or aspirations were also suggested during initial staging, since this may be the only site of metastatic disease and detection would result in a change of stage from limited to extensive. This has been abandoned given the very low incidence of marrow disease in the absence of obvious disease on conventional imaging [18].

FDG-PET/CT

Staging

PET/CT has the potential to provide more accurate staging and prognostic information compared with conventional staging (Fig. 7.11) changing management in up to 25 % of patients, although studies remain limited to relatively small retrospective series [27]. The major value lies in the ability of PET/CT to upstage patients to extensive disease and spare the patient unnecessary therapy. Small cases series show that patients are upstaged in 8–15 % of cases as well as downstaged from extensive to limited disease in 5–10 % [28–31]. In a prospective trial PET/CT was shown to be superior to a conventional staging regimen of CT, bone scintigraphy, and bone marrow analysis, changing stage in 5 of 29 (17 %) subjects [29].

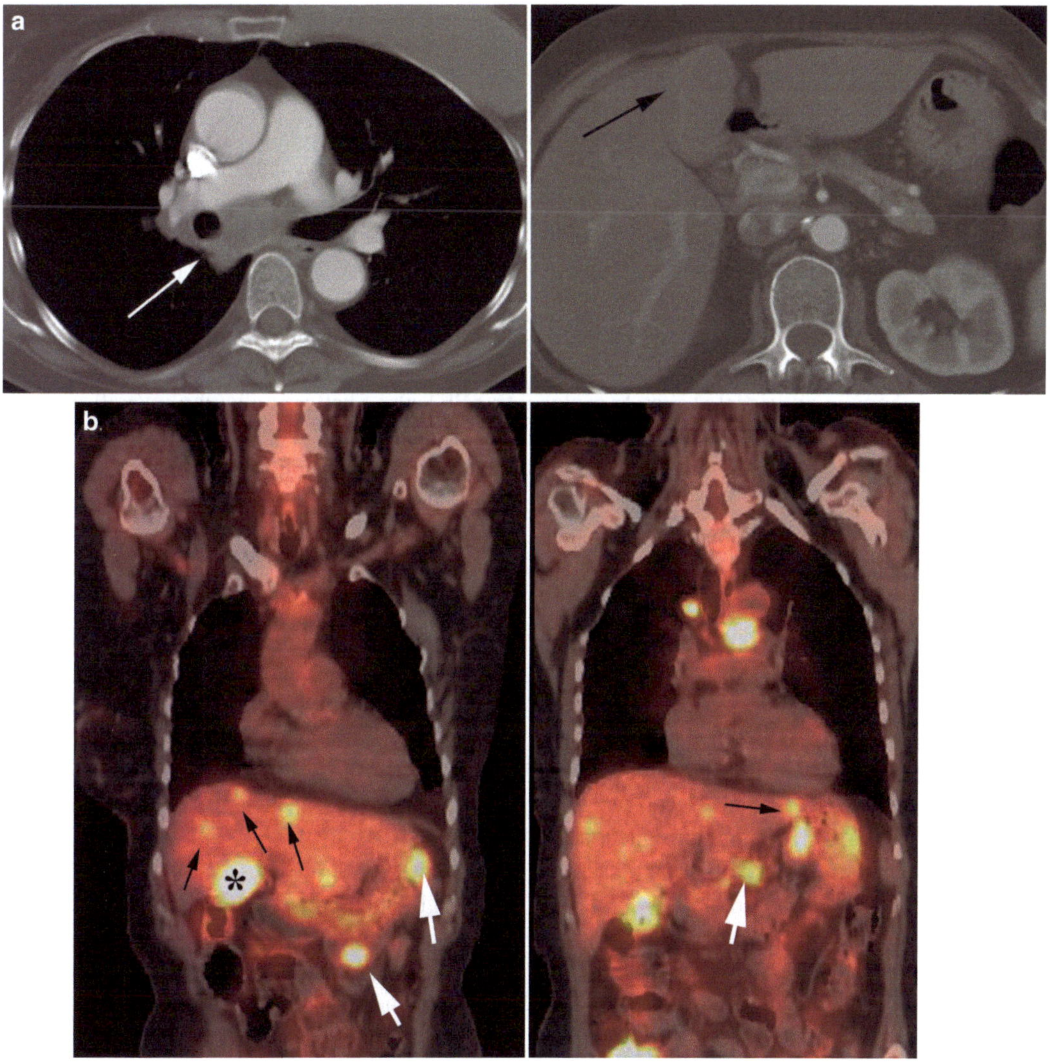

Fig. 7.11 Value of FDG-PET/CT in assessing extent of disease. (**a**) Axial CT images reveal mediastinal adenopathy and solitary hepatic metastasis (*arrows*) as the only sites of disease on conventional staging. (**b**) Coronal FDG-PET/CT images confirm the adenopathy and liver metastasis (*asterisk*) but reveal multiple additional liver metastases (*black arrows*) as well as multiple metastatic nodules in mesentery adjacent to bowel and stomach walls (*white arrows*)

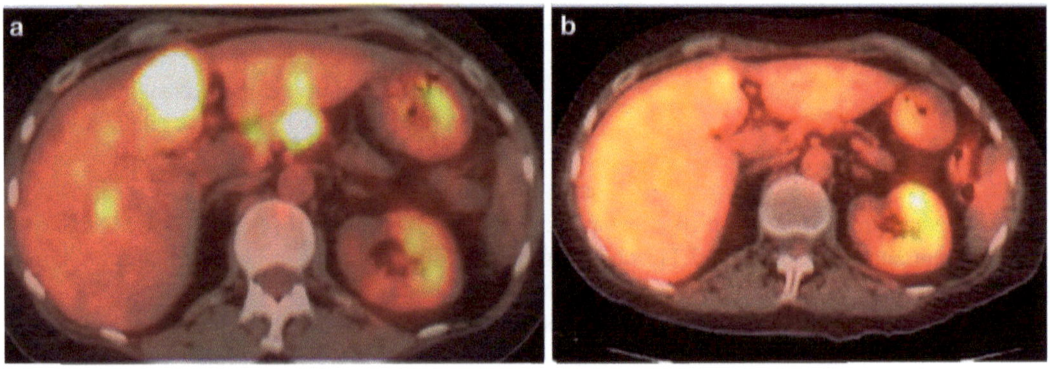

Fig. 7.12 Value of FDG-PET/CT in restaging. (**a**) Axial FDG-PET/CT shows multiple hepatic metastases. (**b**) After four cycles of chemotherapy, only dominant lesion remains metabolically active and has decreased from SUV of 10.4 to 3.6

Treatment Planning

In patients treated with radiation therapy, the field size has important implications both in terms of toxicity and possibility of local failure. The addition of FDG-PET to usual staging allows for better delineation of treatment fields through both the inclusion of otherwise unsuspected sites or exclusion of unaffected nodal stations. This may result in adjustment of the radiation therapy plan in up to 30 % of cases [31–33]. Because of respiratory artifact, it is ultimately incumbent on evaluating sites of uptake based and gross tumor volume based on the CT component to ultimately determine the tumor outline. The effect of such approach is the elimination of elective nodal irradiation with the presumed benefit of higher delivery of radiation to the clinical tumor volume (CTV). It is important to note that such an approach is associated with approximately 10 % rate of nodal recurrence outside of the CTV [33–35], although isolated nodal failure (that without associated distant disease) was 3 % in the study by van Loon.

Prognosis

Other potential uses of PET/CT in SCLC including determination of prognosis and response to therapy remain uncertain [36, 37]. Similar to non-small cell lung cancer, a higher SUV is associated with a poorer prognosis. Using the median SUVmax (8.7) as a cutoff in a cohort of 76 patients, stage-specific survival was increased 15 months for limited disease and 8 months for extensive disease for those with median SUVmax below the median [38]. With regard to post-therapeutic staging, in a retrospective review of 22 subjects using FDG-PET, a post-therapy negative PET was a better predictor of overall survival compared with non-metabolic responders (Fig. 7.12). In addition, metabolic response was a better predictor than anatomic response (Fig. 7.13) [39]. Another small study including 25 subjects suggested that post-therapy PET alters management in approximately 50 %. Unfortunately over 80 % of cases in that study did not have a pretreatment PET for comparison [40]. The utility of FDG-PET as an imaging biomarker in SCLC awaits further confirmation.

Conclusion

Although apparently decreasing in incidence, small cell lung cancer remains associated with a poor prognosis often due to distant metastatic disease at the time of diagnosis. The staging paradigm has shifted to a TNM classification so that appropriate patients may be considered for surgery. The radiologic staging has also changed from a multi-modality approach to one using predominately PET/CT as well as imaging of the brain, preferably MR imaging.

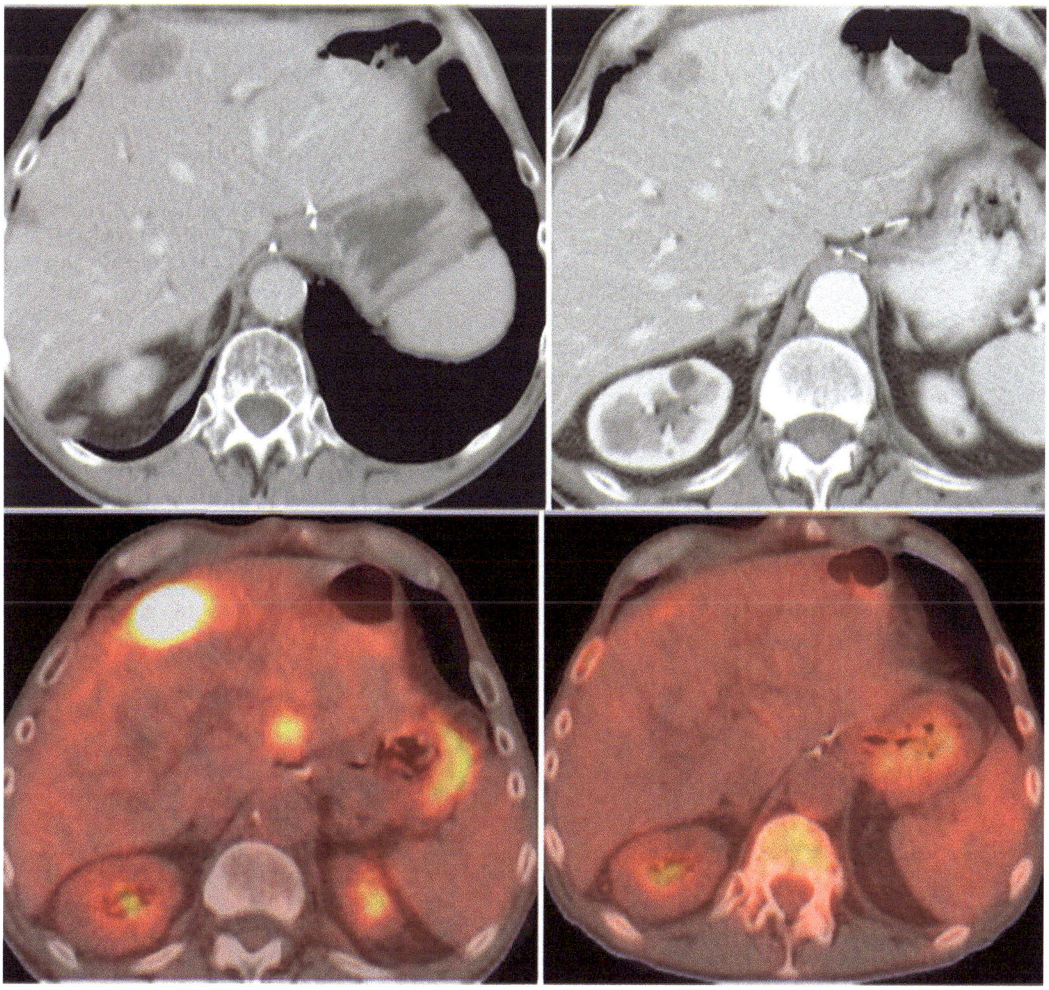

Fig. 7.13 Value of FDG-PET in restaging. Composite image of CT and FDG-PET/CT at two different time points. CT images reveal a decrease in diameter of 50 % which would be termed a partial response to therapy. PET/CT images however reveal a complete metabolic response even with a persistent anatomic abnormality

References

1. Jackman DM, Johnson BE. Small-cell lung cancer. Lancet. 2005;366(9494):1385–96.
2. Sher T, Dy GK, Adjei AA. Small cell lung cancer. Mayo Clin Proc. 2008;83(3):355–67.
3. Crotty E, Patz Jr EF. FDG-PET imaging in patients with paraneoplastic syndromes and suspected small cell lung cancer. J Thorac Imaging. 2001;16(2):89–93.
4. Campling BG, Sarda IR, Baer KA, et al. Secretion of atrial natriuretic peptide and vasopressin by small cell lung cancer. Cancer. 1995;75(10):2442–51.
5. Johnson BE, Chute JP, Rushin J, et al. A prospective study of patients with lung cancer and hyponatremia of malignancy. Am J Respir Crit Care Med. 1997; 156(5):1669–78.
6. Shepherd FA, Laskey J, Evans WK, Goss PE, Johansen E, Khamsi F. Cushing's syndrome associated with ectopic corticotropin production and small-cell lung cancer. J Clin Oncol. 1992;10(1): 21–7.
7. Stewart PM, Gibson S, Crosby SR, et al. ACTH precursors characterize the ectopic ACTH syndrome. Clin Endocrinol (Oxf). 1994;40(2):199–204.
8. Seute T, Leffers P, ten Velde GP, Twijnstra A. Neurologic disorders in 432 consecutive patients with small cell lung carcinoma. Cancer. 2004;100(4):801–6.
9. Toothaker TB, Rubin M. Paraneoplastic neurological syndromes: a review. Neurologist. 2009;15(1): 21–33.
10. Osterlind K, Ihde DC, Ettinger DS, et al. Staging and prognostic factors in small cell carcinoma of the lung. Cancer Treat Rep. 1983;67(1):3–9.

11. Stahel R, Ginsberg R, Havemann K, et al. Staging and prognostic factors in small cell lung cancer: a consensus report. Lung Cancer. 1989;5:119–26.
12. Inoue M, Miyoshi S, Yasumitsu T, et al. Surgical results for small cell lung cancer based on the new TNM staging system. Thoracic Surgery Study Group of Osaka University, Osaka, Japan. Ann Thorac Surg. 2000;70(5):1615–9.
13. Vallières E, Shepherd FA, Crowley J, et al. The IASLC Lung Cancer Staging Project: proposals regarding the relevance of TNM in the pathologic staging of small cell lung cancer in the forthcoming (seventh) edition of the TNM classification for lung cancer. J Thorac Oncol. 2009;4(9):1049–59.
14. Kreisman H, Wolkove N, Quoix E. Small cell lung cancer presenting as a solitary pulmonary nodule. Chest. 1992;101(1):225–31.
15. Pearlberg JL, Sandler MA, Lewis Jr JW, Beute GH, Alpern MB. Small-cell bronchogenic carcinoma: CT evaluation. AJR Am J Roentgenol. 1988;150(2): 265–8.
16. Whitley NO, Mirvis SE. Abdominal CT in the staging of small cell carcinoma of the lung. Crit Rev Diagn Imaging. 1989;29(2):103–16.
17. Mirvis SE, Whitley NO, Aisner J, Moody M, Whitacre M, Whitley JE. Abdominal CT in the staging of small-cell carcinoma of the lung: incidence of metastases and effect on prognosis. AJR Am J Roentgenol. 1987;148(5):845–7.
18. Simon GR, Turrisi A, American College of Chest Physicians. Management of small cell lung cancer: ACCP evidence-based clinical practice guidelines (2nd edition). Chest. 2007;132(3 Suppl):324S–39S.
19. Hirsch FR, Paulson OB, Hansen HH, Larsen SO. Intracranial metastases in small cell carcinoma of the lung. Prognostic aspects. Cancer. 1983;51(3): 529–33.
20. Giannone L, Johnson DH, Hande KR, Greco FA. Favorable prognosis of brain metastases in small cell lung cancer. Ann Intern Med. 1987;106(3):386–9.
21. Seute T, Leffers P, ten Velde GP, Twijnstra A. Detection of brain metastases from small cell lung cancer: consequences of changing imaging techniques (CT versus MRI). Cancer. 2008;112(8):1827–34.
22. Lee HY, Chung JK, Jeong JM, et al. Comparison of FDG-PET findings of brain metastasis from non-small-cell lung cancer and small-cell lung cancer. Ann Nucl Med. 2008;22(4):281–6.
23. Hochstenbag MM, Twijnstra A, Wilmink JT, Wouters EF, ten Velde GP. Asymptomatic brain metastases (BM) in small cell lung cancer (SCLC): MR-imaging is useful at initial diagnosis. J Neurooncol. 2000;48(3):243–8.
24. Dalmau J, Rosenfeld MR. Paraneoplastic syndromes of the CNS. Lancet Neurol. 2008;7(4):327–40.
25. Seute T, Leffers P, ten Velde GP, Twijnstra A. Leptomeningeal metastases from small cell lung carcinoma. Cancer. 2005;104(8):1700–5.
26. Adjei AA, Marks RS, Bonner JA. Current guidelines for the management of small cell lung cancer. Mayo Clin Proc. 1999;74(8):809–16.
27. Azad A, Chionh F, Scott AM, et al. High impact of 18F-FDG-PET on management and prognostic stratification of newly diagnosed small cell lung cancer. Mol Imaging Biol. 2010;12(4):443–51.
28. Niho S, Fujii H, Murakami K, et al. Detection of unsuspected distant metastases and/or regional nodes by FDG-PET [corrected] scan in apparent limited-disease small-cell lung cancer. Lung Cancer. 2007;57(3):328–33.
29. Fischer BM, Mortensen J, Langer SW, et al. A prospective study of PET/CT in initial staging of small-cell lung cancer: comparison with CT, bone scintigraphy and bone marrow analysis. Ann Oncol. 2007;18(2):338–45.
30. Brink I, Schumacher T, Mix M, et al. Impact of [18F] FDG-PET on the primary staging of small-cell lung cancer. Eur J Nucl Med Mol Imaging. 2004;31(12): 1614–20.
31. Bradley JD, Dehdashti F, Mintun MA, Govindan R, Trinkaus K, Siegel BA. Positron emission tomography in limited-stage small-cell lung cancer: a prospective study. J Clin Oncol. 2004;22(16):3248–54.
32. van Loon J, Offermann C, Bosmans G, et al. 18FDG-PET based radiation planning of mediastinal lymph nodes in limited disease small cell lung cancer changes radiotherapy fields: a planning study. Radiother Oncol. 2008;87(1):49–54.
33. van Loon J, De Ruysscher D, Wanders R, et al. Selective nodal irradiation on basis of (18)FDG-PET scans in limited-disease small-cell lung cancer: a prospective study. Int J Radiat Oncol Biol Phys. 2010; 77(2):329–36.
34. Salem A, Abuodeh Y, Khader J. Selective nodal irradiation on basis of (18)FDG-PET scans in limited-disease small-cell lung cancer: a prospective study. In regard to van Loon et al. (Int J Radiat Oncol Biol Phys 2010;77:329–336). Int J Radiat Oncol Biol Phys. 2010;78(5):1606; author reply 1606–7.
35. De Ruysscher D, Bremer RH, Koppe F, et al. Omission of elective node irradiation on basis of CT-scans in patients with limited disease small cell lung cancer: a phase II trial. Radiother Oncol. 2006;80(3):307–12.
36. Kut V, Spies W, Spies S, Gooding W, Argiris A. Staging and monitoring of small cell lung cancer using [18F]fluoro-2-deoxy-D-glucose-positron emission tomography (FDG-PET). Am J Clin Oncol. 2007;30(1):45–50.
37. Fischer BM, Mortensen J, Langer SW, et al. PET/CT imaging in response evaluation of patients with small cell lung cancer. Lung Cancer. 2006;54(1):41–9.
38. Lee YJ, Cho A, Cho BC, et al. High tumor metabolic activity as measured by fluorodeoxyglucose positron emission tomography is associated with poor prognosis in limited and extensive stage small-cell lung cancer. Clin Cancer Res. 2009;15(7):2426–32.
39. Onitilo AA, Engel JM, Demos JM, Mukesh B. Prognostic significance of 18 F-fluorodeoxyglucose—positron emission tomography after treatment in patients with limited stage small cell lung cancer. Clin Med Res. 2008;6(2):72–7.
40. Blum R, MacManus MP, Rischin D, Michael M, Ball D, Hicks RJ. Impact of positron emission tomography on the management of patients with small-cell lung cancer: preliminary experience. Am J Clin Oncol. 2004;27(2):164–71.

Invasive Staging of Non-small Cell Lung Cancer

8

Clayton J. Shamblin, Mario Gomez, and Gerard A. Silvestri

Lung cancer is the leading cause of cancer-related death worldwide, and despite advances in therapy, the 5-year survival rate for all stages combined is approximately 16 % [1]. For these reasons, a careful initial diagnostic evaluation to determine the location and the extent of primary and metastatic disease is critical for the adequate care of patients.

The objective of non-small cell lung cancer (NSCLC) staging in the absence of distal metastases is to evaluate for mediastinal lymph node involvement. Accurate staging of NSCLC is important not only to determine the patient's prognosis but also to decide a treatment plan, as the presence of mediastinal lymph node involvement (N2 disease) is diagnostic for stage IIIA or IIIB lung cancer that suggests inoperability and the need for treatment with chemotherapy, radiation, or both.

Mediastinal lymph node staging is divided into noninvasive (imaging) and invasive staging. Noninvasive techniques include computed tomography (CT), magnetic resonance imaging (MRI), positron emission tomography (PET), and PET-CT. It has been reported that the sensitivity and specificity of CT scanning for identifying mediastinal lymph node metastasis are 51 % (95 % confidence interval (CI), 47–54 %) and 86 % (95 % CI, 84–88 %), respectively, demonstrating that CT scanning has limited ability either to rule in or exclude mediastinal metastasis. Furthermore, the sensitivity and specificity of PET scanning for identifying mediastinal metastasis are 74 % (95 % CI, 69–79 %) and 85 % (95 % CI, 82–88 %), respectively [2]. The combined modality of PET-CT for preoperative staging was evaluated in a prospective randomized trial of conventional staging vs. conventional plus PET-CT with end point being avoidance of futile thoracotomy. Results showed a reduction in futile thoracotomies in the PET-CT group vs. the conventional group (21 % vs. 42 %, respectively) and that one futile thoracotomy was avoided for every 5 PET-CTs performed. Additionally, the diagnostic accuracy and sensitivity were 79 % and 64 %, respectively, compared to 60 % and 32 %, respectively, for conventional staging [3]. These data suggest that PET scanning is more accurate than CT and that the combined modality may provide additional benefit; however, all abnormal scan findings require cytological or histological confirmation of malignancy by invasive techniques, so that patients are not denied the opportunity of potentially curative treatment.

Invasive staging techniques are divided into surgical and nonsurgical procedures including endoscopic and bronchoscopic techniques. Surgical staging includes mediastinoscopy, left anterior mediastinotomy (Chamberlain procedure), and video-assisted thoracoscopic surgery (VATS).

C.J. Shamblin, M.D. • G.A. Silvestri, M.D., M.S. (✉)
Department of Internal Medicine, Division of Pulmonary and Critical Care, Allergy, and Sleep Medicine, Medical University of South Carolina, 96 Jonathan Lucas Street, Suite 812-CSB, MSC 630, Charleston, SC 29425-6300, USA
e-mail: silvestr@musc.edu

M. Gomez, M.D.
Pulmonary and Sleep Center of the Valley, 1604 East 8th Street, Suite A, Weslaco, TX 78596, USA

J.G. Ravenel (ed.), *Lung Cancer Imaging*, Contemporary Medical Imaging,
DOI 10.1007/978-1-60761-620-7_8, © Springer Science+Business Media New York 2013

Nonsurgical staging includes minimally invasive needle biopsy techniques such as transbronchial needle aspiration (TBNA), transthoracic needle aspiration (TTNA), esophageal endoscopic ultrasound-guided fine-needle aspiration (EUS-FNA), and endobronchial ultrasound-guided transbronchial needle aspiration (EBUS-TBNA).

A wide spectrum of factors must be considered when determining the appropriate tests to assess the lymph nodes in NSCLC. These include the sensitivity and specificity of the test, the false-negative and false-positive rates, the morbidity of the procedure, the accessibility of the tumor and suspicious lymph nodes, the requirement of general anesthesia, and the surgical skills required. Knowledge of lymph node nomenclature is frequently helpful in choosing the correct staging procedure [4, 5].

Surgical Techniques of Invasive Mediastinal Staging

Cervical Mediastinoscopy

Cervical mediastinoscopy is considered the "gold standard" for mediastinal staging of NSCLC. It is performed in the operating room under general anesthesia, and in most centers, patients are discharged the same day if they are stable [6, 7]. The procedure involves a small skin incision above the suprasternal notch, insertion of a mediastinoscope alongside the trachea, and biopsy of the mediastinal nodes under direct or video-assisted view. Lymph nodes accessible with this technique include right and left high paratracheal nodes (stations 2R, 2L, 4R, and 4L), pretracheal nodes (stations 1 and 3), and anterior subcarinal nodes (station 7) (Fig. 8.1). Lymph nodes that cannot be biopsied with this approach are posterior subcarinal nodes (station 7), inferior mediastinal nodes (stations 8 and 9), aortopulmonary window (APW) nodes (station 5), and para-aortic nodes (station 6). Rates of morbidity and mortality from this procedure are very low, 0.5–1 % and 0.08 %, respectively [8]. Minor complications include left recurrent nerve injury (0.7–0.9 %), pneumothorax (0.5–0.7 %), wound infection, chylous leak, and phrenic nerve injury. Major complications including bleeding due to injury of major blood vessels (0.1–0.2 %), tracheobronchial injury, and esophageal trauma are rare [9, 10]. A meta-analysis of 19 studies [11] showed that the sensitivity of mediastinoscopy to detect mediastinal node involvement from cancer was 78 %

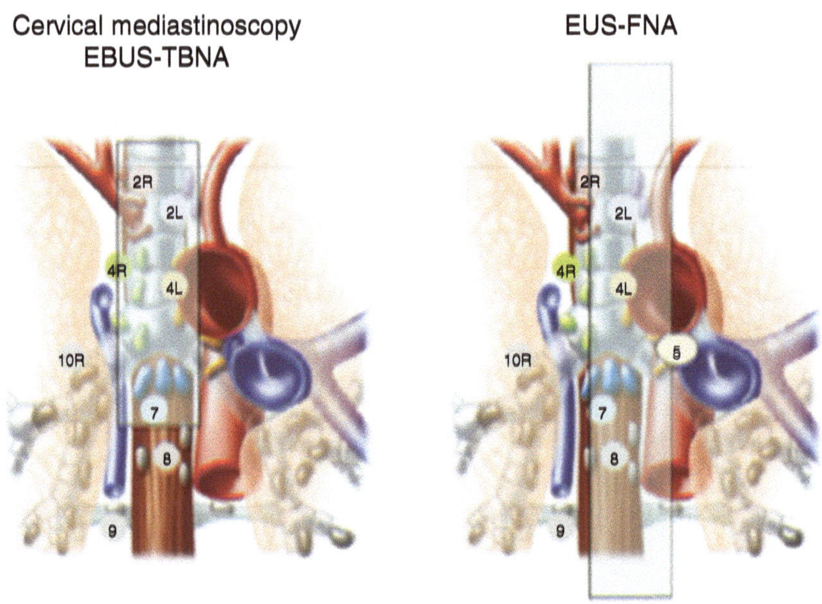

Fig. 8.1 Nodal levels accessible by cervical mediastinoscopy and EBUS-TBNA compared to EUS-FNA (From De Leyn P, et al.: ESTS guidelines for preoperative lymph node staging for non-small cell lung cancer. Eur J Cardiothorac Surg. Jul;32:1–8, 2007, with permission)

and the false-negative rate was 10 %. Some of the false-negative cases (42–57 %) can be explained by the presence of nodes that are not accessible by the mediastinoscope and by the operator skills and quality of dissection and sampling during the procedure. Videomediastinoscopy appears to improve sensitivity to 90 % and decrease false-negative rates to 7 %. The use of extended cervical mediastinoscopy, a procedure that involves directing the mediastinoscope lateral to the aortic arch, allows access to the APW and para-aortic lymph nodes (stations 5 and 6) that are not accessible by standard cervical mediastinoscopy [12], though not many surgeons perform this procedure.

Anterior Mediastinotomy

Left anterior mediastinotomy, or the Chamberlain procedure, is used for evaluation of left upper lobe tumors and lymph nodes located in the anterior mediastinum and APW. It is performed under general anesthesia in the operating room. The patient is placed in supine position and a skin incision is made over the second left intercostal space. The internal mammary artery is identified medially and preserved, and then the scope is inserted. After exploration, biopsies are taken from stations 5 and 6. The sensitivity for detecting mediastinal lymph node involvement of the anterior mediastinum ranges from 63 to 86 % [13, 14], but when it is coupled with standard cervical mediastinoscopy may increase to 87 % [11, 15]. The reported complications are very low including superficial wound infections, bleeding, and pneumothoraces.

Video-Assisted Thoracoscopic Surgery

VATS is performed in the operating room and under general anesthesia through 5–20 mm skin incisions placed at three sites in the intercostal space. The thoracoscope is inserted through one of the lower ports, and forceps are inserted through the other ports. VATS requires double-lumen endotracheal intubation to obtain atelectasis of the ipsilateral lung. As a diagnostic tool, VATS is an alternative to transthoracic needle aspiration of the peripherally located indeterminate pulmonary nodule, with a greater diagnostic yield (100 vs. 80–95 %) [16]. In addition, VATS has been used to access lymph nodes in stations 5, 6, 8, and 9, generally considered out of the reach of standard mediastinoscopy. The sensitivity is 75 % ranging from 37 to 100 %, and the specificity is 100 % [11]. The disadvantage compared with mediastinoscopy is that VATS allows only exploration of the ipsilateral side. Besides mediastinal staging, VATS may provide additional information on tumor status and pleural carcinomatosis and evaluation of pleural effusions.

Minimally Invasive Techniques for Mediastinal Staging

Transbronchial Needle Aspiration

TBNA, also known as Wang needle aspiration, is a bronchoscopic procedure that is performed on an outpatient basis. After using the CT scan to assess the level and size of the lymph node, the needle catheter is passed through the working channel of the bronchoscope, and then it is advanced through the tracheobronchial wall into the lymph node with no direct target visualization. TBNA is most frequently used to assess subcarinal nodes (station 7). Paratracheal nodes may also be biopsied, but they are sometimes more difficult to access due to the angulation required from the bronchoscope and needle. It has been reported that adequate specimens are obtained in 80–90 % of cases. On-site cytological evaluation of the aspirates improves the yield, is cost-effective, and eliminates unnecessary passes during the procedure [17]. A meta-analysis of 17 studies that included 1,339 patients showed that the overall sensitivity for mediastinal staging with TBNA is 78 %, with values ranging from 14 to 100 % [11]. The false-negative rate is approximately 28 % (range, 0–66 %). The specificity and false-positive rates are 100 % and 0 %, respectively [11]. This analysis, however, was not restricted to patients with NSCLC, did not assess study method quality, and did not set out to identify sources of variation in study results. A more recent meta-analysis of five studies accounting for the aforementioned data showed a much lower pooled sensitivity of 39 % (95 % CI, 17–61 %) with specificity of 99 % (95 % CI, 96–100 %) for TBNA [18]. Patients included in the first meta-analysis of TBNA studies had enlarged mediastinal lymph nodes and thus represent a different population when compared to those being considered for surgery that generally have normal-sized or single lymph node station enlargement, which is more representative of the second meta-analysis cited. The high false-negative rate makes TBNA less useful for staging patients with normal-sized nodes. Positive TBNA results demonstrate mediastinal node involvement and can obviate the need for surgical staging. However, negative TBNA results cannot sufficiently exclude mediastinal lymph node involvement and additional staging procedures should be performed.

Transthoracic Needle Aspiration

TTNA is an image-guided procedure commonly performed by a radiologist. Under local anesthesia, a needle is inserted percutaneously most often under CT guidance. Depending on size and location, guidance with conventional fluoroscopy or ultrasound can be performed. The procedure is relatively safe and well tolerated by most patients. Depending on the size of the needle used, core histological biopsies can be obtained in addition to cytological specimen. TTNA can be used for the diagnosis of suspected lung cancer of peripheral parenchymal masses as well as for the diagnosis and staging of the mediastinum. The sensitivity of TTNA for the staging and diagnosis of the mediastinum has been reported to be approximately 90 % (meta-analysis of five studies in 215 patients) [11]. Patients selected for this procedure had extensive mediastinal involvement and lymph nodes more than 1.5 cm in size. Pneumothorax is the most frequent complication (5–60 %), particularly in patients with COPD requiring chest tube insertion in approximately 10 % of patients [11]. Other complications such as hemothorax, hemoptysis, air embolism, or empyema are rare [19]. Implantation of tumor cells at the puncture site is rare and reported to be approximately 1 in 4,000 procedures [20, 21]. Relative contraindications for TTNA include COPD, poor lung function, diffuse pulmonary disease, clotting disorders, pulmonary hypertension, contralateral pneumonectomy, and arteriovenous malformation [22].

Esophageal Endoscopic Ultrasound-Guided Fine-Needle Aspiration

The use of EUS-FNA to stage mediastinal lymph nodes in patients with lung cancer has been reported in the medical literature beginning in the early 1990s [23]. It is an outpatient procedure that is performed under conscious sedation. A 19- or 22-gauge aspiration needle is inserted through a working channel of the endoscope. The needle is then passed through the wall of the esophagus directly into the target using real-time ultrasonography. This is followed by aspiration of the lymph node with direct visualization of the needle. The technique has a minimal risk of infection or bleeding. It is useful for staging of APW (station 5), subcarinal (station 7), esophageal (station 8), and inferior pulmonary ligament (station 9) lymph nodes (Fig. 8.1). Nodes that are anterolateral to the trachea are more difficult to sample because of interference by air in the larger airways. Ultrasonographic properties of lymph nodes indicating possible malignancy include a hypoechoic core, sharp edges, round shape, and a long-axis diameter exceeding 10 mm, though none are reliable enough to forgo biopsy [24–26]. Signs of benign disease include a hyperechoic core (fat), central calcification (remote granulomatous disease), ill-defined edges, a long and narrow shape, and a long-axis diameter up to 10 mm [25, 27, 28]. Histoplasmosis, sarcoidosis, and anthracosilicosis may cause false-positive EUS images [28–30]. A meta-analysis of 18 studies assessed the use of EUS-FNA in the mediastinal staging of 1,201 lung cancer patients [31]. For the detection of malignant mediastinal lymph nodes, the overall sensitivity and specificity were 83 % and 97 %, respectively. False-negative rates have been reported to be 19 % (range, 0 to 61 %) [11]. In addition, it is accepted that nodes that measure less than 1 cm can be successfully sampled using this technique [32, 33]. Among patients with normal-sized lymph nodes seen on CT scans, the sensitivity is 66 % and the false-negative rate is 14 % (specificity, 100 %; false-positive rate, 0 %) [34, 35]. Another advantage of EUS-FNA is that it allows detection of metastatic disease to subdiaphragmatic sites such as the left adrenal gland, celiac lymph nodes, and the liver. Furthermore, the cost of EUS is less than surgical staging procedures. Two studies suggested that EUS may be more cost-effective compared to mediastinoscopy [36, 37], although it was assumed that mediastinoscopy frequently required inpatient hospital admission.

Endobronchial Ultrasound-Guided Transbronchial Needle Aspiration

EBUS-TBNA is a promising modality for mediastinal staging. Initially, EBUS was performed by introducing a catheter with an ultrasound transducer at the tip of the catheter through the working channel of the bronchoscope (radial ultrasound probe). The lymph node was localized with the probe, and the catheter was then withdrawn. The lymph node would then be sampled with TBNA without visualization. More recently, a bronchoscope with a convex ultrasound probe has been developed allowing real-time ultrasound-guided TBNA (linear ultrasound scope, Fig. 8.2) [38]. EBUS-TBNA is performed under local anesthesia and conscious sedation in an outpatient setting. A 22-gauge TBNA needle equipped with an internal sheath is inserted through the working channel of the bronchoscope. The inner diameter of the needle allows the sample of histological cores in some cases. Doppler examination may be used immediately before the biopsy in order to avoid unintended puncture of vessels between the wall of the bronchi and the lesion. Under real-time ultrasonic guidance, the needle is placed in the lesion and suction is applied by a syringe. The needle is moved back and forth inside the lesion. Finally, the needle is retrieved and the internal sheath and the catheter are removed. The aspirated material is smeared onto glass slides, air-dried, and fixed in 95 % alcohol. Dried smears can be evaluated in

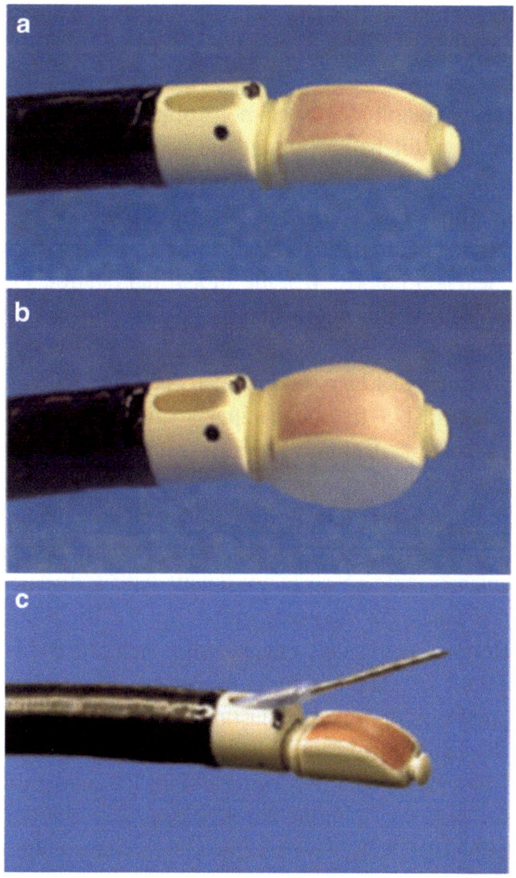

Fig. 8.2 Convex probe endobronchial ultrasound. (**a**) The tip of the convex probe endobronchial ultrasound (Olympus XBF-UC260F-OL8, Olympus, Tokyo, Japan) has a linear curved array ultrasonic transducer of 7.5 MHz. (**b**) The balloon attached to the tip of the bronchoscope is inflated with normal saline. (**c**) A dedicated transbronchial aspiration needle is inserted through the working channel (From Yasufuku K and Fujisawa T: Staging and diagnosis of non-small cell lung cancer: Invasive modalities. Respirology. 12, 173–183, 2007, with permission)

real time by an on-site cytopathologist to confirm adequate cell material, and in a substantial number of cases, a preliminary diagnosis can be made. Histological specimens obtained are fixed in formalin before being sent to the pathology department. EBUS-TBNA can be used to sample the highest mediastinal (station 1), the upper paratracheal (station 2R, 2L), the lower paratracheal (station 4R, 4L), the subcarinal (station 7), as well as the hilar (station 10), the interlobar (station 11), and the lobar (station 12) lymph nodes (Fig. 8.1). A pooled analysis of 12 studies using EBUS for mediastinal staging showed a weighted sensitivity of 93 % (range 79–99 %), false-negative rate of 9 % (range 1–37 %), and specificity of 100 % [39]. The studies using EBUS involved patients with lymph node enlargement, which is consistent with a disease prevalence of approximately 70 %. In 2006, Herth et al. evaluated the performance of EBUS-TBNA in patients with lung cancer and a radiographically normal mediastinum [40]. That study showed an unexpected detection rate of 17 % in 119 lymph nodes 5–10 mm in size. In one out of six patients, a futile thoracotomy was averted using EBUS. This was followed by a study evaluating the accuracy of EBUS-TBNA for staging mediastinal lymph nodes in patients with lung cancer without enlarged lymph nodes on CT and no detectable PET activity in the mediastinum. There was a 9 % prevalence of mediastinal lymph node metastases. The sensitivity, specificity, and negative predictive value were 89 %, 100 %, and 99 %, respectively [41].

Combining EUS-FNA and EBUS-TBNA

Current data suggest that the combination of EUS-FNA and EBUS-TBNA may allow complete access to all mediastinal lymph node stations [42]. Wallace et al. reported that the combination of EUS-FNA and EBUS-TBNA had a higher sensitivity (93 %; 95 % CI, 81–99 %) and negative predictive value (97 %; 95 % CI, 91–99 %) compared with either method alone [43].

Comparing Technologies

With the relatively recent emergence of data supporting nonsurgical invasive techniques including EUS-FNA and EBUS-TBNA for mediastinal lymph node staging in lung cancer, there has been interest in comparing these modalities with their surgical and nonsurgical counterparts. Wallace and coworkers [43] compared the diagnostic accuracy of blind transbronchial needle aspiration, EBUS-TBNA, EUS-FNA, and their combinations. As mentioned previously, the combination of EBUS-TBNA and EUS-FNA was better than either alone, even in scenarios that favored one methodology over another. Additionally, both technologies far outperformed blind TBNA, with EBUS-TBNA detecting 33 % more malignant mediastinal lymph nodes. A recent randomized controlled trial by Annema and coworkers compared minimally invasive endosonography (EBUS-TBNA plus EUS-FNA) followed by surgical staging (if no nodal metastases found) to immediate surgical staging with mediastinoscopy in two hundred forty-one patients over a 2-year period [44]. Results showed that the sensitivity for surgical staging was 79 % (95 % CI, 66–88 %) and for endosonography plus surgical staging, 94 % (95 % CI, 85–98 %). The negative predictive value for surgical staging was 86 % (95 % CI, 76–92 %) and for endosonography and surgical staging, 93 % (95 % CI, 84–97 %). The number of unnecessary thoracotomies was also substantially reduced in the endosonography group as compared to the surgical group (7 % vs. 18 %, respectively). There was no difference in complication rates between the two groups; however, when studied separately the complication rate with endosonography was significantly lower than with surgery (1 % vs. 6 %, *p*-value 0.03). Conclusions from this study suggest that endosonography should be the first step for mediastinal nodal staging.

Table 8.1 summarizes performance characteristics of invasive techniques for mediastinal staging.

Table 8.1 Techniques for mediastinal lymph node staging

Technique	Nodal stations	Accessible sensitivity (%)	Specificity (%)	FP (%)	FN (%)
Cervical mediastinoscopy	1, 2, 3, 4, anterior 7	78 90 (*)	100	0	11 7 (*)
Anterior mediastinotomy	5, 6	75	100	0	6
VATS	5, 6, 8, 9 ipsilateral	75	100	0	7
TBNA	2, 4, 7	39	100	0	8
TTNA	Mediastinal	89	100	0	
EUS-FNA	2, 4, 5, 7, 8, 9	84	99.5	0.4	19
EBUS-NA	1, 2, 4, 7, 10, 11, 12	90	100	0	24

FP false-positive, *FN* false-negative, *VATS* video-assisted thoracoscopic surgery, *TBNA* transbronchial needle aspiration, *TTNA* transthoracic needle aspiration, *EUS-FNA* esophageal endoscopic ultrasound-guided fine-needle aspiration, *EBUS-NA* endobronchial ultrasound-guided transbronchial needle aspiration, * videomediastinoscopy

Source: Detterbeck FC, Jantz MA, Wallace M, et al. Invasive Mediastinal Staging of Lung Cancer: ACCP Evidence-Based Clinical Practice Guidelines (2nd Edition). Chest 2007; 132:202S–220S, with permission

Guidelines for Mediastinal Staging

Guidelines of the American College of Chest Physicians [11] and the European Society of Thoracic Surgery (ESTS) [45] were published in 2007. There has been recent evidence further supporting the increased use of multimodality staging for lung cancer. A cohort study using 7 years of data involving 43,912 patients concluded that multimodality staging is being increasingly used. Additionally, the use of a greater number of staging modalities was associated with a lower risk of death. Trimodality (CT, PET, and invasive staging) vs. single modality (CT only) showed a hazard ratio of 0.49 (99 % CI 0.45–0.54), and trimodality vs. bimodality (CT and PET or CT and invasive staging) showed a hazard ratio of 0.85 (99 % CI 0.77–0.93) [46].

Chest CT is considered the basic imaging modality in lung cancer, but it is not considered accurate enough for mediastinal lymph node staging. Only in patients with extensive mediastinal infiltration of tumor without distant metastases is CT scan assessment sufficient, and there is no need for further invasive confirmation.

For patients with discrete mediastinal lymph node enlargement and no evidence of distant metastases, invasive confirmation is suggested despite of the presence of positive or negative mediastinal nodes on PET scan. If nonmalignant results from a needle technique (EUS-FNA, TBNA, EBUS-TBNA, or TTNA) are obtained, they should be further confirmed by mediastinoscopy, irrespective of whether the findings of a PET scan of the mediastinal nodes are positive or negative. In patients with a normal mediastinum by CT and a central tumor or N1 lymph node enlargement without distant metastases, invasive confirmation is recommended regardless of PET scan mediastinal node status. In general, mediastinoscopy is suggested, but EUS-FNA or EBUS-TBNA may be a reasonable option if nondiagnostic results are followed by mediastinoscopy [47]. This recommendation is likely to change in the next iteration of the guidelines based on the recent randomized controlled trial results showing greater sensitivity for mediastinal nodal metastases and fewer unnecessary thoracotomies with EUS-FNA and EBUS-TBNA. In patients with a peripheral clinical stage I tumor in whom a PET scan shows uptake in the mediastinal nodes (and no distant metastases), invasive staging is recommended. In patients with a left upper lobe cancer in whom invasive mediastinal staging is indicated, the assessment of the APW nodes should be included using one of the following techniques, Chamberlain procedure,

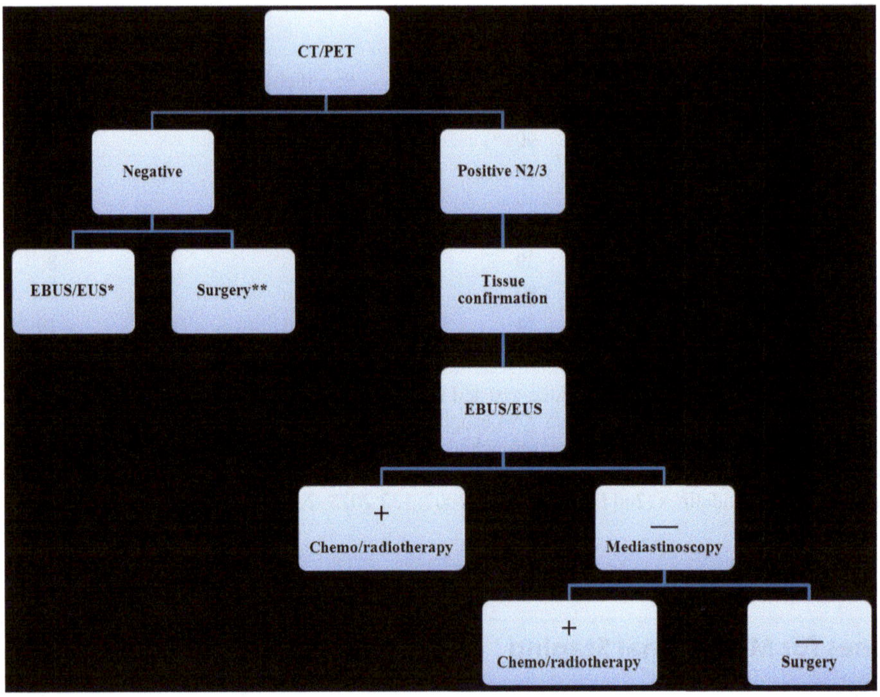

Fig. 8.3 Proposed algorithm for mediastinal staging. *Single asterisk* central tumors, large tumors, enlarged N1 nodes. *Double asterisk* T1a peripheral (Note: because of the 10 % chance of occult metastatic disease to the mediastinum, it is reasonable to invasively stage)

thoracoscopy, extended cervical mediastinoscopy, EUS-FNA, or EBUS-TBNA, if other mediastinal node stations are found to be uninvolved.

A proposed algorithm for mediastinal staging is detailed in Fig. 8.3.

Conclusion

Accurate mediastinal nodal staging is essential for the management of patients with NSCLC in the absence of distant metastases. Imaging studies are not sufficiently reliable, making invasive tests an important part of the staging procedure. Different invasive modalities exist, including surgical and needle-based minimally invasive techniques. These tests should be seen as complementary as they target particular nodal stations and patient groups. Needle techniques are most useful in patients with enlarged mediastinal nodes, while mediastinoscopy remains the "gold standard" in patients with normal-sized nodes though studies are emerging that show that combining EUS and EBUS provides a minimally invasive accurate assessment of the mediastinum in lung cancer.

References

1. American Cancer Society. Cancer facts and figures 2011. Atlanta: American Cancer Society; 2011.
2. Silvestri GA, Gould MK, Margolis ML, et al. Noninvasive staging of non-small cell lung cancer: ACCP evidenced-based clinical practice guidelines (2nd edition). Chest. 2007;132(3 Suppl):178S–201.
3. Fischer B, Lassen U, Mortenson J, et al. Preoperative staging of lung cancer with combined PET-CT. N Engl J Med. 2009;361(1):32–9.
4. Goldstraw P, Crowley J, Chansky K, et al. The IASLC Lung Cancer Staging Project: proposals for the revision of the TNM stage groupings in the forthcoming (seventh) edition of the TNM Classification of malignant tumours. J Thorac Oncol. 2007;2(8):706–14.
5. Mountain CF, Dresler CM. Regional lymph node classification for lung cancer staging. Chest. 1997; 111(6):1718–23.

6. Cybulsky IJ, Bennett WF. Mediastinoscopy as a routine outpatient procedure. Ann Thorac Surg. 1994; 58(1):176–8.
7. Vallières E, Pagé A, Verdant A. Ambulatory mediastinoscopy and anterior mediastinotomy. Ann Thorac Surg. 1991;52(5):1122–6.
8. Passlick B. Initial surgical staging of lung cancer. Lung Cancer. 2003;42 Suppl 1:S21–5.
9. Kirby T, Fell S. Mediastinoscopy. In: Pearson FG, Cooper JD, Deslauriers J, et al., editors. Thoracic surgery. 2nd ed. New York: Churchill Livingstone; 2002. p. 98–103.
10. Semik M, Netz B, Schmidt C, Scheld HH. Surgical exploration of the mediastinum: mediastinoscopy and intraoperative staging. Lung Cancer. 2004;45 Suppl 2:55S–61.
11. Detterbeck FC, Jantz MA, Wallace M, et al. Invasive mediastinal staging of lung cancer: ACCP evidence-based clinical practice guidelines (2nd edition). Chest. 2007;132(3 Suppl):202S–20.
12. Ginsberg RJ, Rice TW, Goldberg M, Waters PF, Schmocker BJ. Extended cervical mediastinoscopy: a single staging procedure for bronchogenic carcinoma of the left upper lobe. J Thorac Cardiovasc Surg. 1987;94(5):673–8.
13. Best LA, Munichor M, Ben-Shakhar M, Lemer J, Lichtig C, Peleg H. The contribution of anterior mediastinotomy in the diagnosis and evaluation of diseases of the mediastinum and lung. Ann Thorac Surg. 1987;43(1):78–81.
14. Pagé A, Nakhlé G, Mercier C, et al. Surgical treatment of bronchogenic carcinoma: the importance of staging in evaluating late survival. Can J Surg. 1987;30(2):96–9.
15. Deneffe G, Lacquet LM, Gyselen A. Cervical mediastinoscopy and anterior mediastinotomy in patients with lung cancer and radiologically normal mediastinum. Eur J Respir Dis. 1983;64(8):613–9.
16. Catarino PA, Goldstraw P. The future in diagnosis and staging of lung cancer: surgical techniques. Respiration. 2006;73(6):717–32.
17. Baram D, Garcia RB, Richman PS. Impact of rapid onsite cytologic evaluation during transbronchial needle aspiration. Chest. 2005;128(2):869–75.
18. Holty JE, Kuschner WG, Gould MK. Accuracy of transbronchial needle aspiration for mediastinal staging of non-small cell lung cancer: a meta-analysis. Thorax. 2005;60(11):949–55.
19. Shaham D. Semi-invasive and invasive procedures for the diagnosis and staging of lung cancer. I. Percutaneous transthoracic needle biopsy. Radiol Clin North Am. 2000;38(3):525–34.
20. Ali Bedirhan M, Turna A. Fine-needle aspiration and tumor seeding. Chest. 2001;120(3):1037–8.
21. Sawabata N, Ohta M, Maeda H. Fine-needle aspiration cytologic technique for lung cancer has a high potential of malignant cell spread through the tract. Chest. 2000;118(4):936–9.
22. Gardner D. vanSonnenberg E, D'Agostino HB, Casola G, Taggart S, May S. CT-guided transthoracic needle biopsy. Cardiovasc Intervent Radiol. 1991; 14(1):17–23.
23. Vincent BD, El-Bayoumi E, Hoffman B, et al. Real-time endobronchial ultrasound-guided transbronchial lymph node aspiration. Ann Thorac Surg. 2008; 85(1):224–30.
24. Faigel DO. EUS in patients with benign and malignant lymphadenopathy. Gastrointest Endosc. 2001; 53(6):593–8.
25. Wiersema MJ, Villman P, Giovannini M, Chang KJ, Wiersema LM. Endosonography-guided fine-needle aspiration biopsy: diagnostic accuracy and complication assessment. Gastroenterology. 1997;112(4): 1087–95.
26. Williams DB, Sahai AV, Aabakken L, et al. Endoscopic ultrasound guided fine needle aspiration biopsy: a large single centre experience. Gut. 1999;44(5): 720–6.
27. Hawes RH, Gress FG, Kesler KA, Cummings OW, Conces Jr DJ. Endoscopic ultrasound versus computed tomography in the evaluation of the mediastinum in patients with non-small-cell lung cancer. Endoscopy. 1994;26(9):784–7.
28. Schuder G, Isringhaus H, Kubale B, Seitz G, Sybrecht GW. Endoscopic ultrasonography of the mediastinum in the diagnosis of bronchial carcinoma. Thorac Cardiovasc Surg. 1991;39(5):299–303.
29. Mishra G, Sahai AV, Penman ID, et al. Endoscopic ultrasonography with fine-needle aspiration: an accurate and simple diagnostic modality for sarcoidosis. Endoscopy. 1999;31:377–82.
30. Wiersema MJ, Chak A, Wiersema LM. Mediastinal histoplasmosis: evaluation with endosonography and endoscopic fine-needle aspiration biopsy. Gastrointest Endosc. 1994;40(1):78–81.
31. Micames C, McCrory D, Pavey DA, Jowell PS, Gress FG. Endoscopic ultrasound-guided fine-needle aspiration for non-small cell lung cancer staging: a systematic review and metaanalysis. Chest. 2007;131(2): 539–48.
32. Fritscher-Ravens A, Soehendra N, Schirrow L, et al. Role of transesophageal endosonography-guided fine-needle aspiration in the diagnosis of lung cancer. Chest. 2000;117(2):339–45.
33. Wallace MB, Silvestri GA, Sahai AV, et al. Endoscopic ultrasound-guided fine needle aspiration for staging patients with carcinoma of the lung. Ann Thorac Surg. 2001;72(6):1861–7.
34. LeBlanc JK, Devereaux BM, Imperiale TF, et al. Endoscopic ultrasound in non-small cell lung cancer and negative mediastinum in computed tomography. Am J Respir Crit Care Med. 2005;171(2):177–82.
35. Wallace MB, Ravenel J, Block MI, et al. Endoscopic ultrasound in lung cancer patients with a normal mediastinum on computed tomography. Ann Thorac Surg. 2004;77(5):1763–8.
36. Aabakken L, Silvestri GA, Hawes R, Reed CE, Marsi V, Hoffman B. Cost-efficacy of endoscopic ultrasonography with fine-needle aspiration vs. mediastinotomy in patients with lung cancer and suspected

mediastinal adenopathy. Endoscopy. 1999;31(9): 707–11.
37. Harewood G, Wiersema MJ, Edell ES, Liebow M. Cost-minimization analysis of alternative diagnostic approaches in a modeled patient with non-small cell lung cancer and subcarinal lymphadenopathy. Mayo Clin Proc. 2002;77(2):155–64.
38. Yasufuku K, Fujisawa T. Staging and diagnosis of non-small cell lung cancer: invasive modalities. Respirology. 2007;12(2):173–83.
39. Gomez M, Silvestri GA. Endobronchial ultrasound for the diagnosis and staging of lung cancer. Proc Am Thorac Soc. 2009;6(2):180–6.
40. Herth FJ, Ernst A, Eberhardt R, et al. Endobronchial ultrasound-guided transbronchial needle aspiration of lymph nodes in the radiologically normal mediastinum. Eur Respir J. 2006;28(5):910–4.
41. Herth FJ, Eberhardt R, Krasnik M, Ernst A. Endobronchial ultrasound-guided transbronchial needle aspiration of lymph nodes in the radiologically and positron emission tomography-normal mediastinum in patients with lung cancer. Chest. 2008;133(4):887–91.
42. Wallace MB, Pascual JM, Raimondo M, et al. Complete "medical mediastinoscopy" under conscious sedation: a prospective blinded comparison of endoscopic and endobronchial ultrasound to bronchoscopic fine needle aspiration for malignant mediastinal lymph nodes [abstract]. Gastrointest Endosc. 2006;63:AB96.
43. Wallace MB, Pascual JM, Raimondo M, et al. Minimally invasive endoscopic staging of suspected lung cancer. JAMA. 2008;299(5):540–6.
44. Annema JT, van Meerbeeck JP, Rintoul RC. Mediastinoscopy vs. endosonography for mediastinal nodal staging of lung cancer: a randomized trial. JAMA. 2010;304(20):2245–52.
45. De Leyn P, Lardinois D, Van Schil PE, et al. ESTS guidelines for preoperative lymph node staging for non-small cell lung cancer. Eur J Cardiothorac Surg. 2007;32(1):1–8.
46. Farjah F, Flum DR, Ramsey SD, Heagerty PJ, Symons RG, Wood DE. Multi-modality mediastinal staging for lung cancer among medicare beneficiaries. J Thorac Oncol. 2009;4(3):355–63.
47. De Leyn P, Lardinois D, Van Schil PE, et al. European trends in preoperative and intraoperative nodal staging: ESTS guidelines. J Thorac Oncol. 2007;2(4): 357–61.

Surgical Treatment for Non-small Cell Lung Cancer

9

Chadrick E. Denlinger

For patients presenting with limited disease, surgical resection remains the most effective method of controlling the primary tumor and provides the best opportunity for long-term survival. Therefore, every patient with NSCLC is assessed for the appropriateness of surgical resection. The surgical goal among patients with limited disease (stages I and II) is complete resection, followed by adjuvant chemotherapy when occult lymph node metastases are discovered with final pathological staging. In addition, patients with limited mediastinal metastatic disease or local invasion (stage IIIA) are considered for surgical resection in many centers.

Despite undergoing complete surgical resections for lung cancer, the expected 5-year survival rates for stages I, II, and III are 60 %, 40 %, and 15 %, respectively, with the vast majority of patients dying from distant metastases rather than local recurrence [1]. The past decades have brought significant progress relating to the preoperative evaluation of patients being considered for surgery, and technological advances have improved surgical options available for the treatment of NSCLC. However, the development of distant metastatic disease despite the assumption of a complete surgical resection leaves a great deal of progress to be made in the evaluation and treatment of NSCLC. This chapter reviews the current surgical treatments available for patients with NSCLC including trends in our surgical paradigm and stage-dependant therapy.

C.E. Denlinger, M.D. (✉)
Division of Cardiothoracic Surgery, Department of Surgery, Medical University of South Carolina, 25 Courtenay Dr., Suite 7018, Charleston, SC 29425, USA
e-mail: denlinge@musc.edu

Historical Perspective

The first surgical resection for lung cancer was performed by Hugh Morriston Davies in 1912 with a procedure involving individual ligation of pulmonary vessels and suture closure of the bronchial stump which is nearly identical to the contemporary surgical procedure. Unfortunately his patient died 8 days later due to inadequate means to manage the postoperative pleural space at that time. The first successful pulmonary resection was not performed until 1933 when Graham and Singer completed a single-stage pneumonectomy for bronchogenic carcinoma. Bunn reported 6 cases in 1929 of successful lobectomies. One case in this series was performed for carcinoma, and five for infectious diseases. An underwater pleural drainage system was developed that allowed for the drainage of pleural fluid while maintaining a negative intrathoracic pressure. This allowed expansion of the remaining lung tissue and minimized the existing pleural space available for the development of an empyema.

With the development of more advanced patient management skills and improved clinical outcomes, surgical resection has become the standard treatment for patients with early stage lung cancer.

J.G. Ravenel (ed.), *Lung Cancer Imaging*, Contemporary Medical Imaging,
DOI 10.1007/978-1-60761-620-7_9, © Springer Science+Business Media New York 2013

Physiological Considerations: Surgeon's Perspective

Two critical components that determine whether a tumor can be successfully surgically resected are the overall medical condition of the patient, including the patient's preoperative pulmonary reserve, and anatomic features of the tumor that determine the extent of resection required. In addition, preoperative studies indicate what type of surgical approach will be necessary to safely perform the procedure. Although there are several means to objectively evaluate the physiological reserve of patients being considered for surgery, an absolutely essential tool remains a thorough clinical history focusing on the daily physical activities tolerated by the patient and determining whether their activity is limited by respiratory difficulties or generalized fatigue. Traditionally, exercise tolerance has been used to stratify patients for the risks of operative mortality and morbidity. This concept was clearly described by Reichel in 1972 by a study that retrospectively compared operative complications and mortality rates with the patients' preoperative exercise capacity measured by a staged treadmill exercise protocol [2].

More recently, more objective studies have been utilized to determine whether adequate pulmonary reserve exists for patients to undergo surgical resection of lung cancers. The most widely utilized objective assessment of pulmonary reserve is the pulmonary function test which includes spirometry and a measure of the oxygen diffusion capacity. The most important pulmonary function components that can be used to risk stratify patients for postoperative pulmonary complications are the forced expiratory volume in 1 second (FEV_1) and the diffusing capacity of carbon monoxide (DLCO). Each of these values is normalized according to the specific patient's age, gender, and height and expressed as a percent predicted value. Calculations are made from the preoperative values and the extent of resection necessary to determine a postoperative predicted FEV_1 and DLCO. Patients with a postoperative predicted FEV_1 or DLCO of less than 40 % are at an increased risk for pulmonary complications following surgery [3]. This understanding of an increased risk for complication is based on studies performed in an era where the standard approach for pulmonary resection was through a thoracotomy. With this surgical approach, the initial postoperative pulmonary function is actually significantly worse than the calculated values due to postoperative pain [4]. Importantly, a more recent study evaluating the risks of pulmonary complications following surgical resections via the less invasive video-assisted thoracoscopic surgery (VATS) approach found that the level of preoperative pulmonary function had very little impact on the risks for postoperative pulmonary complications [5]. Although this study was not adequately powered to determine small differences in operative complication rates, the data suggests that patients with limited pulmonary reserve tolerate surgical resections via a VATS approach better than patients with similar resections being performed through a thoracotomy.

Patients with marginal pulmonary function values are frequently further evaluated with perfusion imaging, especially among patients requiring extensive pulmonary resections for centrally obstructing lesions or for patients with cancers located within regions of the lung that appear particularly diseased. The value of pulmonary perfusion imaging among patients with marginal lung function is to help determine how functional the lung parenchyma is that is being considered for surgical resection. In the setting of a centrally obstructing lesion, the parenchyma to be resected may already have essentially no function because the lung tissue is poorly ventilated. Alternatively, a lung cancer located within a lobe that is particularly diseased may contribute very little to the overall pulmonary function of the patient. A quantitative ventilation perfusion scan can help determine the fraction of pulmonary function being contributed by the region being considered for resection. Unfortunately, the ventilation perfusion scan does not provide specific data regarding each pulmonary lobe because of the obliqueness of the fissure separating the upper and lower lobes of each lung.

A third objective study utilized in patients with marginal spirometry values is a cardiopulmonary stress test which determines the maximal level of oxygen consumption. This study depends on the cardiac and pulmonary physiological reserve as well as the ability of the patient's skeletal muscles to consume oxygen. In essence, the cardiopulmonary stress test objectifies a composite score of the patient's overall level of physical fitness. An individual's vO_2 max falls somewhere on a spectrum of exercise tolerance, and greater values correlate with a lower risk of perioperative pulmonary complications and mortality. Patients with vO_2 max values greater than 20 mL/kg/min are thought to have a low risk for complications, and patients with values less than 10 mL/kg/min are thought to have prohibitive risks for any major pulmonary resection procedure [6]. Clearly, the pulmonary risks of patients with intermediary max vO_2 values fall somewhere in between, and these results need to be interpreted in the context of other clinical and objective data stratifying the patients' operative risks.

Surgical Resection of Non-small Cell Lung Cancer

Pneumonectomy

Historically, the standard operation for patients with bronchogenic carcinoma was a pneumonectomy. This procedure remains the only surgical option for patients with adequate pulmonary reserve with specific anatomical issues related to the tumor that preclude preservation of any of the lesser involved lobe. Common anatomic indications for pneumonectomy are extensive tumor involvement of the mainstem bronchus, adherence of the tumor to the proximal pulmonary artery, or upper lobe tumors that heavily involve the pulmonary artery branches to the lower lobe. Less commonly, more peripherally located tumors may demonstrate extensive invasion across the pulmonary fissure and involve a significant part of the lung parenchyma of both the upper and lower lobes.

The reported operative mortality rate following a pneumonectomy ranges from 5 to 7 % in contemporary series [7–9]. The most frequent postoperative complications are pneumonia, prolonged ventilation, and atrial fibrillation which occur with an incidence of 8 %, 3 %, and 15 %, respectively. Other complications seen less frequently include bronchial stump dehiscence, postpneumonectomy pulmonary edema, and a delayed postpneumonectomy syndrome characterized by the heart and mediastinum shifting into the right chest cavity leading to compression of the left mainstem bronchus against the vertebral column.

Technical Aspects

The standard operative approach for any lung resection, including a pneumonectomy, begins with the induction of general anesthesia and the placement of a double-lumen endotracheal tube with the cuffed bronchial lumen of the tube inserted into the left mainstem bronchus and the tracheal lumen located immediately superior to the tracheal carina. This tube allows for selective ventilation to either the left or right lung while the lung on the operative side is completely deflated which is necessary to visualize the pulmonary hilum. The patient is then positioned in a lateral decubitus position with the operative side up and the table slightly flexed to help widen the intercostal spaces. A standard posterolateral thoracotomy is performed which includes division of the latissimus dorsi muscle but preservation of the serratus anterior muscle. The chest is entered through the fifth intercostal space to provide the optimal exposure to the pulmonary hilum.

A thorough visual and manual exploration of the thoracic cavity and lung are performed to rule out any occult metastatic disease. The inferior pulmonary ligament is divided and the pleurae on both the anterior and posterior aspects of the hilum are divided to expose the pulmonary vasculature and bronchus. Frequently, several hilar lymph nodes are identified and resected for pathological staging as well as to facilitate exposure. In addition, bronchial arterial vessels emanating from the hilum are also divided. The superior and inferior pulmonary veins and pulmonary artery are sequentially dissected circumferentially and typically divided with a stapling device that simultaneously staples the vessel with six rows of staples and cuts the tissue. The mainstem bronchus is also dissected and divided. Intraoperative pathological evaluation is routinely performed to confirm that the bronchial margin is free of disease. In addition, other surgical margins are also evaluated if there is concern for the proximity of the tumor to the line of resection.

Following the procedure, it is the author's preference to place a thoracostomy tube which drains to balanced suction canister that maintains the intrathoracic pressure between +3 and −12 cm H_2O. This helps ensure that the thoracic pressure on the side of the pneumonectomy is properly balanced, thus preventing a shift of the mediastinum either toward or away from the operative side. When this happens, the return of venous blood flow to the heart can be compromised in a situation analogous to a tension pneumothorax. Alternatively, some surgeons prefer to simply not place a thoracostomy tube following the operation and aspirate an appropriate amount of air from the thoracic cavity at the conclusion of the operation to properly position the mediastinum.

Although some authors have described performing a minimally invasive pneumonectomy through either a standard VATS approach or a robotic-assisted procedure, these procedures with smaller incisions have not been widely accepted by most thoracic surgeons [10, 11]. Almost any patient who may be considered for a VATS pneumonectomy also would have anatomy conducive for a sleeve lobectomy. It is preferable to preserve functional lung parenchyma and to minimize the risk for potential complications associated with a vacant hemithorax. Therefore, a sleeve lobectomy is considered a superior option compared to a pneumonectomy even if it requires a thoracotomy rather than a VATS approach.

Immediate postoperative images should demonstrate a normally positioned cardiac silhouette and a vacant thoracic cavity. Over the course of the next several days, the operative side becomes filled with serous fluid (Fig. 9.1), and in the weeks following surgery, the operative hemithorax becomes completely opacified. A significant fall in the intrathoracic fluid level associated with copious expectoration of thin serous fluid may indicate a dehiscence of the bronchial stump which is a serious clinical condition that requires immediate surgical intervention.

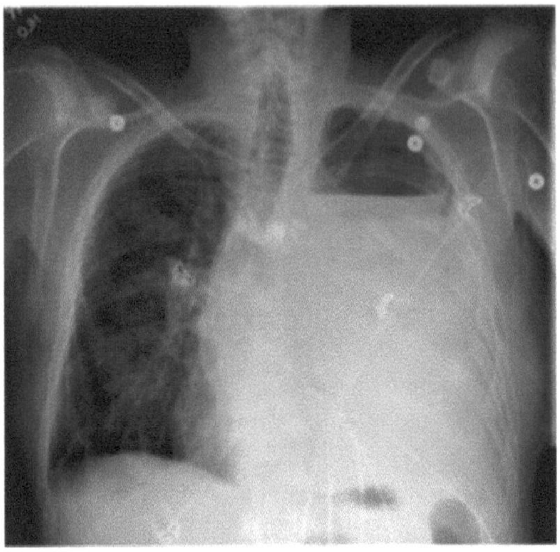

Fig. 9.1 Chest radiograph on postoperative day 3 following a left pneumonectomy. The radiograph demonstrates near complete opacification of the left hemithorax with an air-fluid level near the apex

Postoperative Management

The primary focus of postoperative management for patients who have had a pneumonectomy is preservation and optimizing the function of the remaining lung. Key components of this goal include adequate pain control which is accomplished by the placement of an epidural catheter. In addition, patient-controlled analgesia (PCA) devices are routinely used. The use of PCAs has been shown to both reduce the amount of narcotics used by patients and simultaneously improve their pain control in numerous postoperative settings. Oral narcotic and anti-inflammatory medications are also used. Early mobilization of patients is another important component of patient care following major lung resection surgery. This is generally believed to improve clearance of

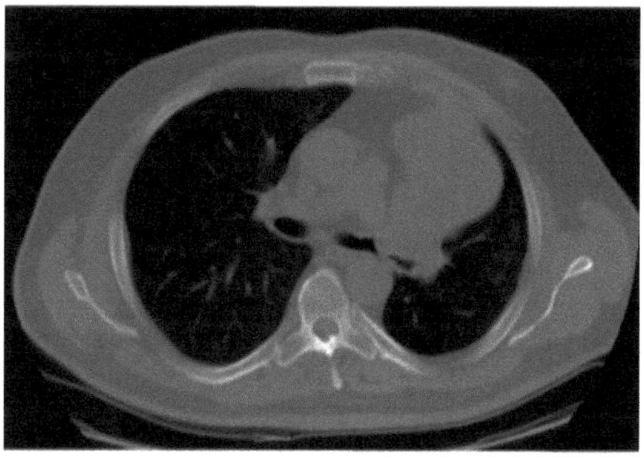

Fig. 9.2 CT image of a large central carcinoid tumor emanating from the left upper lobe bronchus into the left mainstem bronchus. This tumor required a bronchial sleeve resection to achieve negative surgical margins. Note the complete collapse of the left upper lobe resulting from the airway obstruction

pulmonary secretions, and mobilization also reduces the risk of developing deep venous thromboses.

Sleeve Lobectomy

It is always the goal to preserve lung parenchyma and to avoid a complete pneumonectomy if possible. Alternative parenchymal-sparing procedures available to selected patients with centrally located tumors are the bronchial sleeve lobectomy and lobectomy with pulmonary arterioplasty. These procedures are typically performed at larger centers by dedicated thoracic surgeons. The sleeve lobectomy is an option for patients with tumors involving the airway at the bifurcation mainstem bronchus into the upper and lower lobe bronchi on the left (Fig. 9.2) or the bifurcation of the right upper lobe and bronchus intermedius on the right. The tumor is positioned where the involved lobar bronchus cannot simply be divided while achieving negative surgical margins. The sleeve lobectomy included the transection of both the right or left mainstem bronchus and the noninvolved lobar bronchus. A "sleeve" of the mainstem bronchus is then resected on bloc with the surgical specimen, and the remaining lobar bronchus is anastomosed to the transected mainstem bronchus.

Pulmonary Arterioplasty

Pulmonary arterioplasty procedures are another alternative to pneumonectomies for patients with upper lobe tumors that invade the interlobar pulmonary artery supplying the lower lobe. If less than 50 % of the pulmonary artery circumference is involved with tumor, an arterioplasty may be an option. Two other anatomical considerations in patients who may be candidates for a pulmonary arterioplasty are the completeness of the pulmonary fissure and the ability to develop a plane to control the proximal pulmonary artery. This operation is typically performed by first dividing the superior pulmonary vein. Next the upper lobe bronchus is divided. Proximal control of the pulmonary artery is then established. To do this, a plane must be developed between the proximal pulmonary artery and the upper lobe bronchus to facilitate the placement of a clamp. Distal control of the pulmonary artery is established either by placing a temporary ligature around the inferior pulmonary vein or by placing a clamp on the interlobar pulmonary artery. The most challenging part of the operation requires dissecting the upper lobe parenchyma off of the pulmonary artery. This step of the operation is performed from an interior to a superior direction, and a complete pulmonary fissure greatly facilitates the identification of the inferior aspect of the pulmonary artery. As the pulmonary artery is dissected in a superior direction, a patch of the vessel is included en bloc with the surgical specimen where the tumor is densely adherent to the vessel wall. The artery is then reconstructed using a patch of synthetic material or a piece of bovine pericardium. Finally the bronchial stump is sutured closed if it was not initially stapled closed prior to its division. When both the pulmonary artery and the bronchus require repair, an intercostal muscle flap is placed between these two structures to prevent the fatal complication of a pulmonary artery to bronchus fistula.

Lobectomy

Thoracotomy with lobectomy and anatomic division of the lobar arteries, vein, and bronchus is considered the standard treatment for patients with NSCLC for tumors that are amenable to this approach in patients with adequate physiological reserve for this procedure. Traditionally, this operation was performed through a posterolateral thoracotomy as described above. Alternatively, a muscle-sparing thoracotomy can be utilized in relatively thin patients with upper lobe lesions. With this surgical approach, a curvilinear incision is made starting at the axillary hairline and extending inferiorly in the midaxillary line and then curving anteriorly. The latissimus dorsi muscle is retracted posteriorly, but not divided. The serratus anterior muscle is separated in the direction of its fibers which essentially parallels the direction of the underlying ribs. After separation of the intercostal muscles from the rib, exposure is created by spreading the ribs with a chest retractor. Upon entering the chest, the chest visceral and parietal pleural surfaces are examined for evidence of metastatic previously unidentified disease. The lung is also thoroughly palpated to identify additional pulmonary nodules. In the absence of additional malignant disease, the pleura overlying the hilum is divided to expose the underlying pulmonary artery, veins, and bronchus. In addition, any hilar lymph nodes are resected for pathological evaluation. The vascular structures are typically divided outside of the pericardium, but occasionally the pericardium must be opened in order to achieve a negative resection margin.

The pulmonary veins are more accessible and the tissue integrity is greater than that of the pulmonary artery. Therefore, the vein associated with the lobe to be resected is isolated and divided first. The left upper, left lower, and right lower lobes each are associated with a respective single pulmonary vein which carries blood from the lung to the left atrium. Conversely, the right superior pulmonary vein has tributaries from both the right upper lobe and the right middle lobe. Therefore, the right superior pulmonary vein must be dissected more distally during the resection of either the right upper or right middle lobe in order to isolate and divide only the tributaries from the involved lobe. The pulmonary vein is often divided with a linear cutting stapling device that simultaneously creates six lines of staples and divides the tissue in the middle. This leaves three rows of staples on each side of the divided tissue to maintain hemostasis.

The pulmonary artery branches supplying the involved lobe are then dissected. They are then either ligated and cut or divided with a linear cutting stapler. The surgical arterial anatomy of the right lung is fairly consistent. The right upper lobe is supplied by a large truncus anterior branch of the pulmonary artery which is the first branch off of the right main pulmonary artery. A smaller posterior ascending branch supplies the posterior segment of the right upper lobe. The right middle lobe receives either one or two pulmonary artery branches that are located approximately 1 cm distal to the origin of the posterior ascending branch. These branches are located on the anterior aspect of the main pulmonary artery. The pulmonary artery supplying the right lower lobe is normally divided in two places. The superior segmental pulmonary artery is a large branch that is divided individually because it is typically located on the posterior aspect of the main pulmonary artery directly across from the origin of the middle lobe artery. Finally the pulmonary artery supplying the basal segments of the right lower lobe can be divided as a single interlobar trunk at any point distal to the middle lobe branches before it divides into basilar segmental branches.

The arterial anatomy of the left lung is less consistent. Fortunately, the pulmonary surgical anatomy of the left lower lobe is very similar to that of the right lower lobe, and it is controlled in a similar fashion. However, the number and location of pulmonary artery branches to the left upper lobe is greatly variable, and for this reason, a left upper lobectomy is considered by many to be the most technically challenging pulmonary lobe to resect. The left upper lobe may be supplied by as few as two or as many as eight pulmonary artery branches. These branches arise from the main pulmonary artery as it arches around the posterior aspect of the left upper lobe bronchus. This anatomy can be anticipated by closely studying preoperative CT imaging with IV contrast, but small pulmonary artery branches are not always visualized on non-contrast studies.

In most cases, the lobar bronchus is divided last. It is dissected free from the surrounding tissues. The accompanying bronchial arteries are easily controlled with electrocautery. After the bronchus is skeletonized, it is divided with a linear cutting stapler. In some cases, however, the tumor is located with 1.5 cm of the origin of the lobar bronchus. In these circumstances, the bronchus must be divided with a knife, and the bronchial stump is closed with sutures in order to obtain a negative surgical margin.

Video-Assisted Thoracic Surgery

In the past decade, pulmonary resections with VATS have become increasingly popular. Initially VATS procedures involved the utilization of thoracotomy incisions very similar to what was described in the preceding paragraphs. An additional 2 cm incision is made lower in the thoracic cavity for the insertion of a thoracoscope. This approach allows superior visualization of the hilar structures while utilizing a smaller thoracotomy incision. This type of procedure later evolved into what most thoracic surgeons now consider a true VATS operation. With this approach, a 4–7 cm transverse incision is made, centered at the anterior axillary line at the level of the fourth intercostal space. Two smaller incisions are made more posteriorly in the lower thoracic region. In addition to utilizing smaller incisions, another important difference between the VATS approach and a thoracotomy is the lack of rib spreading. The smaller incisions and lack of rib spreading result in substantially less postoperative pain and therefore reduce the risk of several complications likely related to this discomfort.

Although the surgical outcomes of a VATS approach have never been compared to the traditional thoracotomy in a prospective randomized study, numerous retrospective series have demonstrated substantial superiority of the VATS approach. Surgeons comfortable with VATS operations would be unlikely to consider randomizing patients to a VATS or a thoracotomy approach. Prior studies have shown that the VATS approach to pulmonary resections results in a significant reduction in postoperative pain, a shorter length of hospital stay, a reduced incidence of perioperative atrial fibrillation, absence of prolonged air leaks through the chest tubes, and a reduction in the amount of fluid draining through the chest tubes. Importantly, large retrospective studies have also shown that the long-term overall and cancer-specific survival rates are similar or perhaps slightly better following a VATS lobectomy as compared to a traditional thoracotomy with lobectomy [12–15]. However, these studies are commonly criticized for potential selection biases of patients offered with VATS operations. Another criticism of these studies relates to potential differences in the adequacy of mediastinal lymph node assessment and the comprehensive care available to patients treated at centers where VATS procedures are routinely performed compared to centers where only an open approach is available.

Not all lung tumors are amenable to resection with a VATS approach. In general, tumor greater than 6 cm or centrally located tumors still require a thoracotomy. Other relative contraindications to VATS resections are tumor involvement of the chest wall or the presence of left upper lobe tumors in patients with a history of a prior left internal mammary artery (LIMA) coronary artery bypass.

Mediastinal Lymph Node Dissection

An important component of pulmonary resections for lung cancer is a thorough assessment of the mediastinal lymph nodes. By convention, mediastinal lymph nodes have been assigned station numbers according to their anatomic location. Adequate lymph node assessment for right-sided pulmonary resections includes sampling lymph nodes from stations 2R, 4R, 7, 8, 9, and 10, although lymph nodes are not consistently identified at stations 8 or 9. Adequate mediastinal lymph node assessment for patients undergoing left-sided resections includes sampling lymph nodes from stations 5–10.

The identification of mediastinal lymph nodes with evidence of metastatic disease is important for the selection of patients who may benefit from adjuvant chemotherapy and radiation. Recent studies have shown mixed results related to the survival benefits of a complete mediastinal lymph node dissection compared to lymph node sampling [16–19]. The largest multi-institutional randomized trial evaluating this question showed no differences in long-term overall or disease-free survival rates [19]. An important weakness of this study is that it does not reflect our current clinical practice because patients were only randomized in this study after frozen section analysis of sampled lymph nodes was negative for disease. Patients with positive lymph nodes with this initial screen were excluded from randomization in the study. Thus, the oncologic benefit of a complete mediastinal lymph node dissection remains uncertain.

Sublobar Resection

Resection of bronchogenic tumors with less than an anatomic lobectomy is referred to as a sublobar resection. These surgical treatment options are considered for patients with small peripheral lung tumors less than 2 cm. Two distinct types of sublobar resections are a segmentectomy and pulmonary wedge resection. A segmentectomy involves the dissection of airway to the level of the segmental bronchus for its selective division. In addition, the segmental pulmonary artery and vein branches are individually isolated and divided. Occasionally, patients are found to have pleural septations that isolate individual segments. More frequently, however, the identification of segmental boundaries within the pulmonary parenchyma is less clear. Traditionally, these anatomic divisions were identified by bluntly dissecting between the segments while applying gentle traction to fracture the lung tissue. More contemporaneously, segmental boundaries are found by intermittently ventilating the operative lung after the segmental bronchus has been divided. With this maneuver, the lung parenchyma that was supplied by the transected bronchus remains atelectatic and is resected while the aerated lung is left in situ. The pulmonary parenchyma is divided in this operation with a linear cutting stapler device. This operation is essentially the same as a lobectomy, although it is more challenging because it requires a more extensive dissection of the bronchus, artery, and veins more peripherally where these structures become enveloped in lung parenchyma.

Wedge resections are technically simpler operations which may be a suitable option for patients with small peripheral tumors. In this operation the pulmonary nodule is palpated and subsequently removed with a wide margin of normal lung parenchyma using a linear cutting stapler device. During this procedure, individual arteries, veins, or bronchi are identified. The lung tissue is divided in a region peripheral enough that the linear cutting stapler creates a staple line that is both hemostatic and pneumostatic. Although not well supported by objective data, a common recommendation for surgical margins is that a margin should be obtained that is equivalent to the diameter of the tumor being resected.

To date, there has been only one prospective randomized study comparing the outcomes of patients treated with a lobectomy vs. sublobar resections [20]. In this study 276 patients with NSCLC tumors less than 3 cm were randomized to a lobectomy or a sublobar resection (segmentectomy or wedge resection). This study showed a nonsignificant trend toward improved survival among patients treated with a lobectomy ($p=0.09$). However, the local recurrence rate was threefold greater among patients treated with sublobar resections compared to a complete lobectomy ($p=0.008$). There are two common criticisms of this study. First, the study allowed for either a wedge resection or a segmentectomy for the sublobar group, and no distinctions between the two procedures were made in the data analysis. Secondly, the study included patients with tumors up to 3 cm which may have contributed to narrow surgical margins.

In order to address the issue of a higher local recurrence rates among patients treated with sublobar resection, the addition of brachytherapy to the surgical resection margin is being considered.

In December 2009 the American Cooperative of Surgery Oncology Group completed enrollment of a prospective multi-institutional randomized trial of patients treated with sublobar resections with or without the addition of ^{125}I brachytherapy (ACOSOG-Z4032). Further follow-up is necessary as these results mature to determine whether brachytherapy reduces the risk of local recurrence in this patient population.

Several retrospective studies have been completed using more stringent tumor size restrictions for patient eligibility. These studies have not identified any differences in disease-free survival or local recurrence [21–23]. Given the retrospective nature of each of these studies, they have been criticized for selection bias. Enough data has been presented, however, to raise the question of whether a sublobar resection is equivalent to a lobectomy for patients with small peripheral tumors. This question is particularly relevant for tumors comprised primarily of ground glass opacities on preoperative imaging. An ongoing prospective randomized study is currently enrolling patients to examine the oncologic benefits of a lobectomy vs. sublobar resections among patients with tumors less than 2 cm that have adequate pulmonary reserve to undergo a lobectomy (CALBG-140503), and the results of this prospective trial may significantly alter the surgical treatment offered to patients.

Chest Wall Resections

Peripherally located NSCLC tumors may extend beyond the lung parenchyma into the overlying chest wall (Fig. 9.3). These tumors are associated with either localized or referred pain. Tumors located in the superior sulcus of the chest cavity with chest wall involvement are referred to with the eponym "Pancoast tumors," reflecting the initial description of tumors in this location. Historically, patients with Pancoast tumors presented with referred upper extremity pain or motor function abnormalities due to local invasion of the brachial plexus. Currently, any lung tumor with chest wall involvement of the superior sulcus is considered a Pancoast tumor regardless of the presence or absence of any neurological symptoms. Tumors involving lower regions of the chest wall are associated with pain, but motor symptoms are uncommon.

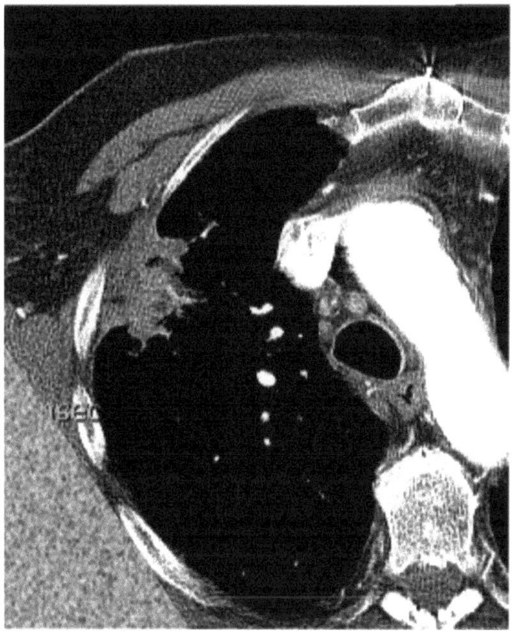

Fig. 9.3 Right upper lobe tumor with chest wall invasion that required an en bloc chest wall resection

According to the current staging system for lung cancers, chest wall involvement classifies tumors T3 lesions. They are resected en bloc with a segment of the infiltrated chest wall. During this operation the adherent chest wall, including ribs and intercostal muscles, is resected en bloc with the adherent lobectomy specimen. When the area of chest wall resection is less than 5 cm or when the resulting chest wall defect is adequately covered by the scapula, no reconstruction is necessary. When a chest wall defect extends inferiorly to the fifth rib posteriorly, the chest wall is typically reconstructed because of the concern of the tip of the scapula falling into the chest cavity after the patient raises their arm above their head.

Two common materials used to reconstruct the chest wall after significant resections are GORE-TEX mesh or methyl methacrylate. The advantage of GORE-TEX reconstruction is that the material remains soft and flexible, leading to greater patient comfort. An advantage of methyl methacrylate is that its rigidity can be used to maintain the normal contour of the body wall. Regardless of the prosthetic material used for reconstruction, these materials are always susceptible to infection and may require subsequent removal.

Summary

Surgery remains the preferred treatment modality for early stage non-small cell lung cancer for patients with adequate physiological reserve. Although the survival benefits of surgery have never been studied prospectively, the expected survival following surgical resection is substantially better than the observed survival among patients who decline any type of treatment modality [24]. Ongoing studies in the future will compare the relative efficacy of surgical resection with other emerging treatment modalities.

References

1. Goldstraw P, Crowley J, Chansky K, et al. The IASLC lung cancer staging project: proposals for the revision of the TNM stage groupings in the forthcoming (seventh) edition of the TNM classification of malignant tumors. J Thorac Oncol. 2007;2(8):707–14.
2. Reichel J. Assessment of operative risk of pneumonectomy. Chest. 1972;62(5):570–6.
3. Ferguson MK. Preoperative assessment of pulmonary risk. Chest. 1999;115(5 Suppl):58S–63.
4. Nakata M, Saeki H, Yokoyama N, Kurita A, Takiyama W, Takashima S. Pulmonary function after lobectomy: video-assisted thoracic surgery versus thoracotomy. Ann Thorac Surg. 2000;70(3):938–41.
5. Berry MF, Villamizar-Ortiz NR, Tong BC, et al. Pulmonary function tests do not predict pulmonary complications after thoracoscopic lobectomy. Ann Thorac Surg. 2010;89(4):1044–51. discussion 1051–2.
6. Brunelli A. Risk assessment for pulmonary resection. Semin Thorac Cardiovasc Surg. 2010;22(1):2–13.
7. Strand TE, Rostand H, Damhuis RA, Norstein J. Risk factors for 30-day mortality after resection of lung cancer and prediction of their magnitude. Thorax. 2007;62(11):991–7.
8. Allen MS, Darling GE, Pechet TT, et al. Morbidity and mortality of major pulmonary resections in patients with early stage lung cancer: initial results of the randomized, prospective ACOSOG Z0030 trial. Ann Thorac Surg. 2006;81(3):1013–9. discussion 1019–20.
9. Dominquez-Ventura A, Allen MS, Cassivi SD, Nichols 3rd FC, Deschamps C, Pairolero PC. Lung cancer in octogenarians: factors affecting morbidity and mortality after pulmonary resection. Ann Thorac Surg. 2006;82(4):1175–9.
10. Spaggiari L, Galeta D. Pneumonectomy for lung cancer: a further step in minimally invasive surgery. Ann Thorac Surg. 2011;91(3):e45–7.
11. Nwogu CE, Yendamuri S, Demmy TL. Does thoracoscopic pneumonectomy for lung cancer affect survival? Ann Thorac Surg. 2010;89(6):s2101–6.
12. Shigemura N, Akashi A, Funaki S, et al. Long-term outcomes after a variety of video-assisted thoracoscopic lobectomy procedures for clinical stage IA lung cancer: a multi-institutional study. J Thorac Cardiovasc Surg. 2006;132(3):507–12.
13. Sugi K, Kaneda Y, Esato K. Video-assisted thorascopic lobectomy achieves a satisfactory long-term prognosis in patients with clinical stage IA lung cancer. World J Surg. 2000;24(1):27–30. discussion 30–1.
14. Kaseda S, Aoki T, Hangai N, Shimizu K. Better pulmonary function and prognosis with video-assisted thoracic surgery than with thoracotomy. Ann Thorac Surg. 2000;70(5):1644–6.
15. Shiraishi T, Shirakusa T, Hiratsuka M, Yamamoto S, Iwasaki A. Video-assisted thoracoscopic surgery lobectomy for C-T1N0M0 primary lung cancer: its impact on locoregional control. Ann Thorac Surg. 2006;82(3):1021–6.
16. Sugi K, Nawata K, Fujita N, et al. Systemic lymph node dissection for clinically diagnosed peripheral non-small cell lung cancer less than 2 cm in diameter. World J Surg. 1998;22(3):290–4. discussion 294–5.
17. Izbicki JR, Passlick B, Pantel K, et al. Effectiveness of radical systemic mediastinal lymphadenectomy in patients with resectable non-small cell lung cancer: results of a prospective randomized trial. Ann Surg. 1998;227(1):138–44.
18. Wu Y, Huang ZF, Wang SY, Yang XN, Ou W. A randomized trial of systematic nodal dissection in resectable non-small cell lung cancer. Lung Cancer. 2002;36(1):1–6.
19. Darling GE, Allen MS, Decker P, et al. Randomized trial of mediastinal lymph node sampling versus complete lymphadenectomy during pulmonary resection in patients with N0 or N1 (less than hilar) non-small cell carcinoma: results of the ACOSOG Z0030 trial. J Thorac Cardiovasc Surg. 2011;141(3):662–70.
20. Ginsberg RJ, Rubinstein LV. Randomized trial of lobectomy versus limited resection for T1N0 non-small cell lung cancer. Lung cancer study group. Ann Thorac Surg. 1995;60(3):615–22.
21. Okada M, Yoshikawa K, Hatta T, et al. Is segmentectomy with lymph node assessment an alternative to lobectomy for non-small cell lung cancer of 2 cm or smaller? Ann Thorac Surg. 2001;71(3):956–60. discussion 961.

22. El-Sherif A, Gooding WE, Santos R, et al. Outcomes of sublobar resection versus lobectomy for stage I non-small cell lung cancer: a 13- year analysis. Ann Thorac Surg. 2006;82(2):408–15. discussion 415–6.
23. Landreneau RJ, Sugarbaker DJ, Mack MJ, et al. Wedge resection versus lobectomy for stage I (T1N0M0) non-small cell lung cancer. J Thorac Cardiovasc Surg. 1997;113(4):691–8. discussion 698–700.
24. Raz DJ, Zell JA, Ou SH, Gandara DR, Anton-Culver H, Jablons DM. Natural history of stage I non-small cell lung cancer: implications for early detection. Chest. 2007;132(1):193–9.

Radiofrequency Ablation of Primary Lung Cancer

10

Ernest M. Scalzetti

The use of heat to ablate malignant neoplasms is a recent development; the first clinical experience with radiofrequency ablation (RFA) of tumors in the lung was reported by Dupuy et al. in 2000 [1] and is supported by successful trials in animals [2–5] as well as by ablate-and-resect trials in human subjects [6–10]. It is the first method of thermal ablation to be applied to lung tumors, followed by microwave, laser, and cryoablation [11]. We are beginning to see reports that document greater than 5-year survival of patients treated for non-small cell lung cancer (NSCLC) with RFA alone, so it appears that this treatment modality can cure lung cancer [12].

There are two possible goals of treatment of lung cancer: cure or palliation. To treat with curative intent, a tumor must be solitary (in case of NSCLC, stage I) or have limited, potentially controllable metastases [13, 14]; in the latter case, RFA might have a role in treating the primary and/or the metastatic sites. Palliation might be undertaken to control symptoms, including pain caused by chest wall invasion [15] or hypertrophic pulmonary osteoarthropathy [16], or to treat hemoptysis in the setting of unresectable lung cancer [17]. The focus of this chapter will be on treating the primary lung cancer. The presentation will describe the appropriate use of this treatment modality, the expected appearance of treated lesions on follow-up imaging, and the current data regarding outcomes.

Patient Selection

At this time, only preliminary data demonstrate equivalence, to say nothing of superiority, of RFA over other established modalities of local control [18]. Therefore, it would be questionable to promote RFA for treatment of a patient with NSCLC rather than surgery or external beam radiation therapy (XRT) unless the patient is not a candidate for either of the other treatment modalities or has been offered them and refused. Ideally, patients should be evaluated in the setting of a multidisciplinary tumor board that includes interventional radiology as well as thoracic surgery, medical oncology, radiation oncology, and pulmonary medicine. This provides a forum for discussion of the relative risks and benefits of all treatment options with the particular patient in mind. The alternative of merely observing a medically inoperable patient who has early-stage NSCLC is not the best approach in most cases [19, 20].

For a patient to be considered for RFA of a lung mass, several conditions must be met. A diagnosis of malignancy must be established before RFA is undertaken. The size of the tumor must be suitable for RFA: although tumors up to 4 cm in greatest dimension can be treated with technical success, given the current state of the

E.M. Scalzetti, M.D. (✉)
Department of Radiology, SUNY Upstate Medical University, 750 E. Adams Street, Syracuse, NY 13104, USA
e-mail: scalzete@upstate.edu

J.G. Ravenel (ed.), *Lung Cancer Imaging*, Contemporary Medical Imaging,
DOI 10.1007/978-1-60761-620-7_10, © Springer Science+Business Media New York 2013

art, lesions of 3 cm or less are most likely to be completely ablated by the treatment [21]. The local anatomy surrounding the tumor must also be considered. Laceration of large pulmonary blood vessels by the needle electrode can lead to death, so it may not be possible to treat some centrally located tumors safely with RFA. Also, the flowing blood in large vessels conducts heat away from the RFA site; portions of the tumor apposed to such vessels may not be treated adequately.

Contraindications to RFA also include coagulopathy, multifocal disease such as bronchioloalveolar cell carcinoma, and the presence of metastatic disease. The last of these may be disregarded if the metastatic disease can be controlled—for example, if there is a solitary brain metastasis that is amenable to resection or radiation therapy. For patients who have pacemakers and implantable defibrillators, arrangements should be made with the cardiologist to prepare the device before RFA and return it to its preexisting mode after RFA [22]. The location of a tumor close to the heart has not been found to increase the risk of cardiac dysrhythmia during RFA [23]. Prior pneumonectomy is not necessarily a contraindication to RFA in the remaining lung [24–26].

Procedural Technique

Once RFA has been selected as the most appropriate therapy for a patient who has biopsy-proven NSCLC, a consultation visit is arranged so that the patient can meet the operator. This provides an opportunity to review the clinical situation with the patient, usually in the presence of family and friends, and for the operator to establish rapport. It also allows time to consider the potential benefits and risks of the procedure, the requirements for immediate post-procedure care, and the expectations for post-procedure imaging to assess response to the treatment. Patients generally find it reassuring to know that RFA generally can be performed as an outpatient procedure in a single session, that it does not preclude additional RFA treatments should they become necessary, and that it will not interfere with chemotherapy or radiation therapy if the clinical circumstances warrant [27]. The procedure may be performed under moderate sedation [28] or general anesthesia, without impact on outcome [29]. Alternatively the procedure may be performed under epidural anesthesia [30]. At the time of the consultation visit, the patient can be advised about the level of pain to expect during the procedure as this may influence the choice of sedation or anesthesia. In general, the closer the treatment site is to the parietal pleura, the more discomfort the patient will experience during RFA.

The RFA procedure itself has two phases. The first phase focuses on accurate placement of the needle electrode and is similar to the initial phase of a CT-guided needle biopsy. Localizing images are made. These images define the current state of the tumor; its size may influence the choice of electrode and its location will determine the approach. These features may have changed substantially in comparison to the pre-procedure diagnostic CT because of the time interval between the scans and because of changes in patient position. After a brief "time-out" to confirm patient identification and tumor location, an appropriate site for placement of the needle electrode is marked on the patient's skin. Grounding pads are applied according to manufacturer's recommendations to complete the electrical circuit during RFA and prevent skin burns. The marked skin site then is prepared and draped using sterile technique, and local anesthetic is administered.

Then the needle electrode is advanced through the chest wall and into the lung. Although ultrasound may be used for imaging guidance of RFA of a peripheral lung mass [31], usually CT is chosen as the imaging modality. Placement of the needle electrode differs from that of a biopsy needle in that the needle electrode must pass to the deep edge of the tumor, or slightly beyond, and must be positioned in the tumor such that the tumor is completely enclosed within the expected treatment volume. Depending on the size of the patient, the dimensions of the gantry of the CT scanner, and the characteristics of the needle electrode, it may not be possible to image the needle electrode while it is in the chest wall. This limitation makes accurate placement of the needle electrode more challenging. It may be helpful, in this

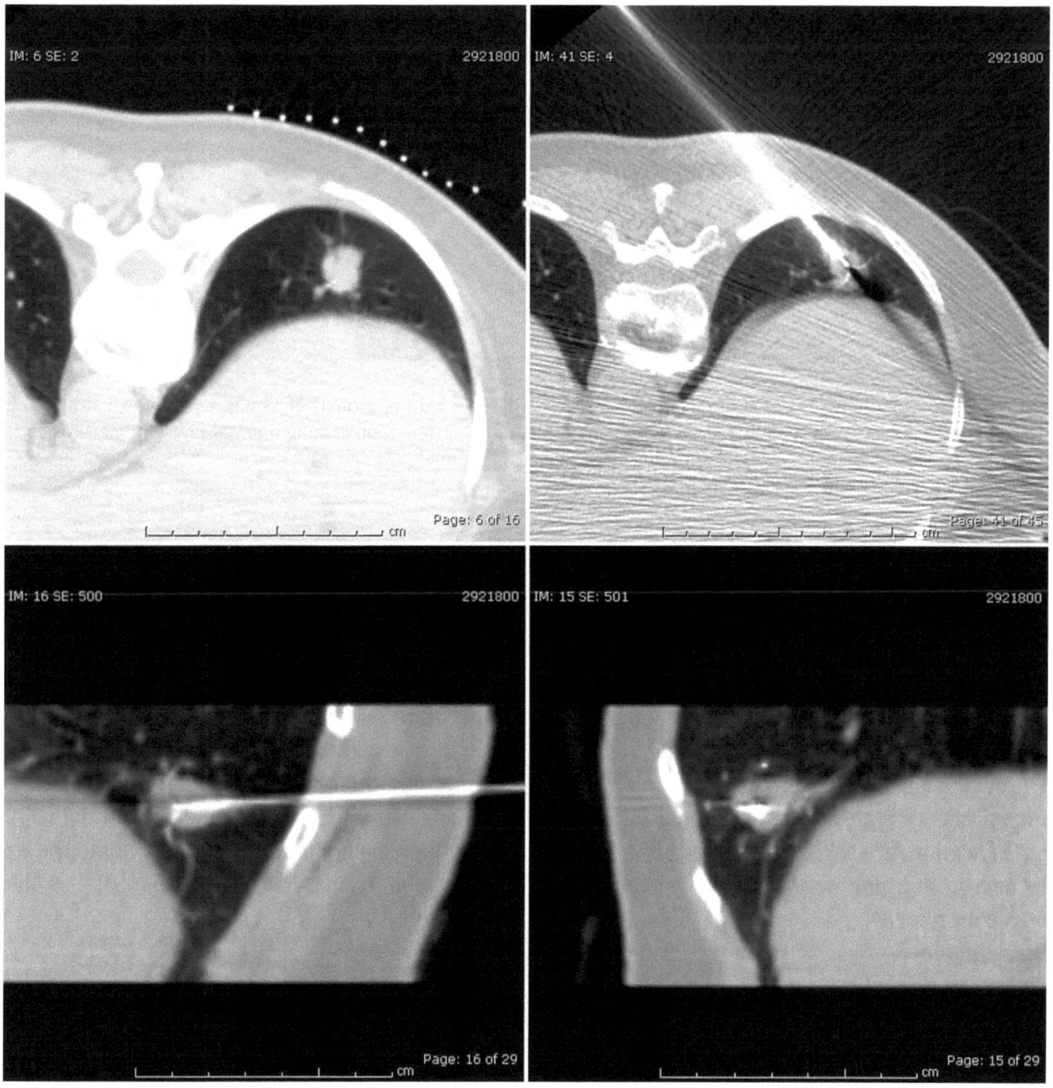

Fig. 10.1 Positioning of the needle electrode. A localizing image shows a biopsy-proven non-small cell lung cancer (NSCLC) in the lower lobe of the right lung (*upper left*). Subsequent CT image in the transverse plane demonstrates a multitined needle electrode deployed in the lesion (*upper right*). Multiplanar assessment of electrode position was obtained in the plane of the needle shaft (*lower left*) and perpendicular to the needle shaft (*lower right*), depicting adequate positioning within the lung nodule

circumstance, to use a paraxial technique in which an accessory needle is positioned in the chest wall, under CT guidance, parallel to the required course of the needle electrode and in the same imaging plane. Care must be taken to ensure that the needle electrode is not advanced too deeply, as unintended but potentially disastrous injury to vital structures may follow.

Once the needle electrode has been advanced into the target lesion, its position relative to the tumor margins must be confirmed in three dimensions. This can be accomplished by obtaining a set of thin-section CT images using helical technique through the tumor and deployed needle electrode. Reformatted images may be created immediately in oblique planes parallel and perpendicular to the shaft of the needle electrode (Fig. 10.1). Although the needle electrode may be adequately positioned in the transverse plane, its craniocaudal position may be unsatisfactory. This

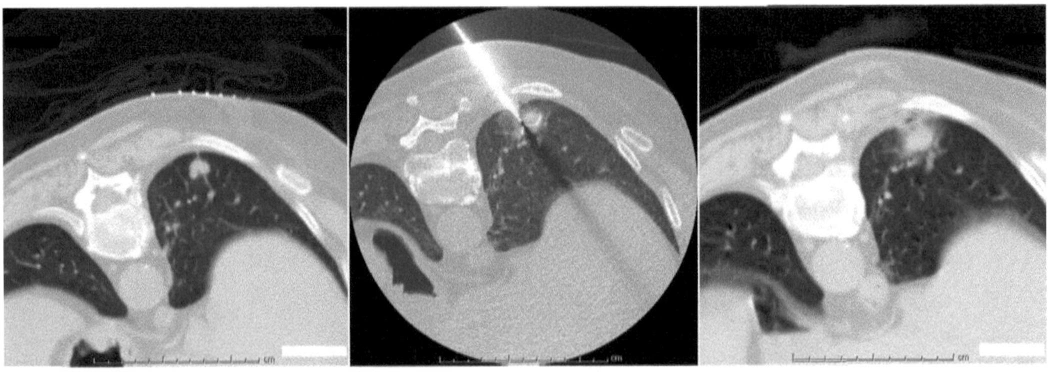

Fig. 10.2 Thermal injury. Prior to radiofrequency ablation (RFA), a biopsy-proven NSCLC is visible in the lower lobe of the right lung (*left*). A multitined needle electrode was placed under CT guidance (*center*). After RFA, a halo of ground-glass opacity is shown around the target lesion, representing thermal injury in the surrounding normal lung (*right*)

would necessitate repositioning of the needle electrode and reevaluating its location.

Once the needle electrode is adequately positioned, the second phase of the procedure, the ablation process, may begin. The treatment protocol will depend on the device's manufacturer. During the ablation the tumor temperature, tissue impedance, or both will be monitored to provide an indication of technical success. For lesions located in the lung periphery, the operator may create a protective pneumothorax; this places an insulating layer of air between the lesion and the chest wall or mediastinum, decreasing the likelihood of intolerable pain or nerve injury [32].

Once target temperature has been achieved and maintained, or tissue impedance increases to indicate coagulation, the ablation is completed. More than one application may be required, depending on the size and shape of the tumor. CT imaging at this point should demonstrate ground-glass opacity surrounding the target lesion, indicating a rim of thermally injured normal lung (Fig. 10.2). If the lung adjacent to any portion of the tumor does not show signs of thermal injury, retreatment at that site should be considered; it appears that a margin of at least 5 mm is necessary to decrease the risk of local recurrence [33]. After the operator is confident that the entire tumor has been treated, the needle electrode can be removed. Post-procedure CT images should be inspected for complications such as pneumothorax, hemothorax, and pulmonary hemorrhage.

The patient then returns to the outpatient unit with orders for follow-up chest radiography and pain control. Typically, we keep our post-RFA patients overnight and discharge them the following morning if they are doing well. Occasionally, if a patient has no adverse effects from the RFA and an adequate support system at home, he or she may be discharged on the same day as the procedure.

Complications

A number of RFA-related procedural complications have been described [34]. Cutaneous burns usually are the result of inadequate grounding and thus are avoidable. However, prolonged treatment times associated with large tumors [35, 36], or treatment of superficial tumors in which the treatment volume includes the skin surface, may lead to burns even under optimal care. Thermal injury may occur in normal tissues adjacent to the tumor, including the esophagus and diaphragm [37]. If the tumor contacts the mediastinal pleura, the possibility of phrenic nerve injury exists [38]; the resulting impairment in diaphragmatic function may be devastating in a patient whose baseline pulmonary function is marginal. Brachial nerve injury also has been described in cases of apical tumors treated with RFA [39]. Thermal osteonecrosis of a rib has been described [40].

Pneumothorax is a common complication, with a reported incidence of 9–63 % in several small series [21, 41–47], and air leaks may be delayed in onset [8, 48] or prolonged [49, 50]. A prolonged air leak may be caused by injury to the visceral pleura; alternatively, a bronchopleural fistula may develop [50–52]. Pleural effusion is another described complication [53]. Pulmonary hemorrhage can be massive if a pulmonary artery is mechanically injured by the needle electrode; this is one complication that can lead to death [54–56]. Pulmonary artery injury also can lead to pseudoaneurysm formation [57]. Systemic air embolization, another potentially fatal complication, poses a risk in RFA as well as needle biopsy [58, 59]. Cerebral microembolization has been observed by ultrasound of the carotid arteries during RFA [60–62] but rarely is associated with clinical findings [63]; a study in an animal model demonstrated this phenomenon in a minority of cases and no evidence of cerebral ischemia [64]. A case of equipment failure, in which an expandable multitined needle electrode could not be withdrawn from the target lesion, has been reported [65]. A case of acute respiratory distress syndrome attributed to RFA of the lung has been described [66]. There is another single case report of pneumomediastinum and subcutaneous emphysema complicating RFA [67]. For several days after RFA, patients may experience a mild flu-like syndrome that has been attributed to tumor lysis; the likelihood of this event is proportional to the volume of the tumor. Infection may supervene in the lung or pleural space [68–70]. Tumor seeding of the needle tract has been described but is rare [71, 72]. Procedural mortality has been reported at a rate of <1 % [35, 42, 44, 53].

Follow-Up Imaging

In the longer term, the treatment site must be monitored to assess response to therapy (Fig. 10.3). Even when the target lesion is coagulated completely, imaging features evolve for 1 year or more [73, 74]. In our institution we recommend that contrast-enhanced CT be performed at 3, 6, and 12 months after RFA, and annually thereafter. At 3 months the treatment site is larger than the original tumor and may be cavitary. There should be no more than a thin rim of contrast enhancement at the margin of the treatment site [74]. Thereafter, the residual opacity at the treatment site should slowly contract, indicating organization and fibrosis [75]. Interestingly, Sharma et al. observed hilar or mediastinal lymph node enlargement on CT scans made 1 month after lung RFA; this nodal enlargement proved to be reversible at 3 and 6 months in all cases indicating that it did not result from metastatic disease [76].

PET imaging with 18F-fluorodeoxyglucose (FDG) may show uptake early after therapy, but the degree of uptake should decline subsequently. A study in a rabbit model suggests that PET scanning should take place no sooner than 1 month after RFA because of reactive changes in the lung surrounding the treatment site [77]. In a clinical trial, the same investigators found that FDG-PET was useful for predicting tumor recurrence at 2 months after RFA [78]. In that study, a standardized uptake value of more than 1.8 at the treatment site, or a standardized uptake value that decreased less than 60 % relative to a pretreatment baseline measurement, suggested the presence of residual malignancy [78]. Akeboshi et al. used FDG-PET and contrast-enhanced CT to follow patients after RFA of lung neoplasms, a minority of which were primary lung cancers [79]. They found that abolition of FDG uptake was both 100 % sensitive and specific for complete response, at both 1 and 3 months after RFA; the performance of CT was indistinguishable from PET at 3 months [79]. Other investigators have found PET-CT, using 18F-FDG, to be useful in predicting local recurrence after RFA [80, 81]. Any CT or PET findings that depart from the expected sequence of events should lead to needle biopsy so that retreatment of incompletely ablated tumors can be undertaken without delay (Fig. 10.4) [82]. One cautionary note regarding PET-CT, uptake of 18F-FDG may occur in the

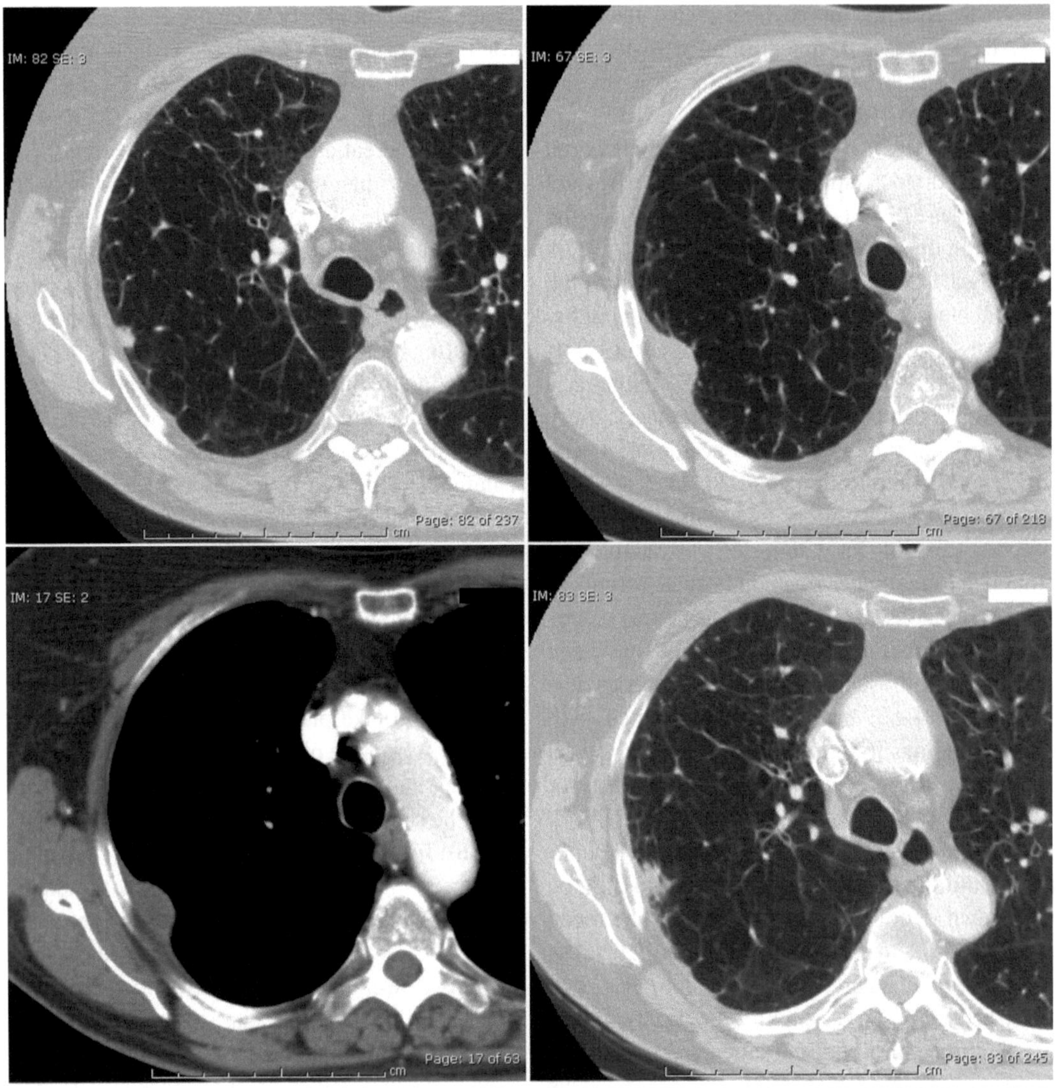

Fig. 10.3 Evolution of post-RFA CT findings. A diagnostic CT scan made before biopsy and RFA reveals a small peripheral lesion in the upper lobe of the right lung (*upper left*). This was found to be a NSCLC and was treated with RFA. Three months later, a contrast-enhanced CT shows a larger, well-defined opacity at the site of RFA (*upper right*); this opacity does not enhance with contrast, suggesting the absence of viable tumor (*lower left*). At 9 months post-RFA, another contrast-enhanced CT scan demonstrates a decrease in the size of the right upper lobe opacity (*lower right*)

needle tract or mediastinal lymph nodes after RFA, unrelated to tumor spread [81].

Another reason to continue to follow these patients is the risk of developing a second primary lung cancer [83]. In general, this risk has been estimated at 2 % per year after successful treatment of NSCLC [84]. However, four of the nine patients we treated for stage IA NSCLC, who survived more than 2 years after RFA, developed a new primary lung cancer; most of the new lesions were also treated with RFA (Fig. 10.5).

Outcomes

A number of reports describe early response of NSCLC to RFA [36, 43, 44, 47, 66, 73, 79, 85–88]. In two studies RFA was followed by resection of

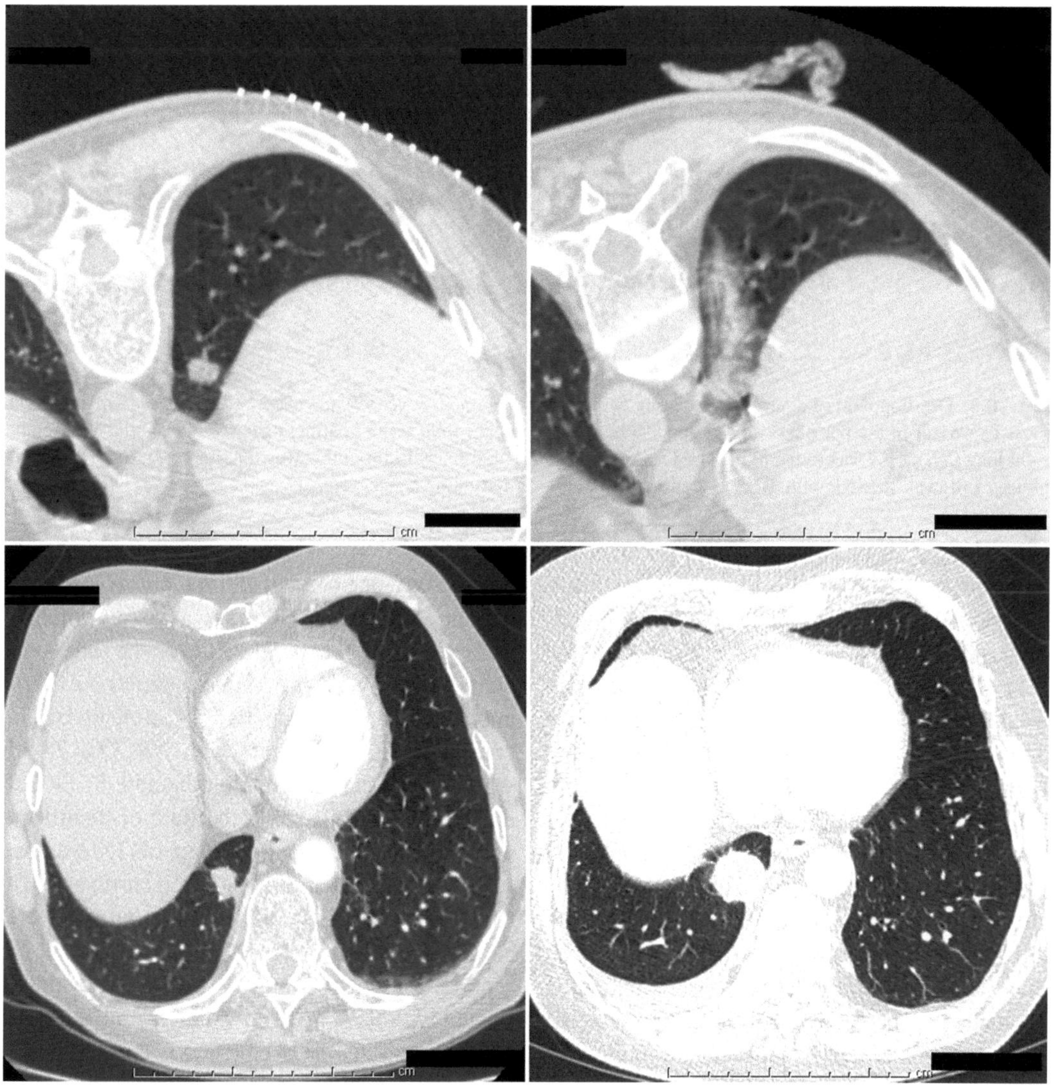

Fig. 10.4 Local recurrence after RFA. A NSCLC is visible in the lower lobe of the right lung on a localizing CT image, just before RFA (*upper left*). Immediately after RFA the lesion is obscured by thermal injury and hemorrhage (*upper right*). Three months later a contrast-enhanced CT shows that the lesion has enlarged slightly and has become more lobulated (*lower left*), although it lacks contrast enhancement (not shown). At 1-year post-RFA, the mass at the treatment site is much larger and is accompanied by a pleural effusion (*lower right*)

the treated tumor, allowing pathologic assessment of the extent of RFA-induced tumor necrosis. One such investigation revealed complete necrosis in 6/9 cases [7]. In another, the complete absence of viable tumor cells was observed in only 3/10 lesions [6]. Hataji et al. reported a patient with recurrent squamous cell carcinoma of the lung, treated with RFA, in whom the tumor was evaluated by autopsy 3 months after treatment; although fibrosis and necrosis were evident in the treatment zone, viable malignant cells were present at the periphery of the tumor [10]. Without question, results determined by pathologic evaluation or clinical follow-up will depend on many factors that remain to be elucidated.

There is little long-term follow-up information in patients who have had RFA as therapy for

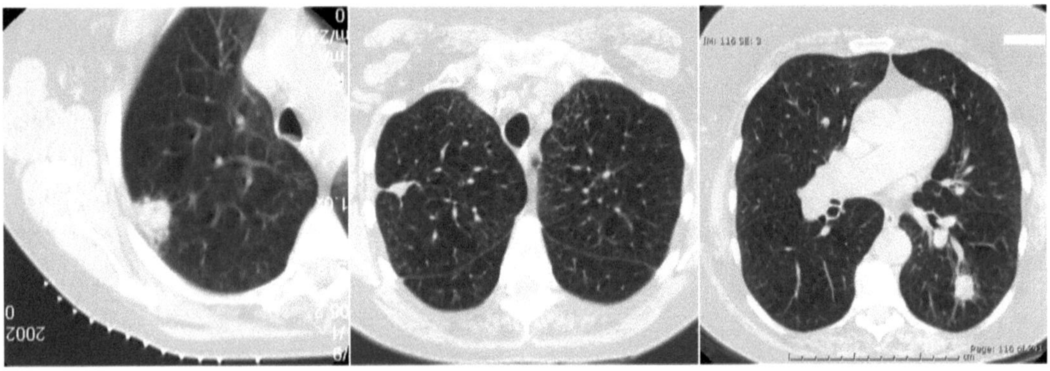

Fig. 10.5 Development of a new primary lung cancer. A mass is present in the periphery of the upper lobe of the right lung (*left*). This was found to be a NSCLC by needle biopsy and was treated with RFA. A surveillance CT obtained 5 years later shows a stable scar in the right upper lobe at the treatment site (*center*), and a new spiculated mass in the left lower lobe representing a new primary lung cancer (*right*)

clinical stage I NSCLC [12, 41]. A small series of 36 patients showed a median survival of 29 months in a medically inoperable population [41]. This compares favorably to the reported results of XRT in a similar population, with a 3-year overall survival approaching 40 % [89]. However, both treatment modalities are evolving: results of stereotactic body radiotherapy recently have become available in this patient population, with an overall 2-year survival of 56 % [90]. One consistent finding is that RFA, as radiation therapy, has less success in treating larger tumors than smaller ones [91]. To emphasize this point, Okuma et al. performed a multivariate analysis on their series of unresectable lung tumors; they found that tumor size of greater than or equal to 2 cm was the only independent risk factor for local progression [92].

Because the efficacy of RFA relative to other treatment modalities has not been demonstrated in the setting of NSCLC and because the procedure can lead to death, the FDA has not approved RFA specifically for treatment of lung cancers. Manufacturers cannot legally market their RFA devices for this indication. Now that several medical centers have had more than 5 years of experience with RFA for NSCLC, single-center reports of efficacy are beginning to appear in the literature [12]. Zemlyak et al. compared RFA and cryoablation to sublobar resection in small numbers of patients with stage I NSCLC. The 3-year survival in the RFA and surgical groups did not differ. Sixty-one percent of the sublobar resection patients were cancer-free at 3 years, whereas 50 % of the RFA patients achieved the same outcome [18]. The largest single-institution experience thus far was reported by Beland et al., consisting of 79 patients with NSCLC, 28 of whom also received radiation therapy; 87 % had clinical stage I disease at the time of treatment, and after an average follow-up of 17 months, 61 % of these had no evidence of recurrence [93]. Consistent with other studies, larger tumors were at increased risk for recurrence [93]. Lanuti et al. report a consecutive series of 31 NSCLC patients treated with RFA, with a median overall survival of 30 months and an overall survival of 78 % at 2 years [69]. A multicenter prospective single-arm clinical trial of RFA of lung tumors that included 33 patients with NSCLC showed an overall survival of 48 % at 2 years (75 % among the subgroup with stage I NSCLC) [94]. Another multicenter prospective single-arm study of RFA in clinical stage I NSCLC, sponsored by the American College of Surgeons Oncology Group (ACOSOG protocol Z4033), has closed to accrual and follow-up data is being collected.

Other Modalities

Two other percutaneous ablative strategies should be mentioned, microwave and cryoablation. Both of these technologies have been studied in solid organs of the abdomen and applied in the lung although data is quite preliminary and theoretical. Microwave refers to the electromagnetic spectrum between infrared radiation and radio waves and functions by creating heat from the agitation of water molecules [95]. The theoretical advantage of microwave over traditional RFA is the ability of both larger volumes and faster heating of tissues as well as a decrease in the heat sink phenomenon [96]. A retrospective study seems to support this data in that size was not predictive of survival following treatment [97]. Cryoablation works on the theory that the formation of ice within the intracellular matrix and subsequent thawing leads to tumor lysis in conjunction with local vascular thrombosis resulting in coagulative necrosis. The theoretical advantage is that there may be less pain than with heat-based technologies [98]. Actual data on cryoablation is sparse; however, it does not appear inferior to RFA [18].

The Future

We will need evidence from additional clinical trials to form a clearer picture of RFA's role in the treatment of patients who suffer from lung cancer. For example, RFA may be viewed not as a competitor to XRT in medically inoperable stage I NSCLC, but as a complementary treatment modality. For tumors with a substantial likelihood of local failure after XRT alone, the two modalities can be combined [99–101]. Also, in cases of local failure of XRT, if restaging demonstrates no other sites of disease, RFA may be used to treat the recurrent tumor. Improvements in RFA treatment protocols may take advantage of animal models [4]. The technology undoubtedly will continue to improve, driven more by applications of RFA in the liver and other anatomic sites where it has specifically been approved for use. These technology advances should include improved design of needle electrodes, the development of treatment planning systems similar to those available for radiation therapy [102], and robotic devices for more accurate placement of needle electrodes in tumors of complex shape.

References

1. Dupuy DE, Zagoria RJ, Akerley W, Mayo-Smith WW, Kavanagh PV, Safran H. Percutaneous radiofrequency ablation of malignancies in the lung. AJR Am J Roentgenol. 2000;174(1):57–9.
2. Goldberg SN, Gazelle GS, Compton CC, Mueller PR, McLoud TC. Radio-frequency tissue ablation of VX2 tumor nodules in the rabbit lung. Acad Radiol. 1996;3(11):929–35.
3. Miao Y, Ni Y, Bosmans H, et al. Radiofrequency ablation for eradication of pulmonary tumor in rabbits. J Surg Res. 2001;99(2):265–71.
4. Ahrar K, Price RE, Wallace MJ, et al. Percutaneous radiofrequency ablation of lung tumors in a large animal model. J Vasc Interv Radiol. 2003;14(8):1037–43.
5. Nomori H, Imazu Y, Watanabe K, et al. Radiofrequency ablation of pulmonary tumors and normal lung tissue in swine and rabbits. Chest. 2005;127(3):973–7.
6. Nguyen CL, Scott WJ, Young NA, Rader T, Giles LR, Goldberg M. Radiofrequency ablation of primary lung cancer: results from an ablate and resect pilot study. Chest. 2005;128(5):3507–11.
7. Ambrogi MC, Fontanini G, Cioni R, Faviana P, Fanucchi O, Mussi A. Biologic effects of radiofrequency thermal ablation on non-small cell lung cancer: results of a pilot study. J Thorac Cardiovasc Surg. 2006;131(5):1002–6.
8. Clasen S, Kettenbach J, Kosan B, et al. Delayed development of pneumothorax after pulmonary radiofrequency ablation. Cardiovasc Intervent Radiol. 2009;32(3):484–90.
9. Jaskolka JD, Kachura JR, Hwang DM, et al. Pathologic assessment of radiofrequency ablation of pulmonary metastases. J Vasc Interv Radiol. 2010;21(11):1689–96.
10. Hataji O, Yamakado K, Nakatsuka A, et al. Radiological and pathological correlation of lung malignant tumors treated with percutaneous radiofrequency ablation. Intern Med. 2005;44(8):865–9.
11. Vogl TJ, Naquib NN, Lehnert T, Nour-Eldin NE. Radiofrequency, microwave and laser ablation of pulmonary neoplasms: clinical studies and technical considerations—review article. Eur J Radiol. 2011;77(2):346–57.
12. Simon CJ, Dupey DE, DiPetrillo TA, et al. Pulmonary radiofrequency ablation: long-term safety and efficacy in 153 patients. Radiology. 2007;243(1):268–75.
13. De Pas TM, de Braud F, Catalano G, et al. Oligometastatic non-small cell lung cancer: a multidisciplinary approach in the positron emission tomographic scan era. Ann Thorac Surg. 2007;83(1):231–4.
14. Khan AJ, Mehta PS, Zusag TW, et al. Long term disease-free survival resulting from combined

modality management of patients presenting with oligometastatic, non-small cell lung carcinoma (NSCLC). Radiother Oncol. 2006;81(2):163–7.
15. Grieco CA, Simon CJ, Mayo-Smith WW, Dipetrillo TA, Ready NE, Dupuy DE. Image-guided percutaneous thermal ablation for the palliative treatment of chest wall masses. Am J Clin Oncol. 2007;30(4):361–7.
16. Kishi K, Nakamura H, Sudo A, et al. Tumor debulking by radiofrequency ablation in hypertrophic pulmonary osteoarthropathy associated with pulmonary carcinoma. Lung Cancer. 2002;38(3):317–20.
17. Baisi A, Raveglia F, De Simone M, Cioffi U. Palliative role of percutaneous radiofrequency ablation for severe hemoptysis in an elderly patient with inoperable lung cancer. J Thorac Cardiovasc Surg. 2010;140(5):1196–7.
18. Zemlyak A, Moore WH, Bilfinger TV. Comparison of survival after sublobar resections and ablative therapies for stage I non-small cell lung cancer. J Am Coll Surg. 2010;211(1):68–72.
19. McGarry RC, Song G, des Rosiers P, Timmerman R. Observation-only management of early stage, medically inoperable lung cancer: poor outcome. Chest. 2002;121(4):1155–8.
20. Raz DJ, Zell JA, Ou SH, Gandara DR, Anton-Culver H, Jablons DM. Natural history of stage I non-small cell lung cancer: implications for early detection. Chest. 2007;132(1):193–9.
21. Ambrogi MC, Lucchi M, Dini P, et al. Percutaneous radiofrequency ablation of lung tumours: results in the mid-term. Eur J Cardiothorac Surg. 2006;30(1):177–83.
22. Donohoo JH, Anderson MT, Mayo-Smith WW. Pacemaker reprogramming after radiofrequency ablation of a lung neoplasm. AJR Am J Roentgenol. 2007;189(4):890–2.
23. Iguchi T, Hiraki T, Gobara H, et al. Percutaneous radiofrequency ablation of lung tumors close to the heart or aorta: evaluation of safety and effectiveness. J Vasc Interv Radiol. 2007;18(6):733–40.
24. Ambrogi MC, Fanucchi O, Lencioni R, Cioni R, Mussi A. Pulmonary radiofrequency ablation in a single lung patient. Thorax. 2006;61(9):828–9.
25. Sofocleous CT, May B, Petre EN, et al. Pulmonary thermal ablation in patients with prior pneumonectomy. AJR Am J Roentgenol. 2011;196(5):W606–12.
26. Hess A, Palussière J, Goyers JF, Guth A, Aupèrin A, de Baère T. Pulmonary radiofrequency ablation in patients with a single lung: feasibility, efficacy, and tolerance. Radiology. 2011;258(2):635–42.
27. Hotta K, Matsuo K, Kiura K, Ueoka H, Tanimoto M. Advances in our understanding of postoperative adjuvant chemotherapy in resectable non-small-cell lung cancer. Curr Opin Oncol. 2006;18(2):144–50.
28. Volpe ML, Piazza O, Palumbo D, et al. Conscious analgosedation for radiofrequency ablation of lung neoplasm. Minerva Anestesiol. 2006;72(3):111–5.
29. Hoffmann RT, Jakobs TF, Lubienski A, et al. Percutaneous radiofrequency ablation of pulmonary tumors—is there a difference between treatment under general anaesthesia and under conscious sedation? Eur J Radiol. 2006;59(2):168–74.
30. Pouliquen C, Kabbani Y, Saignac P, Gékière JP, Palussèire J. Radiofrequency ablation of lung tumours with the patient under thoracic epidural anaesthesia. Cardiovasc Intervent Radiol. 2011;34 Suppl 2:S178–81.
31. Louie J, McGahan JP, Moore EH, Goodnight J, Brock J. Radio frequency ablation of lung metastasis using sonographic guidance. J Ultrasound Med. 2004;23(9):1241–4.
32. Lee EW, Suh RD, Zeidler MR, et al. Radiofrequency ablation of subpleural lung malignancy: reduced pain using an artificially created pneumothorax. Cardiovasc Intervent Radiol. 2009;32(4):833–6.
33. Anderson EM, Lees WR, Gillams AR. Early indicators of treatment success after percutaneous radiofrequency of pulmonary tumors. Cardiovasc Intervent Radiol. 2009;32(3):478–83.
34. Zhu JC, Yan TD, Glenn D, Morris DL. Radiofrequency ablation of lung tumors: feasibility and safety. Ann Thorac Surg. 2009;87(4):1023–8.
35. Sano Y, Kanazawa S, Gobara H, et al. Feasibility of percutaneous radiofrequency ablation for intrathoracic malignancies: a large single-center experience. Cancer. 2007;109(7):1397–405.
36. VanSonnenberg E, Shankar S, Morrison PR, et al. Radiofrequency ablation of thoracic lesions: part 2, initial clinical experience—technical and multidisciplinary considerations in 30 patients. AJR Am J Roentgenol. 2005;184(2):381–90.
37. Mori T, Kawanaka K, Ohba Y, et al. Diaphragm perforation after radio-frequency ablation for metastatic lung cancer. Ann Thorac Cardiovasc Surg. 2010;16(6):426–8.
38. Thornton RH, Solomon SB, Dupuy DE, Bains MS. Phrenic nerve injury resulting from percutaneous ablation of lung malignancy. AJR Am J Roentgenol. 2008;191(2):565–8.
39. Hiraki T, Gobara H, Mimura H, et al. Brachial nerve injury caused by percutaneous radiofrequency ablation of apical lung cancer: a report of four cases. J Vasc Interv Radiol. 2010;21(7):1129–33.
40. Le TX, Andrews RT. Thermal osteonecrosis of the rib after radiofrequency ablation in the thorax. J Vasc Interv Radiol. 2008;19(6):940–4.
41. Ambrogi MC, Dini P, Melfi F, Mussi A. Radiofrequency ablation of inoperable non-small cell lung cancer. J Thorac Oncol. 2007;2(5 Suppl):S2–3.
42. Belfiore G, Moggio G, Tedeschi E, et al. CT-guided radiofrequency ablation: a potential complementary therapy for patients with unresectable primary lung cancer—a preliminary report of 33 patients. AJR Am J Roentgenol. 2004;183(4):1003–11.

43. Cariati M, Giordano G, Midulla M. Radiofrequency ablation of pulmonary lesions. Radiol Med. 2007; 112(2):149–56.
44. de Baère T, Palussière J, Aupérin A, et al. Midterm local efficacy and survival after radiofrequency ablation of lung tumors with minimum follow-up of 1 year: prospective evaluation. Radiology. 2006; 240(2):587–96.
45. Gadaleta C, Catino A, Ranieri G, et al. Radiofrequency thermal ablation of 69 lung neoplasms. J Chemother. 2004;16 Suppl 5:86–9.
46. Gillams AR, Lees WR. Analysis of the factors associated with radiofrequency ablation-induced pneumothorax. Clin Radiol. 2007;62(7):639–44.
47. Pennathur A, Luketich JD, Abbas G, et al. Radiofrequency ablation for the treatment of stage I non-small cell lung cancer in high-risk patients. J Thorac Cardiovasc Surg. 2007;134(4):857–64.
48. Yoshimatsu R, Yamagami T, Terayama K, Matsumoto T, Miura H, Nishimura T. Delayed and recurrent pneumothorax after radiofrequency ablation of lung tumors. Chest. 2009;135(4):1002–9.
49. Yamagami T, Kato T, Hirota T, Yoshimatsu R, Matsumoto T, Nishimura T. Pneumothorax as a complication of percutaneous radiofrequency ablation for lung neoplasms. J Vasc Interv Radiol. 2006;17(10):1625–9.
50. Sakurai J, Hiraki T, Mukai T, et al. Intractable pneumothorax due to bronchopleural fistula after radiofrequency ablation of lung tumors. J Vasc Interv Radiol. 2007;18(1 Pt 1):141–5.
51. Cannella M, Cornelis F, Descat E, et al. Bronchopleural fistula after radiofrequency ablation of lung tumours. Cardiovasc Intervent Radiol. 2011;34 Suppl 2:S171–4.
52. Nachiappan AC, Sharma A, Shepard JA, Lanuti M. Radiofrequency ablation in the lung complicated by positive airway pressure ventilation. Ann Thorac Surg. 2010;89(5):1665–7.
53. Steinke K, Sewell PE, Dupuy D, et al. Pulmonary radiofrequency ablation—an international study survey. Anticancer Res. 2004;24(1):339–43.
54. Vaughn C, Mychaskiw 2nd G, Sewell P. Massive hemorrhage during radiofrequency ablation of a pulmonary neoplasm. Anesth Analg. 2002;94(5): 1149–51.
55. Fattorutto M. Massive hemorrhage during radiofrequency ablation of a pulmonary neoplasm. Anesth Analg. 2003;96(4):1233; author reply 1234.
56. Nour-Eldin NE, Naguib NN, Mack M, Abskharon JE, Vogl TJ. Pulmonary hemorrhage complicating radiofrequency ablation, from mild hemoptysis to life-threatening pattern. Eur Radiol. 2011;21(1):197–204.
57. Sakurai J, Mimura H, Gobara H, Hiraki T, Kanazawa S. Pulmonary artery pseudoaneurysm related to radiofrequency ablation of lung tumor. Cardiovasc Intervent Radiol. 2010;33(2):413–6.
58. Ghaye B, Bruyère PJ, Dondelinger RF. Nonfatal systemic air embolism during percutaneous radiofrequency ablation of a pulmonary metastasis. AJR Am J Roentgenol. 2006;187(3):W327–8.
59. Jeannin A, Saignac P, Palussière J, Gékière JP, Descat E, Lakdja F. Massive systemic air embolism during percutaneous radiofrequency ablation of a primary lung tumor. Anesth Analg. 2009;109(2): 484–6.
60. Yamamoto A, Matsuoka T, Toyoshima M, et al. Assessment of cerebral microembolism during percutaneous radiofrequency ablation of lung tumors using diffusion-weighted imaging. AJR Am J Roentgenol. 2004;183(6):1785–9.
61. Rose SC, Fotoohi M, Levin DL, Harrell JH. Cerebral microembolization during radiofrequency ablation of lung malignancies. J Vasc Interv Radiol. 2002; 13(10):1051–4.
62. Tanigawa N, Kariya S, Kojima H, et al. Cerebral microembolisation during radiofrequency ablation of lung tumours: detection by carotid duplex ultrasound. Br J Radiol. 2009;82(975):249–53.
63. Jin GY, Lee JM, Lee YC, Han YM. Acute cerebral infarction after radiofrequency ablation of an atypical carcinoid pulmonary tumor. AJR Am J Roentgenol. 2004;182(4):990–2.
64. Ahrar K, Stafford RJ, Tinkey PT, et al. Evaluation of cerebral microemboli during radiofrequency ablation of lung tumors in a canine model with use of impedance-controlled devices. J Vasc Interv Radiol. 2007;18(7):929–35.
65. Steinke K, King J, Glenn D, Morris DL. Percutaneous radiofrequency ablation of lung tumors: difficulty withdrawing the hooks resulting in a split needle. Cardiovasc Intervent Radiol. 2003;26(6):583–5.
66. Lee JM, Jin GY, Goldberg SN, et al. Percutaneous radiofrequency ablation for inoperable non-small cell lung cancer and metastases: preliminary report. Radiology. 2004;230(1):125–34.
67. Radvany MG, Allan PF, Frey WC, Banks KP, Malave D. Pulmonary radiofrequency ablation complicated by subcutaneous emphysema and pneumomediastinum treated with fibrin sealant injection. AJR Am J Roentgenol. 2005;185(4):894–8.
68. Okuma T, Matsuoka T, Yamamoto A, et al. Frequency and risk factors of various complications after computed tomography-guided radiofrequency ablation of lung tumors. Cardiovasc Intervent Radiol. 2008;31(1):122–30.
69. Lanuti M, Sharma A, Digumarthy SR, et al. Radiofrequency ablation for treatment of medically inoperable stage I non-small cell lung cancer. J Thorac Cardiovasc Surg. 2009;137(1):160–6.
70. Hiraki T, Gobara H, Mimura H, et al. Aspergilloma in a cavity formed after percutaneous radiofrequency ablation for lung cancer. J Vasc Interv Radiol. 2009;20(11):1499–500.
71. Yamakado K, Akeboshi M, Nakatsuka A, et al. Tumor seeding following lung radiofrequency ablation: a case report. Cardiovasc Intervent Radiol. 2005;28(4):530–2.

72. Hiraki T, Mimura H, Gobara H, et al. Two cases of needle-tract seeding after percutaneous radiofrequency ablation for lung cancer. J Vasc Interv Radiol. 2009;20(3):415–8.
73. Suh RD, Wallace AB, Sheehan RE, Heinze SB, Goldin JG. Unresectable pulmonary malignancies: CT-guided percutaneous radiofrequency ablation—preliminary results. Radiology. 2003;229(3):821–9.
74. Jin GY, Lee JM, Lee YC, Han YM, Lim YS. Primary and secondary lung malignancies treated with percutaneous radiofrequency ablation: evaluation with follow-up helical CT. AJR Am J Roentgenol. 2004;183(4):1013–20.
75. Bojarski JD, Dupuy DE, Mayo-Smith WW. CT imaging findings of pulmonary neoplasms after treatment with radiofrequency ablation: results in 32 tumors. AJR Am J Roentgenol. 2005;185(2):466–71.
76. Sharma A, Digumarthy SR, Kalra MK, Lanuti M, Shepard JA. Reversible locoregional lymph node enlargement after radiofrequency ablation of lung tumors. AJR Am J Roentgenol. 2010;194(5): 1250–6.
77. Okuma T, Matsuoka T, Okamura T, et al. 18F-FDG small-animal PET for monitoring the therapeutic effect of CT-guided radiofrequency ablation on implanted VX2 lung tumors in rabbits. J Nucl Med. 2006;47(8):1351–8.
78. Okuma T, Okamura T, Matsuoka T, et al. Fluorine-18-fluorodeoxyglucose positron emission tomography for assessment of patients with unresectable recurrent or metastatic lung cancers after CT-guided radiofrequency ablation: preliminary results. Ann Nucl Med. 2006;20(2):115–21.
79. Akeboshi M et al. Percutaneous radiofrequency ablation of lung neoplasms: initial therapeutic response. J Vasc Interv Radiol. 2004;15(5):463–70.
80. Singnurkar A, Solomon SB, Gönen M, Larson SM, Schöder H. 18F-FDG PET/CT for the prediction and detection of local recurrence after radiofrequency ablation of malignant lung lesions. J Nucl Med. 2010;51(12):1833–40.
81. Deandreis D, Leboulleux S, Dromain C, et al. Role of FDG PET/CT and chest CT in the follow-up of lung lesions treated with radiofrequency ablation. Radiology. 2011;258(1):270–6.
82. Hiraki T, Mimura H, Gobara H, et al. Repeat radiofrequency ablation for local progression of lung tumors: does it have a role in local tumor control? J Vasc Interv Radiol. 2008;19(5):706–11.
83. Rubins J, Unger M, Colice GL, American College of Chest Physicians. Follow-up and surveillance of the lung cancer patient following curative intent therapy: ACCP evidence-based clinical practice guideline (2nd edition). Chest. 2007;132(3 Suppl): 355S–67S.
84. Rice D, Kim HW, Sabichi A, et al. The risk of second primary tumors after resection of stage I nonsmall cell lung cancer. Ann Thorac Surg. 2003;76(4): 1001–7; discussion 1007–8.
85. Thanos L, Mylona S, Pomoni M, et al. Percutaneous radiofrequency thermal ablation of primary and metastatic lung tumors. Eur J Cardiothorac Surg. 2006; 30(5):797–800.
86. Fernando HC, De Hoyos A, Landreneau RJ, et al. Radiofrequency ablation for the treatment of non-small cell lung cancer in marginal surgical candidates. J Thorac Cardiovasc Surg. 2005;129(3): 639–44.
87. Rossi S, Dore R, Cascina A, et al. Percutaneous computed tomography-guided radiofrequency thermal ablation of small unresectable lung tumours. Eur Respir J. 2006;27(3):556–63.
88. Camacho Romero J, Oliver Goldaracena JM, Rodríquez Caravaca G, Hernando Polo S, Martel Villagrán J, Trapero M. [CT-guided radiofrequency ablation of non-small cell lung cancer]. Med Clin (Barc). 2010;135(13):581–5.
89. Decker RH, Tanoue LT, Colasanto JM, Detterbeck FC, Wilson LD. Evaluation and definitive management of medically inoperable early-stage non-small-cell lung cancer. Part 1: assessment and conventional radiotherapy. Oncology. 2006; 20(7):727–36.
90. Timmerman RD, Kavanagh BD, Cho LC, Papiez L, Xing L. Stereotactic body radiation therapy in multiple organ sites. J Clin Oncol. 2007;25(8):947–52.
91. Steinke K, Glenn D, King J, Morris DL. Percutaneous pulmonary radiofrequency ablation: difficulty achieving complete ablations in big lung lesions. Br J Radiol. 2003;76(910):742–5.
92. Okuma T, Matsuoka T, Yamamoto A, et al. Determinants of local progression after computed tomography-guided percutaneous radiofrequency ablation for unresectable lung tumors: 9-year experience in a single institution. Cardiovasc Intervent Radiol. 2010;33(4):787–93.
93. Beland MD, Wasser EJ, Mayo-Smith WW, Dupuy DE. Primary non-small cell lung cancer: review of frequency, location, and time of recurrence after radiofrequency ablation. Radiology. 2010;254(1): 301–7.
94. Lencioni R, Crocetti L, Cioni R, et al. Response to radiofrequency ablation of pulmonary tumours: a prospective, intention-to-treat, multicentre clinical trial (the RAPTURE study). Lancet Oncol. 2008; 9(7):621–8.
95. Simon CJ, Dupuy DE, Mayo-Smith WW. Microwave ablation: principles and applications. Radiographics. 2005;25 Suppl 1:S69–83.
96. Dupuy DE. Microwave ablation compared with radiofrequency ablation in lung tissue—is microwave not just for popcorn anymore? Radiology. 2009;251(3):617–8.
97. Wolf FJ, Grand DJ, Machan JT, Dipetrillo TA, Mayo-Smith WW, Dupuy DE. Microwave ablation of lung malignancies: effectiveness, CT findings, and safety in 50 patients. Radiology. 2008;247(3): 871–9.

98. Sharma A, Moore WH, Lanuti M, Shepard JA. How I do it: radiofrequency ablation and cryoablation of lung tumors. J Thorac Imaging. 2011;26(2):162–74.
99. Dupuy DE, DiPetrillo T, Gandhi S, et al. Radiofrequency ablation followed by conventional radiotherapy for medically inoperable stage I non-small cell lung cancer. Chest. 2006;129(3):738–45.
100. Grieco CA, Simon CJ, Mayo-Smith WW, DiPetrillo TA, Ready NE, Dupuy DE. Percutaneous image-guided thermal ablation and radiation therapy: outcomes of combined treatment for 41 patients with inoperable stage I/II non-small-cell lung cancer. J Vasc Interv Radiol. 2006;17(7):1117–24.
101. Mukai T, Mimura H, Gobara H. Radiofrequency ablation followed by radiation therapy for large primary lung tumors. Acta Med Okayama. 2007;61(3):177–80.
102. Banovac F, Cheng P, Campos-Nanex E, et al. Radiofrequency ablation of lung tumors in swine assisted by a navigation device with preprocedural volumetric planning. J Vasc Interv Radiol. 2010;21(1):122–9.

Systemic Therapy for Lung Cancer

11

Keisuke Shirai, George R. Simon, and Carol A. Sherman

The benefit of systemic chemotherapy for lung cancer was recognized in the 1980s through multiple trials comparing chemotherapy to best supportive care [1]. The meta-analysis by the Non-small Cell Lung Cancer Cooperative Group demonstrated the benefit of cisplatin-based chemotherapy over best supportive care, with 1.5-month improvement in median overall survival and a 10 % improvement in 1-year survival [1]. Not only response rate and overall survival but also quality of life (QOL) was improved with chemotherapy compared to best supportive care. Based on these experiences, platinum-based doublet chemotherapy has been the standard of care for non-small cell lung cancer (NSCLC). Still, response rates with first-line chemotherapy are modest at 20–40 %, with a median survival time of 8–10 months [2]. Recently molecularly targeted agents have been introduced in the treatment of lung cancer with promising effects.

Currently cancer chemotherapy is administered in an outpatient setting for patients' convenience, QOL, and economical reasons. This is possible with the recent significant improvements in supportive care. Here we discuss the common chemotherapeutic agents employed and new molecularly targeted agents used in lung cancer care.

K. Shirai, M.D. (✉) • C.A. Sherman, M.D.
Division of Hematology/Oncology, Department of Medicine, Medical University of South Carolina, 86 Jonathan Lucas Street, Charleston, SC 29425, USA
e-mail: shirai@musc.edu

G.R. Simon, M.D.
Department of Thoracic/Head & Neck Medical Oncology, MD Anderson Cancer Center, 1400 Holcombe Blvd, Unit# 432, Houston, TX 77030, USA

Non-small Cell Lung Cancer

Advanced Disease

For stage IV and recurrent NSCLC, systemic chemotherapy is the mainstay of treatment. Doublet chemotherapy consisting of a platinum agent (cisplatin or carboplatin) combined with a newer agent is typically employed as first-line therapy. In general, doublet chemotherapy is more active than single-agent chemotherapy and should be offered if a patient's performance status permits [3]. Triplet chemotherapy has failed to improve overall survival over doublet chemotherapy despite increased response rates, and triplet regimens produce increased toxicity [3, 4]. The third-generation chemotherapeutic agents include the taxanes (paclitaxel, docetaxel), gemcitabine, vinorelbine, irinotecan, and pemetrexed, and the various agents have different toxicity profiles. Pemetrexed is indicated only in non-squamous cell lung cancer. These agents are commonly paired with a platinum compound (cisplatin or carboplatin). There is no significant difference in terms of survival benefit among four commonly used platinum-based doublets, paclitaxel + cisplatin, paclitaxel + carboplatin, docetaxel + cisplatin, or gemcitabine + cisplatin, according to the Eastern Cooperative Oncology

J.G. Ravenel (ed.), *Lung Cancer Imaging*, Contemporary Medical Imaging,
DOI 10.1007/978-1-60761-620-7_11, © Springer Science+Business Media New York 2013

Group (ECOG) 1594 study [5]. Other studies also support the comparability of various platinum doublets [6, 7]. One trial, TAX 326, showed docetaxel+cisplatin to be superior to vinorelbine+cisplatin or docetaxel+carboplatin; median survivals were 11.3, 9.9–10.1, and 9.4 months, respectively [8].

Non-platinum doublets have also been studied. Examples of non-platinum regimens are vinorelbine+gemcitabine, paclitaxel+gemcitabine, and docetaxel+gemcitabine. These are commonly used because of favorable toxicity profiles compared to platinum-based regimens, but the 1-year survival rate is more favorable with platinum-based doublets based on a recent meta-analysis [9]. Several recent meta-analyses revealed cisplatin-based regimens to be slightly more active than carboplatin-based regimens [10, 11]. Based on these findings, the current NCCN guidelines recommend using cisplatin instead of carboplatin if a patient's performance status is favorable and if comorbidities are not limiting. The treatment of advanced lung cancer yields only a modest survival benefit, so QOL aspects must be considered. Carboplatin requires less time to infuse than cisplatin since it does not require pre- and post-hydration. Additionally, it is less emetogenic, and it is associated with less renal toxicity, ototoxicity, and neurotoxicity than cisplatin, although it causes more myelosuppression. Therefore, the use of carboplatin may be justified from a QOL point of view. Pemetrexed is a new agent approved in 2004 for the second-line treatment of NSCLC. It showed non-inferiority to docetaxel with a more favorable toxicity profile [12]. Pemetrexed has more recently been studied in combination with platinum agents as another option for first-line treatment specific for non-squamous cell carcinoma [13]. In this study, the importance of histological differences among NSCLC types was observed. Cisplatin+pemetrexed showed a statistically significant OS improvement in non-squamous cell carcinoma patients (11.8 vs. 10.4 months, $p=0.005$), while cisplatin+gemcitabine demonstrated a not statistically significant but favorable trend, in OS with squamous cell carcinoma patients (10.8 vs. 9.4 months, $p=0.05$).

Despite the introduction of newer chemotherapeutic agents, the overall survival of lung cancer patients did not change substantially until recently when molecularly targeted agents were developed. The role of molecularly targeted agents such as bevacizumab, a humanized recombinant monoclonal antibody to vascular endothelial growth factor (VEGF); erlotinib, an oral epidermal growth factor receptor (EGFR) inhibitor; and crizotinib, an oral anaplastic lymphoma kinase (ALK) inhibitor, will be discussed separately.

Maintenance Therapy

How long to continue chemotherapy has been a matter of debate. The benefit of doublet chemotherapy is thought to be maximal at 4 cycles, and usually continuing beyond 4 cycles does not convey significant overall survival benefit but does increase toxicity [14, 15]. Recent studies using single-agent maintenance therapy suggest a benefit in progression-free survival and overall survival by continuing agents such as pemetrexed or erlotinib after 4–6 cycles of standard doublet treatment. The value of maintenance chemotherapy was proven initially by switching chemotherapy to pemetrexed after a standard doublet treatment [16]. In this phase III study, overall survival and progression-free survival were improved significantly by administering pemetrexed after 4 cycles of a platinum doublet compared to placebo. Initial regimens in this study did not contain pemetrexed, so this was called switch maintenance. Subset analysis proved the benefit of maintenance pemetrexed held true only in non-squamous cell carcinoma patients. A recent phase III study showed a similar benefit by continuing with pemetrexed after a pemetrexed-containing induction chemotherapy regimen (pemetrexed+cisplatin) in non-squamous cell carcinoma patients who achieved clinical benefit (complete response, partial response, or stable disease) with induction chemotherapy [17]. Another example of a maintenance strategy is switching to erlotinib after 4 cycles of platinum doublet compared to placebo group [18]. The most significant benefit was seen in patients who had EGFR mutations (HR 0.1). Although the benefit was much smaller, this trend held true even in other subgroups including patients with squamous cell carcinoma.

Bevacizumab, a recombinant humanized monoclonal antibody directed against the VEGF, is also used in maintenance setting in combination with carboplatin and paclitaxel (carboplatin + paclitaxel + bevacizumab followed by bevacizumab only vs. carboplatin + paclitaxel) and showed overall survival benefit (12.3 vs. 10.3 months, $p = 0.013$). Several studies are ongoing to answer the questions whether which agent to continue, bevacizumab and pemetrexed or bevacizumab only.

Salvage Therapy

The goals of second-line/salvage chemotherapy are to improve survival and also minimize or stabilize cancer-related symptoms with acceptable treatment side effects. For patients who have progressed after platinum-based chemotherapy, docetaxel was evaluated compared to best supportive care in TAX 317 [19]. Median overall survival showed a statistically significant improvement (7 vs. 4.6 months), as 1-year survival did (29 % vs. 19 %). Performance status was also better preserved in the docetaxel arm. Subsequently, pemetrexed was tested in a non-inferiority trial compared to docetaxel in the second-line/salvage setting. The overall survival between the two arms was not different, but the toxicity profile of pemetrexed arm was preferable, including less incidence of febrile neutropenia. The landmark trial BR 21, for previously treated advanced NSCLC patients, showed the benefit of erlotinib, an oral tyrosine kinase inhibitor of EGFR, over placebo in terms of overall survival (6.7 vs. 4.7 months) and 1-year survival (31.2 % vs. 21.5 %). A survival benefit was achieved even in male smokers with squamous cell histology (5.5 vs. 3.4 months). The common side effects seen with erlotinib are rash and diarrhea. At present, in the second line setting for EGFR wild type patients, no definitive conclusion has been drawn between erlotinib and chemotherapy. Other chemotherapeutic agents such as gemcitabine, vinorelbine, and irinotecan have also been used in the second-line setting.

Elderly Patients or Patients with Poor Performance Status

Elderly patients are often poorly represented in clinical trials, and in practice they tend to receive single-agent chemotherapy, such as vinorelbine or docetaxel. In the Elderly Lung Cancer Vinorelbine Italian Study (ELVIS) group trial, treatment with vinorelbine demonstrated an improved median survival time of 6.4 vs. 4.8 months in the best supportive care arm [20]. In ECOG 5592 with cisplatin doublets, a subset analysis by age (older than 70 years old vs. younger), there was no difference in terms of response rate (23 % vs. 22 %) or median survival time (8.5 vs. 9.1 months) [21]. All patients had an ECOG performance status of 0–1. This study suggests that for elderly patients with good performance status, standard doublets offer the same benefit as in younger patients. On the other hand, the Multicenter Italian Lung Cancer in the Elderly Study (MILES) did not show a benefit with combination chemotherapy over single agents. This study compared three arms: vinorelbine vs. gemcitabine vs. vinorelbine + gemcitabine [22]. In a subset analysis of ECOG 4599, the benefit of bevacizumab was not observed in the older cohort (older than 70 years old), and increased toxicity was noted [23]. For patients with less favorable performance status or those older than 80 years, single-agent vinorelbine, docetaxel, gemcitabine, or pemetrexed can be used. Erlotinib is also an option [24]. The optimal regimens for these individuals need to be further explored with clinical trials.

Locally Advanced Disease (Stage IIIA, Stage IIIB)

In locally advanced disease including stage IIIA and stage IIIB, cure is not achieved with chemotherapy or radiotherapy alone; combined modality treatment is the standard and yields 5-year survival rates on the order of 10–15 %. Adding chemotherapy sequentially to radiotherapy demonstrated improved overall survival compared to radiotherapy alone [25, 26]. Later, concurrent chemoradiotherapy was proven to be superior to sequential treatment in several studies [27–29]. Cisplatin and etoposide were used in an early SWOG study [29]. Other regimens such as carboplatin and paclitaxel, platinum + pemetrexed, and docetaxel have been used, but the optimal chemotherapy regimen to employ in combination with radiotherapy is not yet defined. The role of chemotherapy in combination with radiotherapy is not only to improve local control as a radiation sensitizer but also to eradicate microscopic disease and decrease the development of distant metastases. In general low-dose weekly chemotherapy trials showed less favorable benefit in terms of overall survival compared to full-dose regimens [30–33]. Therefore, standard full-dose chemotherapy combined with concurrent radiotherapy is recommended for stage IIIA/IIIB patients as long as performance status and comorbidities allow. The addition of surgery to chemoradiotherapy in stage IIIA patients continues to be explored in clinical trials.

Induction or Consolidation Therapy

Although there are several phase II studies which suggested a benefit for the addition of induction or consolidation [34] chemotherapy to concurrent chemoradiotherapy, recent phase III studies showed no benefit with induction or consolidation chemotherapy [35]. The potential benefit of induction or consolidation treatment needs to be further explored.

Early-Stage Lung Cancer

Surgery is the mainstay of treatment for patients with stage I or II disease. Patients found to have minimal IIIA disease at the time of surgery also benefit from resection. Multiple recent trials including the Adjuvant Navelbine International Trialist Association (ANITA) trial [36], the Big Lung Trial (BLT) [37], the International Adjuvant Lung Trial (IALT) [38], and the National Cancer Institute of Canada JBR.10 trial [39] have demonstrated a role for adjuvant chemotherapy in patients with resected stages II and IIIA disease with a prolongation in overall survival. The Adjuvant Lung Project Italy (ALPI) did not show a statistically significant benefit of adjuvant chemotherapy [40]. The Lung Adjuvant Cisplatin Evaluation (LACE) meta-analysis of the above four positive studies plus the negative ALPI trial showed a 5.3 % survival advantage at 5 years with the administration of chemotherapy [41]. For resected stage IB disease, the benefit of adjuvant chemotherapy is still unproven. In the Cancer and Leukemia Group B (CALGB) trial 9633, which was planned specifically for patients with resected stage IB disease, adjuvant chemotherapy consisted of carboplatin and paclitaxel for four cycles. An interim analysis in 2004 [42] showed a benefit in overall survival at 4 years, but an updated analysis in 2006 [43] showed that at 5 years this benefit disappeared. A subsequent unplanned subset analysis showed a benefit in resected stage IB patients with tumor size greater than 4 cm. Based on data provided by the above-noted adjuvant trials and the cisplatin vs. carboplatin (CISCA) meta-analysis [11] in advanced lung cancer, cisplatin-based doublet adjuvant chemotherapy should be offered to all patients with resected stage II or IIIA disease who can tolerate a cisplatin-based regimen. In practice, those patients who cannot tolerate cisplatin because of comorbidities are typically offered carboplatin-based doublet adjuvant chemotherapy.

Molecularly Targeted Agents

With the recent significant progress in molecular biology, several mechanisms of carcinogenesis have been elucidated, including both the activation of oncogenes and the inactivation of tumor suppressor genes. Several key oncogenic driver events have now been elucidated, and targeted agents have been developed against them. Currently, inhibitors against the EGFR pathway, the VEGF signaling pathways, and ALK rearrangements are in common clinical practice.

EGFR tyrosine kinase inhibitors inhibit the EGFR which belongs to a family of four related transmembrane receptors, namely, EGFR HER1,

EGFR HER2, EGFR HER3, and EGFR HER4. EGFR regulates important processes including proliferation, apoptosis, angiogenesis, and invasion. As EGFR is frequently expressed in NSCLC, it has been an important target for the development of new agents [44]. The landmark study BR 21 demonstrated a benefit in overall survival with erlotinib in the second-line setting, and this led to FDA approval of erlotinib in November 2004 [45]. In initial clinical trials of EGFR-TKIs, it was observed that female patients, nonsmokers, patients of Asian ethnicity, and patients with adenocarcinomas had a greater response rate. However, it has now been demonstrated that the EGFR-TKI sensitivity is associated with the presence of activating mutations in the tyrosine kinase domain of EGFR in the NSCLC tumor and not with these clinical characteristics per se [46–48]. However, these mutations occur with higher frequency in women, nonsmokers, adenocarcinoma patients, and patients of Asian ethnicity, thus explaining the higher response rates to treatment with EGFR-TKIs in these patient groups [49]. Importantly, the constitutive EGFR activation caused by these mutations causes oncogene addiction to the EGFR pathway. The presence of the activating mutation in exons 19 and 21 of the EGFR results in an activation of the AKT and STAT pathways without having an effect on ERK/MAP signaling. It has been suggested that EGFR-TKIs affect wild-type and mutant cells differently. Gefitinib triggers apoptosis in tumors harboring EGFR exon 19 or 21 mutations that results in complete or partial response. On the other hand, it induces G1 arrest in EGFR wild-type cells that leads to stable disease. Several mechanisms of acquired resistance have been reported [50, 51].

More recently, several trials have examined the potential role of EGFR-TKIs in the first-line treatment of patients with tumors with activating mutations on the EGFR [52, 53]. These trials showed that the presence of EGFR mutation is a strong predictive marker for improved responses and progression-free survival with EGFR-TKI vs. chemotherapy.

EGFR mutations significantly predict for an increased response both to EGFR-TKI therapy and to chemotherapy in patients with advanced lung adenocarcinoma, thereby making the presence of EGFR mutations a powerful prognostic and predictive marker in NSCLC. Mok et al. randomized previously untreated patients with advanced-stage NSCLC with a high likelihood of carrying EGFR mutations (adenocarcinoma, never or light smokers) to receive gefitinib or cytotoxic chemotherapy [54]. The 12-month rates of progression-free survival were 24.9 % with gefitinib and 6.7 % with carboplatin and paclitaxel. Patients with EGFR mutations treated with gefitinib had superior PFS ($p<0.001$), whereas PFS was superior in patients negative for the mutation who received carboplatin–paclitaxel ($p<0.001$). No significant differences in OS were noted which could be attributed to the crossover treatments offered to patients after their initial treatment. EGFR mutation status was a strong predictive biomarker for improved PFS and overall response rate with gefitinib vs. carboplatin–paclitaxel demonstrating that a molecular-defined population would benefit most from first-line gefitinib. Interestingly this trial, also known as the IPASS trial, demonstrated that the presence of an EGFR mutation is associated with a higher response rate to chemotherapy as well (when compared to EGFR wild-type patients) and is therefore a favorable prognostic factor regardless of treatment. The common side effects associated with these agents are rash and diarrhea. Toxicity is usually mild and controllable with adjunctive therapy or dose adjustment. Interstitial pneumonitis is a rare but sometimes fatal toxicity. An EGFR antibody, cetuximab, which is approved for use in head and neck and colon cancer, is also under investigation in combination with platinum-based doublets in lung cancer.

Angiogenesis, the growth of new blood vessels, is a targeted mechanism of interest for several types of solid tumors, including lung cancer. VEGF is an important signaling protein involved in both vasculogenesis (the de novo formation of the embryonic circulatory system) and angiogenesis (the growth of blood vessels from preexisting vasculature). VEGF also enhances microvascular permeability. The FDA has approved bevacizumab, a humanized recombinant monoclonal antibody to VEGF, for the treatment of metastatic colon and lung cancer. In a randomized phase II trial, bevacizumab in combination with carboplatin and paclitaxel improved overall response rate and time to progression, but major hemoptysis was observed in patients with squamous cell histology, tumor necrosis and cavitation, and disease location close to major blood vessels [55]. Because of these cases of severe and sometimes fatal hemoptysis in patients with squamous cell carcinoma and a general increased risk of bleeding, patients with squamous cell carcinoma, patients with brain metastases, and patients who were on active anticoagulation were excluded from the ECOG 4599 study that led to FDA approval of this agent in October 2006. This study demonstrated an improvement in median overall survival with bevacizumab, carboplatin, and paclitaxel compared to carboplatin and paclitaxel alone (12.3 vs. 10.3 months) in patients with metastatic lung cancer [56]. However, a trial conducted in Europe, often known as the AVAiL trial, compared the addition of bevacizumab to cisplatin and gemcitabine to cisplatin and gemcitabine alone. This trial confirmed the progression-free survival benefit of bevacizumab when combined with cisplatin plus gemcitabine (HR 0.75). However, the progression-free survival benefit did not translate into a significant overall survival benefit [57]. Bevacizumab has a unique side effect profile including hypertension, proteinuria, bleeding, delayed wound healing, and increase in thromboembolic events. Administering bevacizumab only to patients with non-squamous histology can abrogate the bleeding effects, and it is currently approved only for patients with non-squamous histology.

A number of specific genetic lesions (i.e., KRAS, ALK, BRAF, MET, PGDFR, PIK3CA, HER2) driving tumor proliferation have been identified in primary lung adenocarcinomas. Inhibition of these oncogenic drivers in NSCLC patients harboring these mutated pathways is a matter of active and ongoing investigation. More recently the inhibition of ALK in patients with NSCLC has led to the FDA approval of crizotinib in patients that harbor ALK translocations. ALK is an oncogene that induces cell transformation in vitro and in vivo. Translocation of ALK usually with echinoderm microtubule-associated protein-like 4 (EML4), in NSCLC, results in an abnormal fusion gene. The translocation produces an ongoing activation of an intercellular tyrosine kinase, which then leads to proliferation and cancer propagation [58]. In NSCLC carrying this translocation, this is the sole driver of the malignancy [59]. Treatment of patients with ALK rearrangements with crizotinib, an inhibitor of the ALK tyrosine kinase, results in response rates in the vicinity of 60 % and estimated probability of 6-month progression-free survival of 72 % [60]. *ALK* rearrangements and *EGFR* mutations seem to be usually mutually exclusive while mainly occurring in patients with the same clinical characteristics, namely, younger patients, never or light smokers, and patients with adenocarcinoma. Interestingly, the group of patients with *ALK* rearrangements tends to have a slightly higher proportion of males compared with those who have EGFR mutations. Importantly, patients with *ALK* rearrangements do not respond to EGFR-TKI treatment [61].

Molecularly targeted agents have already changed the landscape of NSCLC therapeutics, and their optimal use, in terms of timing, sequence, and selection of patients most likely to benefit from them, remains the subject of ongoing trials. Several newer agents targeting novel oncogenic drivers are also a subject of active investigation.

Small Cell Lung Cancer

The mainstay of treatment for small cell lung cancer patients is systemic chemotherapy, because of the early development of hematogenous metastases and a rapid growth rate in this tumor type. Before the introduction of chemotherapy, the median survival of small cell lung cancer patients was dismal: 12 weeks for limited-stage disease and 5 weeks for extensive-stage disease [62]. Small cell lung cancer tends to respond rapidly and dramatically to chemotherapy, so treatment is typically offered even to patients with poor performance status who may rapidly improve with response to therapy. Compared to NSCLC, available agents for small cell lung cancer are limited. The most commonly used regimen is a combination of cisplatin (or carboplatin) and etoposide based on a phase III trial [63].

Limited-Stage Disease

Small cell lung cancer was initially divided into two categories, limited-stage disease and extensive-stage disease, according to the Veterans Administration Lung Cancer Study Group (VALCSG) staging system. They are based on the feasibility of administering radiotherapy. If disease is confined to one hemithorax and a radiation treatment field can be set up in a single port, then the disease is classified as limited stage. For limited-stage small cell lung cancer, the benefit of combining chemotherapy and radiation therapy has been proven [64]. The median survival of patients with limited-stage small cell lung cancer treated with chemotherapy and radiation is 20–28 months.

The preferred timing of the addition of radiation treatment to chemotherapy remains to be elucidated although earlier treatment is thought to be better. Although small cell lung cancer is aggressive, limited-stage disease should be treated with curative intent with concurrent chemoradiotherapy. A prompt referral to radiation oncology is key, to allow treatment planning while chemotherapy is initiated. As mentioned above cisplatin and etoposide are the most commonly used regimens. It can be administered at full dose with concurrent radiotherapy.

Extensive-Stage Disease

Despite high response rates and improved survival with chemotherapy, extensive-stage disease patients are not considered curable. The median survival of extensive-stage disease patients improves to 9–13 months with systemic chemotherapy. Cisplatin or carboplatin and etoposide are commonly used regimens. The difference, a slightly better response rate with cisplatin over carboplatin seen in limited-stage disease, is not seen in extensive-stage disease. Alternative regimens that have been used include cisplatin or carboplatin with irinotecan. There are at least two phase III studies, one from Japan and one from Europe, demonstrating the superiority of platinum and irinotecan over platinum and etoposide [65, 66]. This benefit, however, has not been confirmed in studies in the United States [67, 68]. Bevacizumab combined with cisplatin and etoposide demonstrated an overall response rate of 69 % in ECOG 3501, a phase II trial [69, 70]. To determine whether the addition of bevacizumab to chemotherapy would be superior to chemotherapy alone would require a randomized phase III trial.

Prophylactic Cranial Irradiation

Either limited- or extensive-stage disease patients who achieve a response to chemotherapy should be offered prophylactic cranial irradiation (PCI) which reduces the rate of brain metastasis and improves overall survival [71, 72].

Salvage Therapy

Topotecan, irinotecan, paclitaxel, docetaxel, gemcitabine, and vinorelbine are active agents which have been tested in phase II trials [73]. For chemotherapy-sensitive disease in which a patient achieves a response and does not have disease progression for at least 3 months after stopping treatment, topotecan is the drug of choice. Topotecan is FDA approved for this indication. In a phase II trial, amrubicin, a synthetic anthracycline derivative, showed promising results as a second-line single agent, but in an international phase III trial, OS benefit was not confirmed despite improvement in response, progression-free survival, and symptom control [74, 75]. Several molecularly targeted agents including gefitinib, imatinib, and thalidomide have been tested in small cell lung cancer, but none of these have proven to be effective.

Future Directions

Many clinically relevant questions have yet to be answered such as how best to combine chemotherapy with surgery and radiation therapy, how to select patients who are most likely to benefit from a given regimen, and how to minimize toxicity and cost. It is important to find a means to select the most appropriate candidates for each treatment and to find the best sequence of combined modality therapy to maximize the benefit achieved.

Despite intense efforts, we do not yet have a reliable way to predict response to chemotherapeutic agents. Some promising studies have been published, including one which demonstrated the utility of using excision repair cross-complementation group 1 (ERCC1) to predict the response to cisplatin [76]. DNA microarray technique is also promising as a means to find subsets of patients who will respond to certain agents. A specific gene signature may be useful to predict response to therapeutic agents. The acquisition of a fuller understanding of how and when to use these therapeutic agents holds great potential to help us further decrease morbidity and mortality from lung cancer. Although much remains to be elucidated, promising early phase data in preclinical and clinical settings suggest the possibility that ongoing and future investigations will translate into a major positive improvement in survival for patients with this disease.

References

1. Chemotherapy in non-small cell lung cancer: a meta-analysis using updated data on individual patients from 52 randomised clinical trials. Non-small Cell Lung Cancer Collaborative Group. BMJ. 1995; 311(7010):899–909.
2. Pfister DG, Johnson DH, Azzoli CG, et al. American Society of Clinical Oncology treatment of unresectable non-small-cell lung cancer guideline: update 2003. J Clin Oncol. 2004;22(2):330–53.
3. Socinski MA, Crowell R, Hensing TE, et al. Treatment of non-small cell lung cancer, stage IV: ACCP evidence-based clinical practice guidelines (2nd edition). Chest. 2007;132(3 Suppl):277S–89S.
4. Delbaldo C, Michiels S, Syz N, Soria JC, Le Chevalier T, Pignon JP. Benefits of adding a drug to a single-agent or a 2-agent chemotherapy regimen in advanced non-small-cell lung cancer: a meta-analysis. JAMA. 2004;292(4):470–84.
5. Schiller JH, Harrington D, Belani CP. Comparison of four chemotherapy regimens for advanced non-small-cell lung cancer. N Engl J Med. 2002;346(2):92–8.
6. Scagliotti GV, De Marinis F, Rinaldi M, et al. Phase III randomized trial comparing three platinum-based doublets in advanced non-small-cell lung cancer. J Clin Oncol. 2002;20(21):4285–91.
7. Kelly K, Crowley J, Bunn Jr PA. Randomized phase III trial of paclitaxel plus carboplatin versus vinorelbine plus cisplatin in the treatment of patients with advanced non-small-cell lung cancer: a Southwest Oncology Group trial. J Clin Oncol. 2001;19(13):3210–8.
8. Fossella F, Pereira JR, von Pawel J, et al. Randomized, multinational, phase III study of docetaxel plus platinum combinations versus vinorelbine plus cisplatin for advanced non-small-cell lung cancer: the TAX 326 study group. J Clin Oncol. 2003;21(16):3016–24.
9. D'Addario G, Pintilie M, Leighl NB, Feld R, Cerny T, Shepherd FA. Platinum-based versus non-platinum-based chemotherapy in advanced non-small-cell lung cancer: a meta-analysis of the published literature. J Clin Oncol. 2005;23(13):2926–36.
10. Hotta K, Matsuo K, Ueoka H, Kiura K, Tabata M, Tanimoto M. Meta-analysis of randomized clinical trials comparing Cisplatin to Carboplatin in patients with advanced non-small-cell lung cancer. J Clin Oncol. 2004;22(19):3852–9.
11. Ardizzoni A, Boni L, Tiseo M, et al. Cisplatin- versus carboplatin-based chemotherapy in first-line treatment of advanced non-small-cell lung cancer: an individual patient data meta-analysis. J Natl Cancer Inst. 2007;99(11):847–57.
12. Hanna N, Shepherd FA, Fossella FV, et al. Randomized phase III trial of pemetrexed versus docetaxel in patients with non-small-cell lung cancer previously treated with chemotherapy. J Clin Oncol. 2004;22(9): 1589–97.
13. Scagliotti GV, Parikh P, von Pawel J, Biesma B, Vansteenkiste J, Manegold C, Serwatowski P, Gatzemeier U, Digumarti R, Zukin M, Lee JS, Mellemgaard A, Park K, Patil S, Rolski J, Goksel T, de Marinis F, Simms L, Sugarman KP, Gandara D. Phase III study comparing cisplatin plus gemcitabine with cisplatin plus pemetrexed in chemotherapy-naive patients with advanced-stage non-small-cell lung cancer. J Clin Oncol. 2008 Jul 20;26(21):3543–51. doi: 10.1200/JCO.2007.15.0375. Epub 2008 May 27. PubMed PMID: 18506025.
14. Socinski MA, Schell MJ, Peterman A, et al. Phase III trial comparing a defined duration of therapy versus continuous therapy followed by second-line therapy in advanced-stage IIIB/IV non-small-cell lung cancer. J Clin Oncol. 2002;20(5):1335–43.

15. Socinski MA, Stinchcombe TE. Duration of first-line chemotherapy in advanced non small-cell lung cancer: less is more in the era of effective subsequent therapies. J Clin Oncol. 2007;25(33):5155–7.
16. Ciuleanu T, Brodowicz T, Zielinski C, et al. Maintenance pemetrexed plus best supportive care versus placebo plus best supportive care for non-small-cell lung cancer: a randomised, double-blind, phase 3 study. Lancet. 2009;374(9699):1432–40.
17. Paz-Ares L, de Marinis F, Dediu M, et al. Maintenance therapy with pemetrexed plus best supportive care versus placebo plus best supportive care after induction therapy with pemetrexed plus cisplatin for advanced non-squamous non-small-cell lung cancer (PARAMOUNT): a double-blind, phase 3, randomised controlled trial. Lancet Oncol. 2012;13(3): 247–55.
18. Cappuzzo F, Ciuleanu T, Stelmakh L, et al. Erlotinib as maintenance treatment in advanced non-small-cell lung cancer: a multicentre, randomised, placebo-controlled phase 3 study. Lancet Oncol. 2010;11(6): 521–9.
19. Shepherd FA, Dancey J, Ramlau R, et al. Prospective randomized trial of docetaxel versus best supportive care in patients with non-small-cell lung cancer previously treated with platinum-based chemotherapy. J Clin Oncol. 2000;18(10):2095–103.
20. Effects of vinorelbine on quality of life and survival of elderly patients with advanced non-small-cell lung cancer. The Elderly Lung Cancer Vinorelbine Italian Study Group. J Natl Cancer Inst. 1999;91(1):66–72.
21. Langer CJ, Manola J, Bernardo P, et al. Cisplatin-based therapy for elderly patients with advanced non-small-cell lung cancer: implications of Eastern Cooperative Oncology Group 5592, a randomized trial. J Natl Cancer Inst. 2002;94(3):173–81.
22. Gridelli C, Perrone F, Gallo C, et al. Chemotherapy for elderly patients with advanced non-small-cell lung cancer: the Multicenter Italian Lung Cancer in the Elderly Study (MILES) phase III randomized trial. J Natl Cancer Inst. 2003;95(5):362–72.
23. Ramalingam SS, Dahlberg SE, Langer CJ. Outcomes for elderly advanced stage non-small cell lung cancer (NSCLC) patients (pts) treated with bevacizumab (B) in combination with carboplatin (C) and paclitaxel (P): analysis of Eastern Cooperative Oncology Group (ECOG) 4599 study. J Clin Oncol. 2008;26(1):60–5.
24. Jackman DM, Lucca J, Fidias P, et al. Phase II study of the EGFR tyrosine kinase erlotinib in patients > 70 years of age with previously untreated advanced non-small cell lung carcinoma. J Clin Oncol. 2005; 23(16S):7148.
25. Dillman RO, Herndon J, Seagren SL, Eaton Jr WL, Green MR. Improved survival in stage III non-small-cell lung cancer: seven-year follow-up of cancer and leukemia group B (CALGB) 8433 trial. J Natl Cancer Inst. 1996;88(17):1210–5.
26. Sause WT, Scott C, Taylor S, et al. Radiation Therapy Oncology Group (RTOG) 88-08 and Eastern Cooperative Oncology Group (ECOG) 4588: preliminary results of a phase III trial in regionally advanced, unresectable non-small-cell lung cancer. J Natl Cancer Inst. 1995;87(3):198–205.
27. Furuse K, Fukuoka M, Kawahara M, et al. Phase III study of concurrent versus sequential thoracic radiotherapy in combination with mitomycin, vindesine, and cisplatin in unresectable stage III non-small-cell lung cancer. J Clin Oncol. 1999;17(9):2692–9.
28. Curran WJ Jr, Paulus R, Langer CJ, Komaki R, Lee JS, Hauser S, Movsas B, Wasserman T, Rosenthal SA, Gore E, Machtay M, Sause W, Cox JD. Sequential vs. concurrent chemoradiation for stage III non-small cell lung cancer: randomized phase III trial RTOG 9410. J Natl Cancer Inst. 2011 Oct 5;103(19):1452–60. doi:10.1093/jnci/djr325. Epub 2011 Sep 8. Erratum in: J Natl Cancer Inst. 2012 Jan 4;104(1):79. PubMed PMID: 21903745; PubMed Central PMCID: PMC3186782.
29. Albain KS, Crowley JJ, Turrisi 3rd AT, et al. Concurrent cisplatin, etoposide, and chest radiotherapy in pathologic stage IIIB non-small-cell lung cancer: a Southwest Oncology Group phase II study, SWOG 9019. J Clin Oncol. 2002;20(16):3454–60.
30. Clamon G, Herndon J, Cooper R, Chang AY, Rosenman J, Green MR. Radiosensitization with carboplatin for patients with unresectable stage III non-small-cell lung cancer: a phase III trial of the Cancer and Leukemia Group B and the Eastern Cooperative Oncology Group. J Clin Oncol. 1999;17(1):4–11.
31. Huber RM, Flentie M, Schmidt M, et al. Simultaneous chemoradiotherapy compared with radiotherapy alone after induction chemotherapy in inoperable stage IIIA or IIIB non-small-cell lung cancer: study CTRT99/97 by the Bronchial Carcinoma Therapy Group. J Clin Oncol. 2006;24(27):4397–404.
32. Vokes EE et al. Induction chemotherapy followed by chemoradiotherapy compared with chemoradiotherapy alone for regionally advanced unresectable stage III non-small-cell lung cancer: Cancer and Leukemia Group B. J Clin Oncol. 2007;25(13):1698–704.
33. Wang L, Wu S, Ou G, et al. Randomized phase II study of concurrent cisplatin/etoposide or paclitaxel/carboplatin and thoracic radiotherapy in patients with stage III non-small cell lung cancer. Lung Cancer. 2012;77(1):89–96.
34. Gandara DR, Chansky K, Albain KS, et al. Long-term survival with concurrent chemoradiation therapy followed by consolidation docetaxel in stage IIIB non-small-cell lung cancer: a phase II Southwest Oncology Group Study (S9504). Clin Lung Cancer. 2006;8(2): 116–21.
35. Hanna NH, Neubauer M, Ansari R, et al. Phase III trial of cisplatin (P) plus etoposide (E) plus concurrent chest radiation (XRT) with or without consolidation docetaxel (D) in patients (pts) with inoperable stage III non-small cell lung cancer (NSCLC): HOG LUN 01-24/USO-023. Proc Am Soc Clin Oncol. 2007; 25:387s (abstr 7512).

36. Douillard JY, Rosell R, De Lena M, et al. Adjuvant vinorelbine plus cisplatin versus observation in patients with completely resected stage IB–IIIA non-small cell lung cancer (Adjuvant Navelbine International Trialist Association [ANITA]): a randomised controlled trial. Lancet Oncol. 2006;7(9):719–27.
37. Waller D, Peake MD, Stephens RJ, et al. Chemotherapy for patients with non-small cell lung cancer: the surgical setting of the Big Lung Trial. Eur J Cardiothorac Surg. 2004;26(1):173–82.
38. Arriagada R, Bergman B, Dunant A, et al. Cisplatin-based adjuvant chemotherapy in patients with completely resected non-small-cell lung cancer. N Engl J Med. 2004;350(4):351–60.
39. Winton T, Livingston R, Johnson D, et al. Vinorelbine plus cisplatin vs. observation in resected non-small-cell lung cancer. N Engl J Med. 2005;352(25):2589–97.
40. Scagliotti GV, Fossati R, Torri V, et al. Randomized study of adjuvant chemotherapy for completely resected stage I, II, or IIIA non-small-cell lung cancer. J Natl Cancer Inst. 2003;95(19):1453–61.
41. Pignon JP, Tribodet H, Scagliotti GV, et al. Lung adjuvant cisplatin evaluation (LACE): a pooled analysis of five randomized clinical trials including 4,584 patients. J Clin Oncol. 2006;24(18S):7008.
42. Strauss GM, Herndon J, Maddaus MA, et al. Randomized clinical trial of adjuvant chemotherapy with paclitaxel and carboplatin following resection in stage IB non-small cell lung cancer (NSCLC): report of Cancer and Leukemia Group B (CALGB) Protocol 9633. J Clin Oncol. 2004;22(14S):7019.
43. Strauss GM, Herndon J, Maddaus MA, et al. Adjuvant chemotherapy in stage IB non-small cell lung cancer (NSCLC): update of Cancer and Leukemia Group B (CALGB) Protocol 9633. J Clin Oncol. 2006; 24(18S):7007.
44. Rusch V, Klimstra D, Venkatraman E, Pisters PW, Langenfeld J, Dmitrovsky E. Overexpression of the epidermal growth factor receptor and its ligand transforming growth factor alpha is frequent in resectable non-small cell lung cancer but does not predict tumor progression. Clin Cancer Res. 1997;3(4):515–22.
45. Shepherd FA, Rodriques Pereira J, Ciuleanu T, et al. Erlotinib in previously treated non-small-cell lung cancer. N Engl J Med. 2005;353(2):123–32.
46. Rosell R, Moran T, Queralt C, et al. Screening for epidermal growth factor receptor mutations in lung cancer. N Engl J Med. 2009;361(10):958–67.
47. Lynch TJ, Bell DW, Sordella R, et al. Activating mutations in the epidermal growth factor receptor underlying responsiveness of non-small-cell lung cancer to gefitinib. N Engl J Med. 2004; 350(21):2129–39.
48. Paez JG, Jänne PA, Lee JC, et al. EGFR mutations in lung cancer: correlation with clinical response to gefitinib therapy. Science. 2004;304(5676):1497–500.
49. Pao W, Miller V, Zakowski M, et al. EGF receptor gene mutations are common in lung cancers from "never smokers" and are associated with sensitivity of tumors to gefitinib and erlotinib. Proc Natl Acad Sci U S A. 2004;101(36):13306–11.
50. Pao W, Miller VA, Politi KA, et al. Acquired resistance of lung adenocarcinomas to gefitinib or erlotinib is associated with a second mutation in the EGFR kinase domain. PLoS Med. 2005;2(3):e73.
51. Engelman JA, Zejnullahu K, Mitsudomi T, et al. MET amplification leads to gefitinib resistance in lung cancer by activating ERBB3 signaling. Science. 2007; 316(5827):1039–43.
52. Mitsudomi T, Morita S, Yatabe Y, et al. Gefitinib versus cisplatin plus docetaxel in patients with non-small-cell lung cancer harbouring mutations of the epidermal growth factor receptor (WJTOG3405): an open label, randomised phase 3 trial. Lancet Oncol. 2010;11(2):121–8.
53. Maemondo M, Inoue A, Kobayashi K, et al. Gefitinib or chemotherapy for non-small-cell lung cancer with mutated EGFR. N Engl J Med. 2010;362(25): 2380–8.
54. Mok TS, Wu YL, Thongprasert S, et al. Gefitinib or carboplatin-paclitaxel in pulmonary adenocarcinoma. N Engl J Med. 2009;361(10):947–57.
55. Johnson DH, Fehrenbacher L, Novotny WF, et al. Randomized phase II trial comparing bevacizumab plus carboplatin and paclitaxel with carboplatin and paclitaxel alone in previously untreated locally advanced or metastatic non-small-cell lung cancer. J Clin Oncol. 2004;22(11):2184–91.
56. Sandler A, Gray R, Perry MC, et al. Paclitaxel-carboplatin alone or with bevacizumab for non-small-cell lung cancer. N Engl J Med. 2006;355(24): 2542–50.
57. Reck M, von Pawel J, Zatloukal P, et al. Overall survival with cisplatin-gemcitabine and bevacizumab or placebo as first-line therapy for nonsquamous non-small-cell lung cancer: results from a randomised phase III trial (AVAiL). Ann Oncol. 2010;21(9): 1804–9.
58. Horn L, Pao W. EML4-ALK: honing in on a new target in non-small-cell lung cancer. J Clin Oncol. 2009;27(26):4232–5.
59. Soda M, Choi YL, Enomoto M, et al. Identification of the transforming EML4-ALK fusion gene in non-small-cell lung cancer. Nature. 2007;448(7153): 561–6.
60. Kwak EL, Bang YJ, Camidge DR, et al. Anaplastic lymphoma kinase inhibition in non-small-cell lung cancer. N Engl J Med. 2010;363(18):1693–703.
61. Shaw AT, Yeap BY, Mino-Kenudson M, et al. Clinical features and outcome of patients with non-small-cell lung cancer who harbor EML4-ALK. J Clin Oncol. 2009;27(26):4247–53.
62. Hyde L, Wolf J, McCracken S, Yesner R. Natural course of inoperable lung cancer. Chest. 1973;64(3): 309–12.
63. Roth BJ, Johnson DH, Einhorn LH, et al. Randomized study of cyclophosphamide, doxorubicin, and vincristine versus etoposide and cisplatin versus alternation of these two regimens in extensive small-cell lung

cancer: a phase III trial of the Southeastern Cancer Study Group. J Clin Oncol. 1992;10(2):282–91.
64. Turrisi AT, Sherman CA. The treatment of limited small cell lung cancer: a report of the progress made and future prospects. Eur J Cancer. 2002;38(2): 279–91.
65. Noda K, Nishiwaki Y, Kawahara M, et al. Irinotecan plus cisplatin compared with etoposide plus cisplatin for extensive small-cell lung cancer. N Engl J Med. 2002;346(2):85–91.
66. Hermes A, Bergman B, Bremnes R, et al. A randomized phase III trial of irinotecan plus carboplatin versus etoposide plus carboplatin in patients with small cell lung cancer, extensive disease (SCLC-ED): IRIS-Study. J Clin Oncol. 2007;25(18S):7010.
67. Hanna N, Bunn Jr PA, Langer C, et al. Randomized phase III trial comparing irinotecan/cisplatin with etoposide/cisplatin in patients with previously untreated extensive-stage disease small-cell lung cancer. J Clin Oncol. 2006;24(13):2038–43.
68. Natale RB, Lara PN, Chansky K, et al. S0124: a randomized phase III trial comparing irinotecan/cisplatin (IP) with etoposide/cisplatin (EP) in patients (pts) with previously untreated extensive stage small cell lung cancer (E-SCLC). J Clin Oncol. 2008; 26:7512.
69. Sandler A, Szwaric S, Dowlati A, Moore DF, Schiller JH. A phase II study of cisplatin (P) plus etoposide (E) plus bevacizumab (B) for previously untreated extensive stage small cell lung cancer (SCLC) (E3501): a trial of the Eastern Cooperative Oncology Group. J Clin Oncol. 2007;25(18S):7564.
70. Sandler A. Bevacizumab in non small cell lung cancer. Clin Cancer Res. 2007;13(15 Pt 2):s4613–6.
71. Aupérin A, Arriagada R, Pignon JP, et al. Prophylactic cranial irradiation for patients with small-cell lung cancer in complete remission. Prophylactic Cranial Irradiation Overview Collaborative Group. N Engl J Med. 1999;341(7):476–84.
72. Slotman B, Faivre-Finn C, Kramer G, et al. Prophylactic cranial irradiation in extensive small-cell lung cancer. N Engl J Med. 2007;357(7):664–72.
73. Kelly K. New chemotherapy agents for small cell lung cancer. Chest. 2000;117(4 Suppl 1):156S–62S.
74. Onoda S, Masuda N, Seto T, et al. Phase II trial of amrubicin for treatment of refractory or relapsed small-cell lung cancer: Thoracic Oncology Research Group Study 0301. J Clin Oncol. 2006;24(34): 5448–53.
75. Jotte R, Von Pawel J, Spigel DR. Randomized phase III trial of amrubicin versus topotecan (Topo) as second-line treatment for small cell lung cancer (SCLC). Journal of Clinical Oncology, 2011 ASCO Annual Meeting Proceedings (Post-Meeting Edition). Vol 29, No 15_suppl (May 20 Supplement), 2011: 7000.
76. Grenader T, Shavit L. DNA repair by ERCC1 in non-small-cell lung cancer. N Engl J Med. 2006; 355(24):2591; author reply 2591.

Radiotherapy in Lung Cancer

12

S. Lewis Cooper and Anand Sharma

External beam radiation therapy (EBRT) is an important component in the management of lung cancer. Radiotherapy would be required at some point in the treatment of small cell lung cancer (SCLC) and non-small cell lung cancer (NSCLC) in 50–60 % of patients [1]. Technical advances made in radiation planning and delivery such as 3D conformal radiotherapy (3DCRT), intensity modulated radiotherapy (IMRT), image-guided radiotherapy (IGRT), and stereotactic body radiotherapy (SBRT) have transformed the role of RT in the management of lung cancer, particularly in the last decade. RT is used as definitive therapy in medically inoperable NSCLC (3DCRT, SBRT), as multimodality therapy in locally advanced (stage III) NSCLC and limited stage SCLC, neoadjuvant and adjuvant in stage IIIA NSCLC, palliative treatment of metastasis in stage IV lung cancer, and for prophylactic cranial irradiation (PCI) in both SCLC and NSCLC [2]. Modern techniques of accurate target delineation and normal tissue avoidance have significantly improved chances of locoregional control of disease as well as reduced normal tissue toxicity.

Definitive Radiotherapy in Medically Inoperable NSCLC

In patients with early stage (I and II) NSCLC who are technically resectable at presentation, lobectomy or pneumonectomy and pathologic mediastinal nodal staging offer the best overall survival. Based on data from the Surveillance, Epidemiology, and End Results (SEER) program of the National Cancer Institute, 30 % of patients with localized NSCLC did not undergo surgical treatment. High rate of comorbid medical illness, poor baseline pulmonary function, advanced age, poor performance status, and patient decision are the most common reasons among this patient population [3]. These patients are treated with definitive RT and more recently, selected patients are treated with SBRT. Five-year survival rates in surgically treated stage IA, IB, and II NSCLC reach 80 %, 50 %, and 35 %, respectively. Five-year survival with conventional RT in this group ranges from 10 to 42 %. Local recurrence and distant failure dominate the causes of failure [4]. Isolated nodal failures are uncommon.

RT dose escalation has been evaluated by several investigators. The University of Michigan lung cancer dose escalation study in stage I NSCLC patients concluded that doses of radiation of 92.4 and 102.9 Gy can be delivered safely to limited lung volumes with minimal toxicity and 2- and 3-year freedom from local progression, overall survival and cause-specific survival rates of 82 % and 68 %, 54 % and 33 %, and 76

S.L. Cooper, M.D. • A. Sharma, M.D. (✉)
Department of Radiation Oncology, Medical University of South Carolina, 169 Ashley Avenue, Charleston, SC 26425, USA
e-mail: sharmaak@musc.edu

J.G. Ravenel (ed.), *Lung Cancer Imaging*, Contemporary Medical Imaging,
DOI 10.1007/978-1-60761-620-7_12, © Springer Science+Business Media New York 2013

% and 48 %, respectively [5]. Urbanic et al. reported 37 % local failure rate for medically inoperable lung cancer patients treated with 3DCRT to 80.5 Gy in 7 weeks [6]. RTOG conducted a phase I–II dose escalation study using three-dimensional conformal radiotherapy in patients with inoperable non-small cell lung carcinoma. For patients receiving RT alone or radiation following induction chemotherapy, data from RTOG 9311 established that doses of 83.8 Gy using three-dimensional conformal RT techniques were tolerable, with excess mortality observed at 90.3 Gy. Elective nodal failure occurred in less than 10 % of patients [7].

Stereotactic Body Radiotherapy

Recent developments in IGRT are ushering in a new era of radiotherapy for lung cancer. Positron emission tomography-computed tomography (PET-CT) has been shown to improve targeting accuracy in 25–50 % of cases. Daily on-board imaging reduces treatment setup uncertainty and provides information about daily organ motion and variations in anatomy. Image-guided stereotactic radiotherapy can achieve local control rates exceeding 90 % through the use of focused, hypofractionated, highly biologically effective doses (Figs. 12.1 and 12.2) [8]. Four-dimensional CT scans and abdominal compression are frequently used to account for lung motion and reduce superior to inferior tumor excursion which is critical in treating tight radiation fields adequately [9].

Timmerman et al. published results of a phase I study in medically inoperable stage I NSCLC treated with extracranial stereotactic radioablation. Patients with comorbid medical problems that precluded thoracotomy and with clinically staged T1 or T2 (tumor size 7 cm or less) N0M0 biopsy confirmed NSCLC were included. Patients with T1 vs. T2 tumors underwent independent dose escalations. Both T-stage groups ultimately reached and tolerated 20 Gy per fraction for 3 fractions (total: 60 Gy) [10]. Treatments were completed in 12 days. A phase II study by the same group included 70 T1 and T2 medically inoperable NSCLC patients [11]. Kaplan–Meier local control at 2 years was 95 %. Median overall survival was 32.6 months and 2-year overall survival was 54.7 %. Grade 3–5 toxicity occurred in a total of 14 patients. Patients treated for tumors in the peripheral lung had 2-year freedom from severe toxicity of 83 % compared with only 54 % for patients with central tumors. An important observation from this study was that SBRT of centrally located lesions is associated with increased risk of toxicity and that appropriate patient selection is very important (Fig. 12.3).

Onishi and colleagues published results from the Japanese multi-institutional study of hypofractionated stereotactic radiotherapy (HypoFXSRT) for 257 patients with stage I NSCLC [12]. A total dose of 18–75 Gy at the isocenter was administered in 1–22 fractions. The median calculated biological effective dose (BED) was 111 Gy (range: 57–180 Gy). At a median follow-up of 38 months, local recurrence rate was 8.4 % for a BED of 100 Gy or more compared with 42.9 % for less than 100 Gy ($p<0.001$). The 5-year overall survival rate of medically operable patients was 70.8 % among those treated with a BED of 100 Gy or more compared with 30.2 % among those treated with less than 100 Gy ($p<0.05$). BED is a function of total dose and RT fraction size for a given α/β ratio. Early results of hypofractionated SBRT are promising with limited acute toxicity in selected T1 and T2 inoperable NSCLC (Table 12.1).

As the encouraging results of SBRT for early stage lung cancer from Timmerman et al. and the Japanese became available, the interest in SBRT has grown rapidly. RTOG 02-36 investigated 54 Gy in 3 fractions for patients with clinically staged T1 or T2a (less than 5 cm in diameter), N0M0 NSCLC, and comorbid conditions precluding surgery. Tumors within 2 cm of the proximal bronchial tree were not allowed. The 3-year primary tumor control rate was 97.6 % and the 3-year local-regional control rate was 87.2 % [13]. The use of SBRT in centrally located tumors is being further investigated in RTOG 0813.

A population-based study in the Netherlands found that as the use of SBRT became available

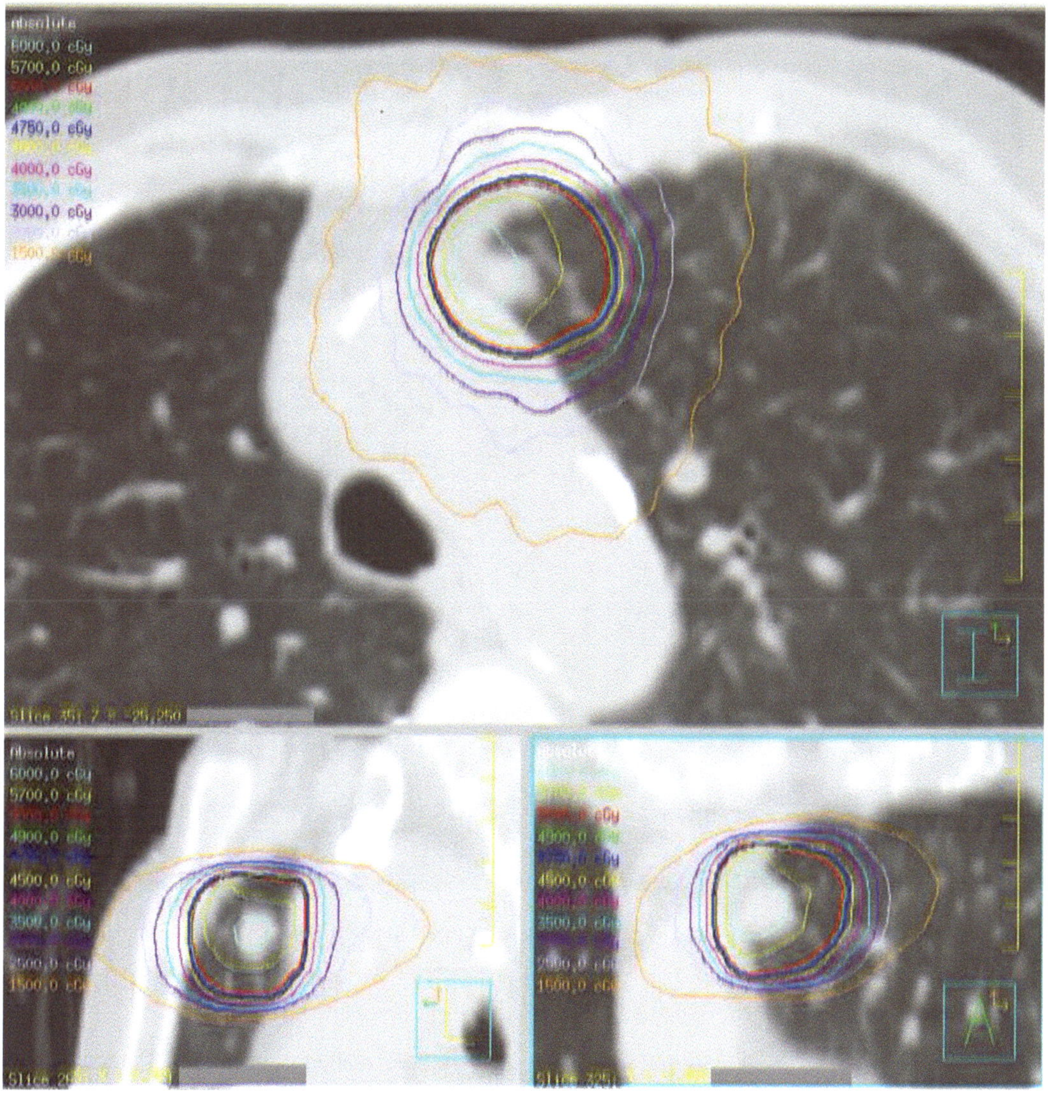

Fig. 12.1 SBRT plan delivering 50 Gy in 5 fractions to a cT1aN0M0 NSCLC of the left upper lobe. A 4D CT was done at the time of simulation and the tumor contoured at all phases of the breathing cycle to generate an internal target volume (ITV). The treatment was delivered free breathing with prescription dose being delivered to the ITV with daily image guidance with cone beam CT (CBCT)

in 2002–2004 and was widely used in 2005–2007, the percentage of patients with stage I NSCLC choosing no active treatment declined and the median survival improved for all patients [23]. Another single institution study compared patients with clinical T1 or T2N0M0 NSCLC who received wedge resection or SBRT. The overall survival was higher in those who received wedge resection, but cause-specific survival was identical and the SBRT patients had reduced local recurrence [24]. RTOG is currently evaluating the role of SBRT in the treatment of patients with operable stage I/II NSCLC in a phase II study (RTOG 06-18). In addition, two phase III randomized trials (NCT00687986 and NCT00840749) will randomize patients with early stage NSCLC to surgical resection or SBRT. As results from current trials become available the role of SBRT in NSCLC will continue to evolve.

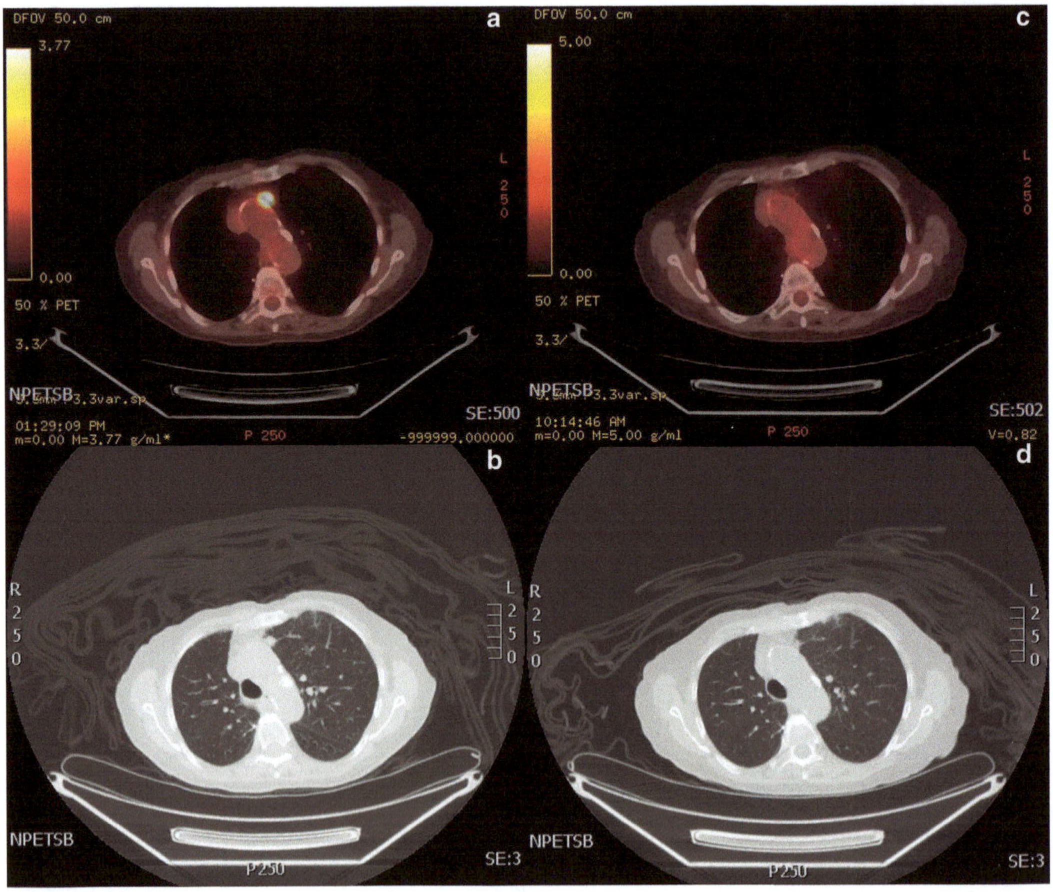

Fig. 12.2 PET-CT (**a**) and CT (**b**) images of a left upper lobe cT1aN0M0 NSCLC prior to SBRT and then 3 months after treatment (**c**, **d**)

Combined Modality Therapy

Non-small Cell Lung Cancer

Resectable NSCLC

Neoadjuvant chemoradiotherapy (CRT) is utilized in certain instances including superior sulcus tumors and selected stage IIIA (N2) disease. In Southwest Oncology Group (SWOG) trial, 9,416 patients with clinical T3–4, N0–1 superior sulcus NSCLC received two cycles of cisplatin and etoposide concurrently with radiation (45 Gy). Patients with stable or responding disease underwent thoracotomy. After completion of neoadjuvant therapy, 80 % underwent thoracotomy and 76 % had complete resection. A complete response or minimal microscopic disease was seen in 65 % of thoracotomy specimens. Five-year survival was 44 % for all patients and 54 % after complete resection [25]. This was a significant improvement over resection rates with RT and surgery of 50 %.

SWOG-8805 confirmed the feasibility of concurrent cisplatin/etoposide plus chest radiotherapy followed by surgery for stage III NSCLC. Intergroup 0139 showed that induction CRT followed by surgical resection for resectable stage III NSCLC patients improved progression-free survival compared to CRT alone [26]. The lack of survival benefit (27 % vs. 20 %) was largely attributed to excess mortality related to right pneumonectomy. The subgroup of patients receiving lobectomy had significantly improved

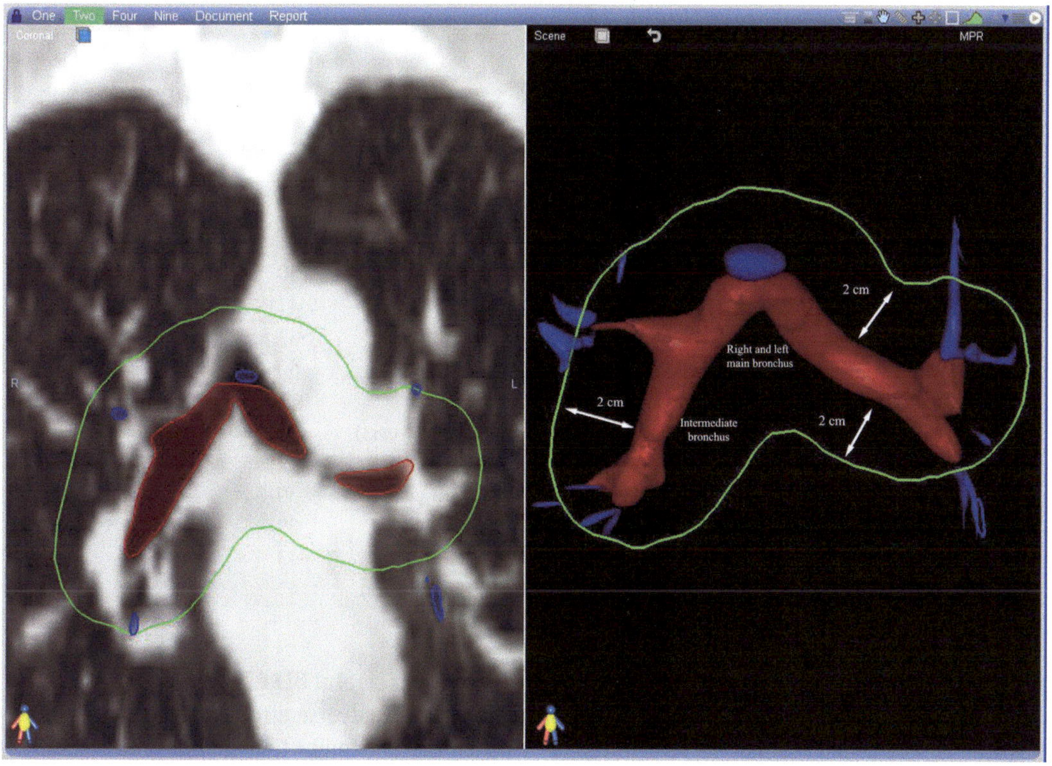

Fig. 12.3 Coronal CT image with the proximal bronchial tree (carina, right and left main bronchi, right and left upper lobe bronchi, intermedius bronchus, right middle lobe bronchus, lingular bronchus, and right and left lower lobe bronchi all contoured in *red*) with a 2 cm expansion (in *green*) to produce the zone of the proximal bronchial tree. Bronchioles distal to the proximal bronchial tree are contoured in *blue*. The contours are shown in 3D to the right. Tumors in the zone of the proximal bronchial tree are at risk for increased toxicity when treated with SBRT to large fractional doses (i.e., 60 Gy in 3 fractions)

5-year survival (36 % vs. 18 %) compared to CRT alone. It appears that induction CRT followed by surgery may benefit resectable stage IIIA patients who do not need pneumonectomy. RTOG 04-12 is further evaluating the role of neoadjuvant CRT by comparing induction chemotherapy with induction CRT followed by surgery and consolidation chemotherapy for resectable stage IIIA NSCLC.

Unresectable NSCLC

Concurrent CRT is the standard of care in locally advanced, unresectable NSCLC. RT alone is used for patients who are not candidates for chemotherapy due to poor Karnofsky performance status (KPS), old age, or medical comorbidities. Poor outcomes are obtained in such patients treated with RT alone. The role of chemotherapy in locally advanced NSCLC was established with the publication of a randomized trial (CALGB-8433) of induction chemotherapy plus high-dose radiation vs. radiation alone in stage III NSCLC by Dillman et al. [27]. In patients with stage III NSCLC, induction chemotherapy with cisplatin and vinblastine before radiation significantly improved median survival (by about 4 months) and doubled the number of long-term survivors, as compared to radiation therapy alone. A 7-year update confirmed these results [28]. RTOG 88-08 conducted a phase III trial comparing standard radiation therapy, induction chemotherapy followed by standard radiation therapy, and twice-daily radiation therapy in patients with surgically unresectable stage II, IIIA, or IIIB NSCLC. Patients were required to have a KPS of 70 or more and less than 5 % weight loss. Ninety-five percent of enrolled patients were stage III. The chemotherapy plus

Table 12.1 Results of SBRT in NSCLC

Results of SBRT in NSCLC			
Author	Treatment	Local control	Single fraction equivalent dose (Gy)
North America/Europe			
Timmerman et al. [13]	18 Gy×3	97.6 % (3 years)	50
Timmerman et al. [11]	20–22 Gy×3	95 % (2+ years)	56–62
Baumann et al. [14]	15 Gy×3	80 % (3 years)	41
Fritz et al. [15]	30 Gy×1	80 % (3 years)	30
Nyman et al. [16]	15 Gy×3	80 % (crude)	41
Zimmermann et al. [17]	12.5 Gy×3	87 % (3 years)	43.5
Timmerman et al. [10]	18–24 Gy×3	90 % (2 years)	50–68
Asia			
Matsuo et al. [18]	12 Gy×4	86.8 % (3 years)	43
Xia et al. [19]	5 Gy×10	95 % (3 years)	32
Hara et al. [20]	30–34 Gy×1	80 % (3 years)	30–34
Onimaru et al. [21]	6 Gy×8	70 % (3 years)	35
Nagata et al. [22]	12 Gy×4	94 % (3 years)	43
Onimaru et al. [21]	7.5 Gy×8	100 % (3 years)	47

radiotherapy arm was statistically superior to the other two treatment arms [29]. Mature results of this trial reported that median survival for standard radiation, CRT, and hyperfractionated radiotherapy was 11.4, 13.2, and 12 months, respectively. The respective 5-year survivals were 5 % for standard RT, 8 % for chemotherapy followed by radiation therapy, and 6 % for hyperfractionated (HFX) RT [30].

RTOG conducted a phase III randomized trial (RTOG 94-10) comparing sequential and concurrent chemotherapy with daily and hyperfractionated RT. Five-year survival was 10 % for sequential chemotherapy, 16 % for concurrent daily RT, and 13 % for concurrent HFX RT [31]. A French randomized trial of sequential and concurrent reported that 2-, 3-, and 4-year survival rates were better in the concurrent arm (39 %, 25 %, and 21 %, respectively) than in the sequential arm (26 %, 19 %, and 14 %, respectively). Although the results were not statistically significant, the trend favored the concurrent CRT arm [32]. Finally, a meta-analysis of concurrent vs. sequential CRT for locally advanced NSCLC revealed a 5.7 % overall survival benefit to concurrent CRT at 5 years [33].

Concurrent CRT with daily RT is the current standard of treatment for unresectable NSCLC (Fig. 12.4). Doses of radiation range from 60 to 70 Gy with careful 3D CT guided planning with a low risk of adverse effects. RTOG 01-17 established the maximum tolerated dose of radiotherapy in the setting of concurrent chemotherapy as 74 Gy [34]. However, RTOG 06-17, which compares high (74 Gy) and low (60 Gy) radiotherapy as well as the addition of cetuximab to carboplatin and taxol, recently closed the high-dose arm due to futility. Thus, the optimum dose of radiotherapy in the setting of concurrent chemotherapy is unclear. Optimum results also depend on timely completion of RT. Machtay et al. evaluated effect of overall treatment time on outcomes after concurrent CRT for locally advanced NSCLC treated on RTOG trials. In multivariate analysis of treatment time as a continuous variable, prolonged treatment time was significantly associated with poorer survival ($p=0.02$), indicating a 2 % increase in the risk of death for each day of prolongation in therapy [35].

Small Cell Lung Cancer

Limited Stage Small Cell Lung Cancer

The standard of care for limited stage small cell lung cancer (LS-SCLC) is chemoradiotherapy followed by PCI in patients with complete response to local treatment in the chest. SCLC is

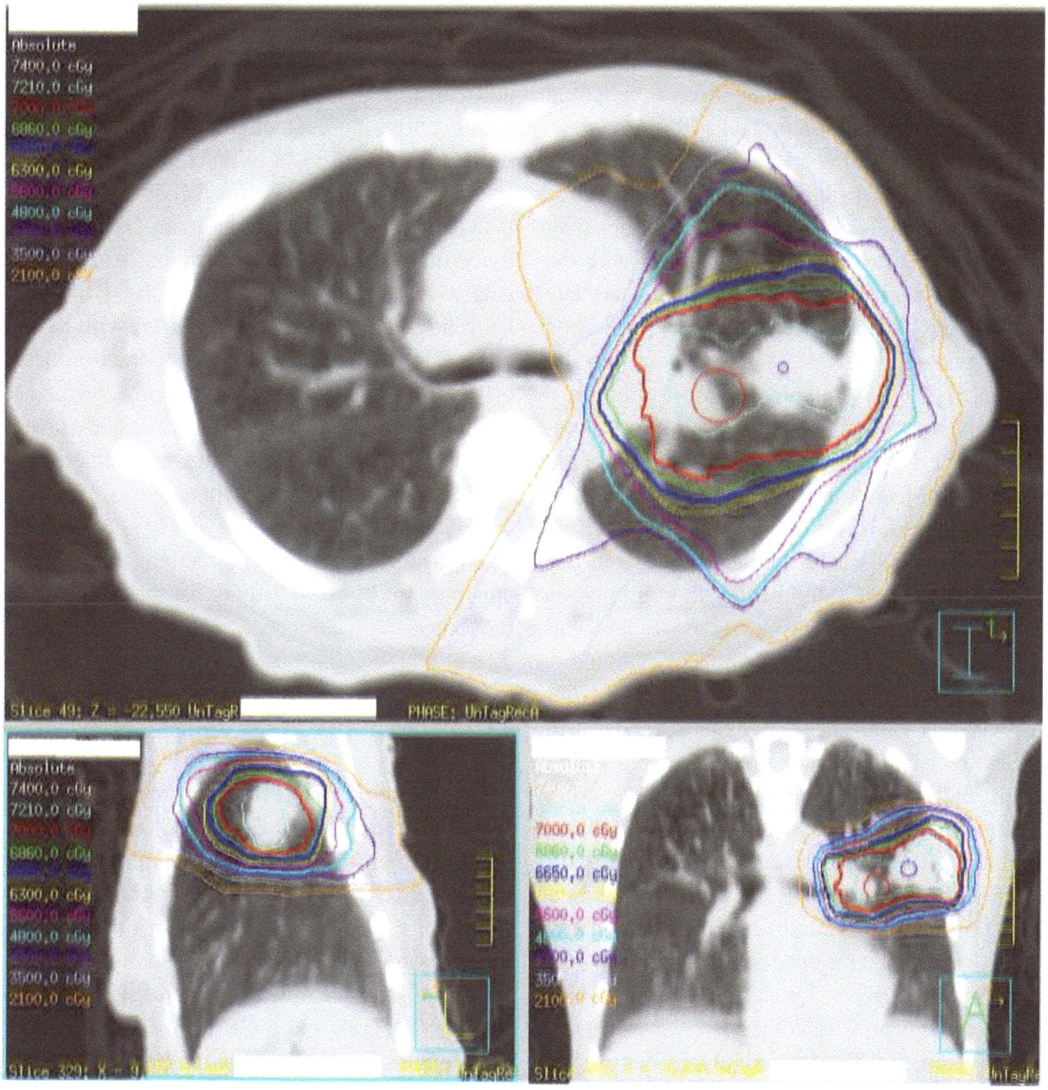

Fig. 12.4 A 3D conformal radiotherapy (3DCRT) plan for an elderly woman with a cT2aN1M0 adenocarcinoma of the left upper lobe. A 4D CT was done at the time of simulation and the tumor contoured at all phases of the breathing cycle to generate an ITV. An additional expansion was then added for setup uncertainty to generate the planning target volume (PTV). The prescription dose was 70 Gy in 35 fractions

characterized by its propensity for early metastasis and rapid doubling time [36]. SCLC is considered a systemic disease; therefore, the role of chemotherapy is very important. Perry et al. evaluated the role of thoracic RT (TRT) in a prospective, randomized trial [37]. Patients were randomly assigned to receive initial radiotherapy pluschemotherapy, delayed radiotherapy plus chemotherapy, or chemotherapy alone. Chemotherapy was given every 3 weeks for 18 months. The radiotherapy comprised 40 Gy in 4 weeks,followed by a 10 Gy "boost" directed against residual disease. All patients received prophylactic whole brain radiation. The addition of thoracic radiotherapy to combination chemotherapy improved both complete response rates and survival, with increased but acceptable toxicity. Several meta-analyses have confirmed the benefit of RT in LS-SCLC. Pignon in a 1992 meta-analysis showed a 14 % reduction in mortality rate and

5.4 % improvement in overall survival at 3 years [38]. Warde et al. published another meta-analysis that revealed 5.4 % overall survival benefit at 2 years with the addition of TRT [39].

The optimal timing of TRT was studied in a NCI-Canada study that randomized LS-SCLC patients to early TRT (40 Gy in 15 fractions over 3 weeks to the primary site) concurrent with the first cycle of chemotherapy (week 3) and late TRT patients who received the same radiation concurrent with the last cycle of chemotherapy (week 15) [40]. Median progression-free survival was 15.4 months in the early TRT group compared to 11.8 months in the late radiation group ($p=0.036$). Median overall survival was 21.2 vs. 16 months, favoring the early RT group ($p=0.008$). A phase III study of concurrent vs. sequential thoracic radiotherapy in combination with cisplatin and etoposide for LS-SCLC was conducted by the Japan Clinical Oncology Group. TRT consisted of 45 Gy over 3 weeks (1.5 Gy twice daily). All patients received four cycles of cisplatin plus etoposide every 3 weeks (sequential arm) or 4 weeks (concurrent arm). TRT was begun on day 2 of the first cycle of chemotherapy in the concurrent arm and after the fourth cycle in the sequential arm. Median survival time was 19.7 months in the sequential arm vs. 27.2 months in the concurrent arm. The 2-, 3-, and 5-year survival rates for patients who received sequential radiotherapy were 35.1 %, 20.2 %, and 18.3 %, respectively, as opposed to 54.4 %, 29.8 %, and 23.7 %, respectively, for the patients who received concurrent RT [41].

The optimum dose and fractionation of TRT had not yet been determined. Due to rapid tumor repopulation, accelerated and hyperfractionated RT has been evaluated. A prospective, randomized phase III study (Intergroup 0096) compared twice-daily RT with once-daily thoracic radiotherapy in limited small-cell lung cancer treated concurrently with cisplatin and etoposide. Patients were assigned to receive a total of 45 Gy of concurrent TRT, given either twice daily over a 3-week period or once daily over a period of 5 weeks beginning with first cycle of chemotherapy. After a median follow-up of almost 8 years, 2- and 5-year OS was 47 % and 26 % for twice-daily arm compared to 41 % and 16 % for once-daily arm, respectively. Grade 3 esophagitis was significantly more frequent in the twice-daily group at 27 % vs. 11 % [42]. This study has been criticized because 45 Gy in 1.8 Gy daily fractions is not biologically equivalent to 45 Gy in 1.5 Gy twice-daily fractions. The duration of treatment is also shorter by 2 weeks in the BID arm. Currently, patients are either treated with twice-daily RT to 45 Gy in 1.5 Gy per fraction or to 60 Gy in 2 Gy daily fractions with concurrent chemotherapy. CALGB 30610 is currently investigating the optimal dose and fractionation in LS-SCLC and randomizes patients to 45 Gy at 1.5 Gy twice-daily fractions, 70 Gy at 2 Gy daily fractions, or 61.2 Gy at 1.8 fractions daily with a concomitant boost of 1.8 Gy for the last 9 treatment days.

Extensive Stage SCLC

Chemotherapy alone is the mainstay of treatment in extensive stage SCLC (ES-SCLC) and RT is utilized either for PCI in good responders [43] or for palliative treatment in bone or brain metastasis or for relief of airway or superior vena cava obstruction. The role of consolidative TRT in ES-SCLC was examined in patients with a CR or PR in the thorax and a CR at distant sites after three cycles of cisplatin and etoposide. Patients were randomized to four additional cycles of cisplatin and etoposide or 54 Gy in 36 fractions TRT over 18 treatment days with carboplatin and etoposide followed by two cycles of cisplatin and etoposide. All patients received PCI. Five-year survival was improved in the TRT arm at 9.1 % vs. 3.7 % in the chemotherapy alone arm [44]. However, thoracic RT is not widely accepted in ES-SCLC. RTOG 09-37 is a phase II trial that further examines the role of RT in ES-SCLC by randomizing patients with up to 1–4 sites of extracranial metastatic disease and partial or complete response after 4–6 cycles of platinum-based chemotherapy to PCI alone or PCI and consolidative extracranial irradiation.

Adjuvant Radiotherapy in NSCLC

The use of adjuvant RT in completely resected NSCLC remains controversial. Lung Cancer Study Group (LCSG) 773 assessed the effect of mediastinal RT (50 Gy in 5–5.5 weeks) following resection of stage II and III squamous cell carcinoma of lung. A marked reduction in local relapse as first site of failure from 41 to 3 % was observed for patients receiving postoperative RT (PORT), but this was without survival benefit. A subgroup analysis of N2 patients revealed a trend towards a survival benefit.

A meta-analysis of PORT [45] showed that there was a 21 % relative increase in the risk of death in patients treated with PORT, equivalent to an absolute detriment of 7 % at 2 years, reducing overall survival from 55 to 48 %. Subgroup analyses suggested that this adverse effect was greatest for patients with stage I/II, N0–N1 disease. For those with stage III, N2 disease, there was no clear evidence of an adverse effect. This detriment was presumably due to increase in intercurrent deaths. Results of this analysis were widely criticized for many reasons including methodological issues and including series with outdated RT modality, technique, and inappropriate radiation dose and fractionation [46]. A Mayo Clinic retrospective review to determine the local recurrence and survival rates for patients with N2 disease undergoing complete surgical resection with or without PORT revealed that actuarial 4-year local recurrence rate was 60 %, compared with 17 % for PORT ($p<0.0001$) [47]. The actuarial 4-year survival rate was 22 % for treatment with surgery alone, compared with 43 % for treatment with PORT. Recent studies using modern RT have failed to show a detrimental effect of PORT [48]. A phase III trial of adjuvant radiotherapy in NSCLC with pathological stage I randomized pathologic staged IA and IB patients to PORT or observation. Local recurrence rate was 2.2 % in the RT group compared to 23 % in the observation group. Overall 5-year survival (Kaplan–Meier) showed a positive trend in the treated group: 67 % vs. 58 %. Treatment-related toxicity was acceptable [49].

Recently, the Adjuvant Navelbine International Trialist Association (ANITA) randomized trial analyzed the results of patients receiving PORT in the phase III randomized trial of adjuvant chemotherapy following surgery. Approximately 30 % of patients received PORT. They concluded that PORT had a beneficial effect in the pathologic N2 subgroup of patients [50]. The European Organization for the Research and Treatment of Cancer (EORTC) is launching a large randomized trial to further evaluate the role of adjuvant RT in N2 disease. Adjuvant RT is advisable for positive/close margins of resection in T1–T2 N0–1 disease. Mediastinal RT to 50 Gy in 1.8–2 Gy per fraction using 3D conformal RT may be considered for selected pathologic N2 patients, particularly with multi-station nodal involvement (Fig. 12.5). An excellent review by Bogart et al. can provide further insights [46].

Palliative Radiotherapy

Radiation therapy is very effective in palliating symptoms of metastatic lung cancer [51]. Symptoms of pain from bone metastasis, chest wall invasion by primary tumor, and radicular pain from nerve root invasion can be palliated by RT. Prompt radiotherapy for spinal cord compression, superior vena cava syndrome, and brain metastasis can help relieve symptoms or preempt development of more serious effects. Brain metastases are usually treated with surgery, whole brain RT (WBRT), and/or stereotactic radiosurgery (SRS). Optimal treatment of brain metastases depends on age, primary site, control of the primary, interval to development of brain metastases, disease-free interval, number of brain metastases, presence of extracranial metastases, KPS, treatment of brain metastases, and recursive partitioning analysis (RPA) class. A phase III randomized trial of WBRT with or without SRS boost for patients with 1–3 brain metastases (RTOG 95-08) concluded that WBRT and stereotactic boost treatment improved functional autonomy (KPS) for all patients and survival for patients with a single unresectable brain metastasis [52]. In a randomized trial of surgery followed

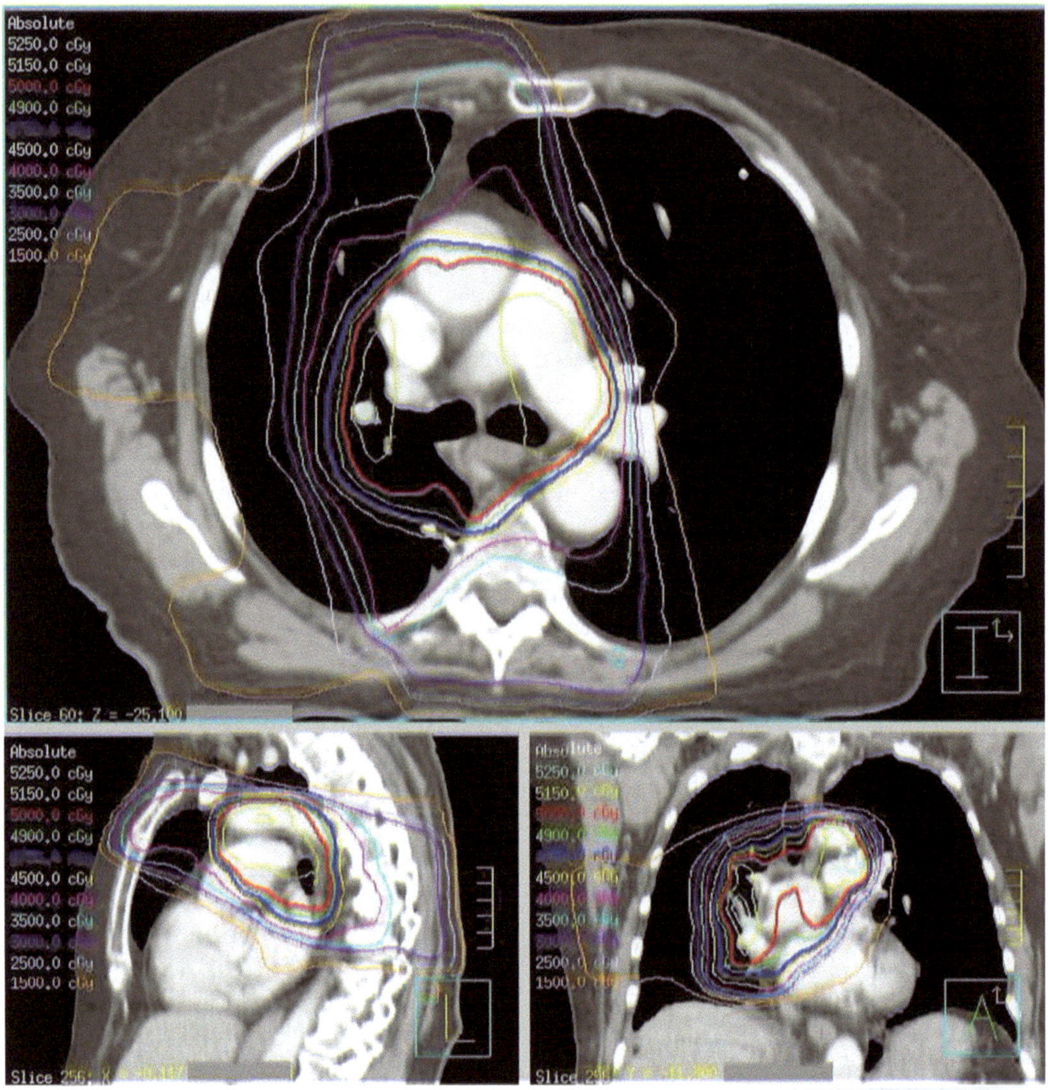

Fig. 12.5 A 3DCRT plan in a gentleman with locally advanced NSCLC who had pT2aN2M0 disease after lobectomy and mediastinal lymph node dissection. He received four cycles of adjuvant chemotherapy (carboplatin and pemetrexed) prior to radiotherapy. The prescription dose was 50 Gy in 25 fractions

by WBRT compared to WBRT alone in the treatment of single metastases to the brain, Patchell et al. concluded that patients with a single metastasis to the brain who receive treatment with surgical resection plus radiotherapy live longer, have fewer recurrences of cancer in the brain, and have a better quality of life than similar patients treated with radiotherapy alone [53]. Another randomized trial by the same group compared postoperative WBRT with surgery alone. Patients with single metastases to the brain who received treatment with surgical resection and postoperative radiotherapy had fewer recurrences of cancer in the brain and were less likely to die of neurologic causes than similar patients treated with surgical resection alone [54]. The RTOG is currently conducting a phase III randomized, double blind, placebo-controlled trial of Memantine for prevention of cognitive dysfunction in patients receiving WBRT (RTOG 06-14).

Other examples of palliation include relief of airway obstruction to improve symptoms of dyspnea or prevention of recurrent post-obstructive pneumonia. RT is also very effective in treating hemoptysis arising from ulcerative lesions in the lung. Sometimes, endobronchial bleeding lesions are treated with intraluminal brachytherapy in single or multiple fractions. The usual radiotherapy dose for palliation ranges from 37.5 Gy in 15 fractions to 20 Gy in 5 fractions given daily, 5 days a week. The type and duration of treatment depends on the KPS of the patient and type and status of the cancer.

A randomized trial of single treatment with 8 Gy compared to 30 Gy in 10 fractions was conducted in patients with painful bone metastases [55]. Both regimens were equivalent in terms of pain and narcotic relief at 3 months and were well tolerated with few adverse effects. A meta-analysis of fractionated radiotherapy trials for the palliation of painful bone metastases showed no significant difference in complete and overall pain relief between single and multi-fraction palliative RT for bone metastases [56].

Prophylactic Cranial Irradiation

The brain is an important site of disease failure in lung cancer and is associated with poor prognosis. Overall CNS failure after potentially curative local therapy ranges from 21 to 54 % [57, 58]. Brain metastases are common in adenocarcinoma, large cell carcinoma, and locally advanced disease. Stuschke et al. treated patients with stage III NSCLC with PCI and reduced the rate of brain metastases as first site of relapse from 30 to 8 % at 4 years ($p=0.005$) and overall brain relapse from 54 to 13 % ($p<0.0001$) [57]. The late toxicity to normal brain was acceptable. RTOG conducted a phase III randomized trial (RTOG 02-14) of PCI compared to observation in patients with stage III NSCLC with stable extracranial disease 4 months after completion of their initial treatment. The study was closed early due to slow accrual. There was no difference in overall survival or disease-free survival at 1 year, but rates of brain metastasis at 1 year were significantly lower in the PCI arm (7.7 % vs. 18 %) [59]. Currently, PCI is not recommended for patients with NSCLC outside of a clinical trial.

Brain metastases are common in SCLC. Arriagada et al. conducted a prospective study of PCI compared to no PCI in 300 patients with SCLC in complete remission. The 2-year cumulative rate of brain metastasis as an isolated first site of relapse was 45 % in the control group and 19 % in the treatment group ($p<10(-6)$). The total 2-year rate of brain metastasis was 67 % and 40 %, respectively (relative risk $=0.35$; $p<10(-13)$). The 2-year overall survival rate was 21.5 % in the control group and 29 % in the treatment group (relative risk $=0.83$; $p=0.14$). There were no significant differences between the two groups in terms of neuropsychological function or abnormalities indicated by brain CT scans [60]. A meta-analysis of seven randomized trials of PCI in SCLC showed that PCI improved both overall survival (5.4 % at 3 years) and disease-free survival among patients with SCLC in complete remission [61]. RTOG 02-12 compared 25 Gy in 10 fractions to 36 Gy (18 daily fractions or 24 twice-daily fractions) of PCI in patients with limited stage SCLC in complete remission. The 2-year incidence of brain metastases and overall survival were the same in both arms and 25 Gy is considered the standard for PCI in limited stage SCLC [62].

Slotman and colleagues recently published results of a phase III randomized trial of PCI in ES-SCLC patients who had a response to chemotherapy [43]. The primary end point was the time to symptomatic brain metastases. Several dose and fractionation schedules were allowed and the one most commonly used was 20 Gy in 5 fractions. The cumulative risk of brain metastases within 1 year was 14.6 % in the irradiation group and 40.4 % in the control group. Irradiation was associated with an increase in median disease-free survival from 12.0 to 14.7 weeks and in median overall survival from 5.4 to 6.7 months after randomization (Fig. 12.6). The 1-year survival rate was 27.1 % in the irradiation group and 13.3 % in the control group.

Toxicity of Radiation Therapy

Radiation therapy delivered either alone or in combination with chemotherapy or surgery may cause both acute and late side effects due to the

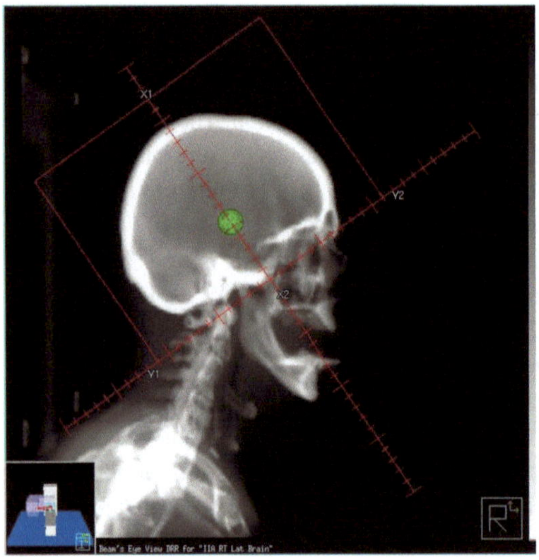

Fig. 12.6 A typical field used for prophylactic cranial irradiation in a patient with extensive stage SCLC who had a partial response to chemotherapy. The prescription dose was 25 Gy in 10 fractions

effect of RT on normal tissue and organ systems. Recent advances in imaging, technique, and delivery of RT such as IGRT and IMRT have improved target accuracy and normal tissue avoidance, but increased heterogeneity can lead to increased "hotspots" in surrounding tissues. Most common acute side effects of thoracic RT (during and up to 3 months following treatment) include fatigue, radiation dermatitis (usually in RT portals), dyspnea, and esophagitis. Late effects include radiation pneumonitis (RP), esophageal stricture/perforation, risk of rib fracture, cardiac toxicity (including pericardial disease, valvular disease, and myocardial infarction), spinal cord injury, and brachial plexopathy.

Esophagitis leads to pain in swallowing and poor oral intake leading to dehydration, electrolyte imbalance, and weight loss. Approximately 50–70 % patients receiving concomitant chemoradiotherapy develop grade 1 or 2 esophageal toxicity. A retrospective study of predictors of radiation-induced esophageal toxicity in patients with NSCLC treated with three-dimensional conformal radiotherapy showed that concurrent chemotherapy and the maximal esophageal point dose (58 Gy) were significantly associated with a risk of grade 3–5 esophageal toxicity [63]. Esophagitis is treated with diet modifications, mucositis rinses, antacids, and pain medications. Esophageal strictures are managed by dilatations.

Radiation pneumonitis (RP) is inflammation of the lungs as a result of radiation. It usually manifests itself 2 weeks to 6 months after completion of RT. Symptoms include dyspnea on exertion, cough, and low grade fever. RP is an interstitial pulmonary inflammation that can develop in as many as 5–15 % of patients with thoracic irradiation (Fig. 12.7). Classical RP involves direct toxic injury to endothelial and epithelial cells from the radiation, resulting initially in an acute alveolitis. This process leads to an accumulation of inflammatory and immune effector cells within the alveolar walls and spaces. The accumulation of leukocytes distorts the normal alveolar structures and results in the release of lymphokines and monokines. The alveolar macrophage is thought to play a central role in the subsequent development of chronic inflammation. Sporadic RP results in an "out-of-field" response. This is thought to be an immunologically mediated process resulting in bilateral lymphocytic alveolitis. The severity of RP may range from asymptomatic X-ray changes to severe respiratory compromise requiring ventilator support. Some of the factors determining risk and degree of RP include prior lung disease, history of lung resection, volume of lung treated and dose (mean lung dose [MLD]), chemotherapy, and performance status.

Several investigators have published data regarding predictors of RP. Bradley and colleagues reviewed data from RTOG 9311 and their institutional dataset and concluded that there was greater risk of RP due to inferior lung irradiation and increasing normal lung mean dose [64]. A prospective study showed that MLD, V20, and V30 (volume of lung receiving 20 Gy and 30 Gy, respectively) were associated with severe RP [65]. Another investigator concluded V10 and V13 as the best predictors of RP risk, with a decrease in predictive value above those volumes [66]. Borst et al. looked at pulmonary function changes after radiotherapy in NSCLC patients with long-term disease-free survival and suggested that a significant decrease in pulmonary

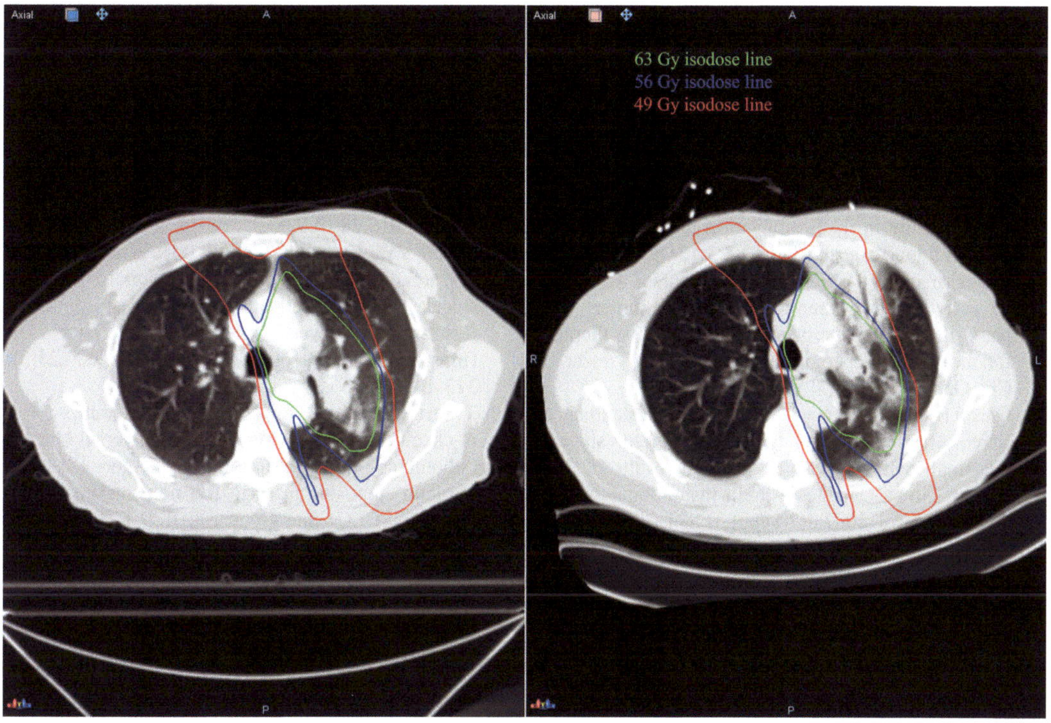

Fig. 12.7 A follow-up CT (on the *right*) revealing radiation pneumonitis in a patient who had received chemoradiotherapy for a stage IIIA NSCLC was fused with the planning CT (on the *left*). Contours were then created from the plan isodose lines demonstrating pneumonitis within the radiation field

function was observed 3 months after RT. No recovery in pulmonary function was seen at 18 and 36 months after RT. The decrease in pulmonary function was dependent on the MLD, and patients with chronic obstructive pulmonary disease had larger reductions in the PFTs [67]. Most recently, the QUANTEC (quantitative analyses of normal tissue effects in the clinic) group recommended maintaining V20 ≤ 30–35 % and MLD ≤ 20–23 Gy to limit the risk of RP to ≤20 % [68]. Treatment of RP is steroids, oxygen, antibiotics for infection, and ventilator support if needed.

References

1. Tyldesley S, Boyd C, Schulze K, Walker H, Mackilop WJ. Estimating the need for radiotherapy for lung cancer: an evidence-based, epidemiologic approach. Int J Radiat Oncol Biol Phys. 2001;49(4):973–85.
2. Kong FM, Zhao L, Hayman JA. The role of radiation therapy in thoracic tumors. Hematol Oncol Clin North Am. 2006;20(2):363–400.
3. Decker RH, Tanoue LT, Colasanto JM, Detterbeck FC, Wilson LD. Evaluation and definitive management of medically inoperable early-stage non-small-cell lung cancer. Part 1: assessment and conventional radiotherapy. Oncology (Williston Park). 2006;20(7): 727–36.
4. Zimmermann FB, Bamberg M, Molls M, Jeremic B. Radiation therapy alone in early stage non-small cell lung cancer. Semin Surg Oncol. 2003;21:91–7.
5. Narayan S, Henning GT, Ten Haken RK, Sullivan MA, Martel MK, Hayman JA. Results following treatment to doses of 92.4 or 102.9 Gy on a phase I dose escalation study for non-small cell lung cancer. Lung Cancer. 2004;44(1):79–88.
6. Urbanic JJ, Turrisi AT, Sharma AK, et al. Conformal high dose external radiation therapy, 80.5 Gy, alone for medically inoperable non-small cell lung cancer: a retrospective analysis. J Thorac Oncol. 2006;1(2): 112–9.
7. Bradley J, Graham MV, Winter K, et al. Toxicity and outcome results of RTOG 9311: a phase I-II dose-escalation study using three-dimensional conformal radiotherapy in patients with inoperable non-small-cell lung carcinoma. Int J Radiat Oncol Biol Phys. 2005;61:318–28.
8. Chang JY, Dong L, Liu H, et al. Image-guided radiation therapy for non-small cell lung cancer. J Thorac Oncol. 2008;3(2):177–86.

9. Heinzerling JH, Anderson JF, Papiez L, et al. Four-dimensional computed tomography scan analysis of tumor and organ motion at varying levels of abdominal compression during stereotactic treatment of lung and liver. Int J Radiat Oncol Biol Phys. 2008;70(5):1571–8.
10. Timmerman R, Papiez L, McGarry R, et al. Extracranial stereotactic radioablation: results of a phase I study in medically inoperable stage I non-small cell lung cancer. Chest. 2003;124(5):1946–55.
11. Timmerman R, McGarry R, Tiannoutsos C, et al. Excessive toxicity when treating central tumors in a phase II study of stereotactic body radiation therapy for medically inoperable early-stage lung cancer. J Clin Oncol. 2006;24(30):4833–9.
12. Onishi H, Shirato H, Nagata Y, et al. Hypofractionated stereotactic radiotherapy (HypoFXSRT) for stage I non-small cell lung cancer: updated results of 257 patients in a Japanese multi-institutional study. J Thorac Oncol. 2007;2(7 Suppl 3):S94–100.
13. Timmerman R, Paulus R, Galvin J, et al. Stereotactic body radiation therapy for inoperable early stage lung cancer. JAMA. 2010;303:1070–6.
14. Baumann P, Nyman J, Lax I, et al. Factors important for efficacy of stereotactic body radiotherapy of medically inoperable stage I lung cancer. A retrospective analysis of patients treated in the Nordic countries. Acta Oncol. 2006;45(7):787–95.
15. Fritz P, Kraus HJ, Muhlnickel W, et al. Stereotactic, single-dose irradiation of stage I non-small cell lung cancer and lung metastases. Radiat Oncol. 2006;1:30.
16. Nyman J, Johansson KA, Hulten U, et al. Stereotactic hypofractionated radiotherapy for stage I non-small cell lung cancer—mature results for medically inoperable patients. Lung Cancer. 2006;51(1):97–103.
17. Zimmermann FB, Geinitz H, Schill S, et al. Stereotactoc hypofractionated radiation therapy for stage I non-small cell lung cancer. Lung Cancer. 2005;48(1):107–14.
18. Matsuo Y, Shibuya K, Nagata Y, et al. Prognostic factors in stereotactic body radiotherapy for non-small-cell lung cancer. Int J Radiat Oncol Biol Phys. 2011;79(4):1104–11.
19. Xia T, Li H, Sun Q, et al. Promising clinical outcome of stereotactic body radiotherapy for patients with inoperable stage I/II non-small cell-lung cancer. Int J Radiat Oncol Biol Phys. 2006;66(1):117–25.
20. Hara R, Itami J, Aruga T, et al. Clinical outcomes of single-fraction stereotactic radiation therapy of lung tumors. Cancer. 2006;106(6):1347–52.
21. Onimaru R, Shirato H, Shimizu S, et al. Tolerance of organs at risk in small-volume, hypofractionated, image-guided radiotherapy for primary and metastatic lung cancers. Int J Radiat Oncol Biol Phys. 2003; 56(1):126–35.
22. Nagata Y, Takayama K, Matsuo Y, et al. Clinical outcomes of a phase I/II study of 48 Gy of stereotactic body radiotherapy in 4 fractions for primary lung cancer using a stereotactic body frame. Int J Radiat Oncol Biol Phys. 2005;63(5):1427–31.
23. Palma D, Visser O, Lagerwaard FJ, Belderbos J, Slotman BJ, Senan S. Impact of introducing stereotactic lung radiotherapy for elderly patients with stage I non-small-cell lung cancer: a population-based time-trend analysis. J Clin Oncol. 2010;28(35):5153–9.
24. Grills IS, Mangona VS, Welsh R, et al. Outcomes after stereotactic lung radiotherapy or wedge resection for stage I non-small-cell lung cancer. J Clin Oncol. 2010;28(6):928–35.
25. Rusch VW, Giroux DJ, Kraut MJ, et al. Induction chemoradiation and surgical resection for superior sulcus non-small-cell lung carcinomas: long-term results of Southwest Oncology Group Trial 9416 (Intergroup Trial 0160). J Clin Oncol. 2007;25(3):313–8.
26. Turrisi AT, Scott C, Rusch V, et al. Randomized trial of chemoradiotherapy to 61 Gy [no S] versus chemoradiotherapy to 45 Gy followed by surgery [S] using cisplatin etoposide in stage IIIa non-small cell lung cancer (NSCLC): intergroup trial 0139, RTOG (9309). Int J Radiat Oncol Biol Phys. 2003;57:S125–6.
27. Dillman RO, Seagren SL, Propert KJ, et al. A randomized trial of induction chemotherapy plus high-dose radiation versus radiation alone in stage III non-small-cell lung cancer. N Engl J Med. 1990; 323:940–5.
28. Dillman RO, Herndon J, Seagren SL, et al. Improved survival in stage III non-small-cell lung cancer: seven-year follow-up of cancer and leukemia group B (CALGB) 8433 trial. J Natl Cancer Inst. 1996;88:1210–5.
29. Sause WT, Scott C, Taylor S, et al. Radiation Therapy Oncology Group (RTOG) 88–08 and Eastern Cooperative Oncology Group (ECOG) 4588: preliminary results of a phase III trial in regionally advanced, unresectable non-small-cell lung cancer. J Natl Cancer Inst. 1995;87:198–205.
30. Sause W, Kolesar P, Taylor S, et al. Final results of phase III trial in regionally advanced unresectable non-small cell lung cancer: Radiation Therapy Oncology Group, Eastern Cooperative Oncology Group, and Southwest Oncology Group. Chest. 2000; 117:358–64.
31. Curran W, Paulus R, Langer C, et al. Sequential vs concurrent chemoradiation for stage III non-small cell lung cancer: randomized phase III trial RTOG 9410. J Natl Cancer Inst. 2011;103:1–9.
32. Fournel P, Robinet G, Thomas P, et al. Randomized phase III trial of sequential chemoradiotherapy compared with concurrent chemoradiotherapy in locally advanced non-small-cell lung cancer: Groupe Lyon-Saint-Etienne d'Oncologie Thoracique-Groupe Francais de Pneumo-Cancerologie NPC 95–01 Study. J Clin Oncol. 2005;23(25):5910–7.
33. Auperin A, Le Pechoux C, Rolland E, et al. Meta-analysis of concomitant versus sequential radiochemotherapy in locally advanced non-small-cell lung cancer. J Clin Oncol. 2010;28(13):2181–90.
34. Bradley J, Moughan J, Graham MV, et al. A phase I/II radiation dose escalation study with concurrent

chemotherapy for patients with inoperable stages I to III non-small-cell lung cancer: phase I results of RTOG 0117. Int J Radiat Oncol Biol Phys. 2010;77:367–72.
35. Machtay M, Hsu C, Komaki R, et al. Effect of overall treatment time on outcomes after concurrent chemo-radiation for locally advanced non-small-cell lung carcinoma: analysis of the Radiation Therapy Oncology Group (RTOG) experience. Int J Radiat Oncol Biol Phys. 2005;63:667–71.
36. Simon G, Ginsberg RJ, Ruckdeschel JC. Small-cell lung cancer. Chest Surg Clin N Am. 2001;11(1):165–88; ix.
37. Perry MC, Eaton WL, Propert KJ, et al. Chemotherapy with or without radiation therapy in limited small-cell carcinoma of the lung. N Engl J Med. 1987;316(15):912–8.
38. Pignon JP, Arriagada R, Ihde DC, et al. A meta-analysis of thoracic radiotherapy for small-cell lung cancer. N Engl J Med. 1992;327(23):1618–24.
39. Warde P, Payne D. Does thoracic irradiation improve survival and local control in limited-stage small-cell carcinoma of the lung? A meta-analysis. J Clin Oncol. 1992;10(6):890–5.
40. Murray N, Coy P, Pater JL, et al. Importance of timing for thoracic irradiation in the combined modality treatment of limited-stage small-cell lung cancer. The National Cancer Institute of Canada Clinical Trials Group. J Clin Oncol. 1993;11(2):336–44.
41. Takada M, Fukuoka M, Kawahara M, et al. Phase III study of concurrent versus sequential thoracic radiotherapy in combination with cisplatin and etoposide for limited-stage small-cell lung cancer: results of the Japan Clinical Oncology Group Study 9104. J Clin Oncol. 2002;20(14):3054–60.
42. Turrisi III AT, Kim K, Blum R, et al. Twice-daily compared with once-daily thoracic radiotherapy in limited small-cell lung cancer treated concurrently with cisplatin and etoposide. N Engl J Med. 1999;340(4):265–71.
43. Slotman B, Faivre-Finn C, Kramer G, et al. Prophylactic cranial irradiation in extensive small-cell lung cancer. N Engl J Med. 2007;357(7):664–72.
44. Jeremic B, Shibamoto Y, Nikolic N, et al. Role of radiation therapy in the combined-modality treatment of patients with extensive disease small-cell lung cancer: a randomized study. J Clin Oncol. 1999;17:2092–9.
45. Postoperative radiotherapy in non-small-cell lung cancer: systematic review and meta-analysis of individual patient data from nine randomised controlled trials. PORT Meta-analysis Trialists Group. Lancet. 1998;352:257–63.
46. Bogart JA, Aronowitz JN. Localized non-small cell lung cancer: adjuvant radiotherapy in the era of effective systemic therapy. Clin Cancer Res. 2005; 11(13 Pt 2):5004s–10s.
47. Sawyer TE, Bonner JA, Gould PM, et al. The impact of surgical adjuvant thoracic radiation therapy for patients with nonsmall cell lung carcinoma with ipsilateral mediastinal lymph node involvement. Cancer. 1997;80:1399–408.
48. Machtay M, Lee JH, Shrager JB, Kaiser LR, Glatstein E. Risk of death from intercurrent disease is not excessively increased by modern postoperative radiotherapy for high-risk resected non-small-cell lung carcinoma. J Clin Oncol. 2001;9(19):3912–7.
49. Trodella L, Granone P, Valente S, et al. Adjuvant radiotherapy in non-small cell lung cancer with pathological stage I: definitive results of a phase III randomized trial. Radiother Oncol. 2002;62(1):11–9.
50. Douillard JY, Rosell R, De Lena M, et al. Impact of postoperative radiation therapy on survival in patients with complete resection and stage I, II, or IIIA non-small-cell lung cancer treated with adjuvant chemotherapy: the adjuvant Navelbine International Trialist Association (ANITA) Randomized Trial. Int J Radiat Oncol Biol Phys. 2008;72(3):695–701.
51. Konski AS, Feigenberg S, Chow E. Palliative radiation therapy. Semin Oncol. 2005;32(2):156–64.
52. Andrews DW, Scott CB, Sperduto PW, et al. Whole brain radiation therapy with or without stereotactic radiosurgery boost for patients with one to three brain metastases: phase III results of the RTOG 9508 randomised trial. Lancet. 2004;363(9422):1665–72.
53. Patchell RA, Tibbs PA, Walsh JW, et al. A randomized trial of surgery in the treatment of single metastases to the brain. N Engl J Med. 1990;322(8):494–500.
54. Patchell RA, Tibbs PA, Regine WF, et al. Postoperative radiotherapy in the treatment of single metastases to the brain: a randomized trial. JAMA. 1998;280(17): 1485–9.
55. Hartsell WF, Scott CB, Bruner DW, et al. Randomized trial of short- versus long-course radiotherapy for palliation of painful bone metastases. J Natl Cancer Inst. 2005;97(11):798–804.
56. Wu JS, Wong R, Johnston M, Bezjak A, Whelan T, Cancer Care Ontario Practice Guidelines Initiative Supportive Care Group. Meta-analysis of dose-fractionation radiotherapy trials for the palliation of painful bone metastases. Int J Radiat Oncol Biol Phys. 2003;55(3):594–605.
57. Stuschke M, Eberhardt W, Pottgen C, et al. Prophylactic cranial irradiation in locally advanced non-small-cell lung cancer after multimodality treatment: long-term follow-up and investigations of late neuropsychologic effects. J Clin Oncol. 1999;17(9): 2700–9.
58. Andre F, Grunenwald D, Pujol JL, et al. Patterns of relapse of N2 nonsmall-cell lung carcinoma patients treated with preoperative chemotherapy: should prophylactic cranial irradiation be reconsidered? Cancer. 2001;91(12):2394–400.
59. Gore EM, Bae K, Wong SJ, et al. Phase III comparison of prophylactic cranial irradiation versus observation in patients with locally advanced non-small-cell lung cancer: primary analysis of radiation therapy oncology group study RTOG 0214. J Clin Oncol. 2010;29(3):272–8.

60. Arriagada R, Le Chevalier T, Borie F, et al. Prophylactic cranial irradiation for patients with small-cell lung cancer in complete remission. J Natl Cancer Inst. 1995;87(3):183–90.
61. Aupérin A, Arriagada R, Pignon JP, et al. Prophylactic cranial irradiation for patients with small-cell lung cancer in complete remission. Prophylactic Cranial Irradiation Overview Collaborative Group. N Engl J Med. 1999;341(7):476–84.
62. Le Péchoux C, Dunant A, Senan S, et al. Stand-dose versus higher-dose prophylactic cranial irradiation (PCI) in patients with limited-stage small-cell lung cancer in complete remission after chemotherapy and thoracic radiotherapy (PCI 99–01, EORTC 22003-08004, RTOG 0212, and IFCT 99–01): a randomised clinical trial. Lancet Oncol. 2009;10(5):467–74.
63. Singh AK, Lockett MA, Bradley JD. Predictors of radiation-induced esophageal toxicity in patients with non-small-cell lung cancer treated with three-dimensional conformal radiotherapy. Int J Radiat Oncol Biol Phys. 2003;55(2):337–41.
64. Bradley JD, Hope A, El Naga I, et al. A nomogram to predict radiation pneumonitis, derived from a combined analysis of RTOG 9311 and institutional data. Int J Radiat Oncol Biol Phys. 2007;69(4):985–92.
65. Claude L, Pérol D, Ginestet C, et al. A prospective study on radiation pneumonitis following conformal radiation therapy in non-small-cell lung cancer: clinical and dosimetric factors analysis. Radiother Oncol. 2004;71(2):175–81.
66. Schallenkamp JM, Miller RC, Brinkmann DH, et al. Incidence of radiation pneumonitis after thoracic irradiation: dose-volume correlates. Int J Radiat Oncol Biol Phys. 2007;67(2):410–6.
67. Borst GR, De Jaeger K, Belderbos JS, Burgers SA, Lebesque JV. Pulmonary function changes after radiotherapy in non-small-cell lung cancer patients with long-term disease-free survival. Int J Radiat Oncol Biol Phys. 2005;62(3):639–44.
68. Marks LB, Bentzen SM, Deasy JO, et al. Radiation dose-volume effects in the lung. Int J Radiat Oncol Biol Phys. 2010;76(3 Suppl):S70–6.

Imaging the Chest Following Radiation Therapy

13

Jeffrey P. Kanne and J. David Godwin

External beam radiation therapy is used in the treatment of pulmonary, mediastinal, and chest wall malignancies, including primarily lung carcinoma, breast carcinoma, and lymphoma. Radiation therapy may be used alone or in conjunction with chemotherapy, surgery, or both, for either palliation or cure.

The lung is the primary dose-limiting structure in the chest, and radiation-induced lung injury resulting in pneumonitis, fibrosis, or both markedly limits the total dose of radiation that can be safely administered. Additionally, radiation pneumonitis can be one of the most severe complications of total body radiation therapy.

Imaging plays a central role in the follow-up of patients treated for lung carcinoma. Computed tomography (CT) and chest radiography are used to assess for recurrent neoplasm and response to therapy, and they help identify and characterize complications related to surgery, radiation therapy, and systemic chemotherapy. The imaging features of radiation-induced lung injury can be fairly specific, and recognition of these findings can aid in distinguishing recurrent neoplasm or infection from radiation pneumonitis or radiation fibrosis.

The incidence of radiation-induced lung disease ranges greatly among reported series. One review of 18 studies comprising 5,534 patients reported before 1992 found symptomatic radiation pneumonitis in 7 % (range 1–34 %) following radiation therapy for mesothelioma, Hodgkin lymphoma, or carcinoma of the lung or the breast [1]. Another review of 24 series comprising 1,911 patients found the incidence of symptomatic pneumonitis to be 8 % [2]. However, differences in treatment protocols, variable follow-up intervals, and different criteria defining radiation-induced lung injury prevent direct comparisons among institutions. Moreover, patient deaths early after treatment and before radiation injury has become symptomatic may lead to an underestimation of its true incidence [1].

Predisposing Factors

Factors that increase the risk of radiation-induced lung injury include the technique of delivering the radiation, previous radiation treatment, concurrent chemotherapy, corticosteroid withdrawal, preexisting lung disease, and variations in genetic susceptibility.

The total dose of radiation absorbed is a critical factor. The dose–response relationship is stronger for radiation fibrosis than for acute radiation pneumonitis. With total doses up to 30 Gy, symptomatic lung injury is rare, whereas it is

J.P. Kanne, M.D. (✉)
Department of Radiology, University of Wisconsin School of Medicine and Public Health,
600 Highland Ave, MC 3252, Madison, WI 53792, USA
e-mail: kanne@wisc.edu

J.D. Godwin, M.D.
Department of Radiology, University of Washington, Seattle, WA, USA
e-mail: godwin@u.washington.edu

J.G. Ravenel (ed.), *Lung Cancer Imaging*, Contemporary Medical Imaging,
DOI 10.1007/978-1-60761-620-7_13,

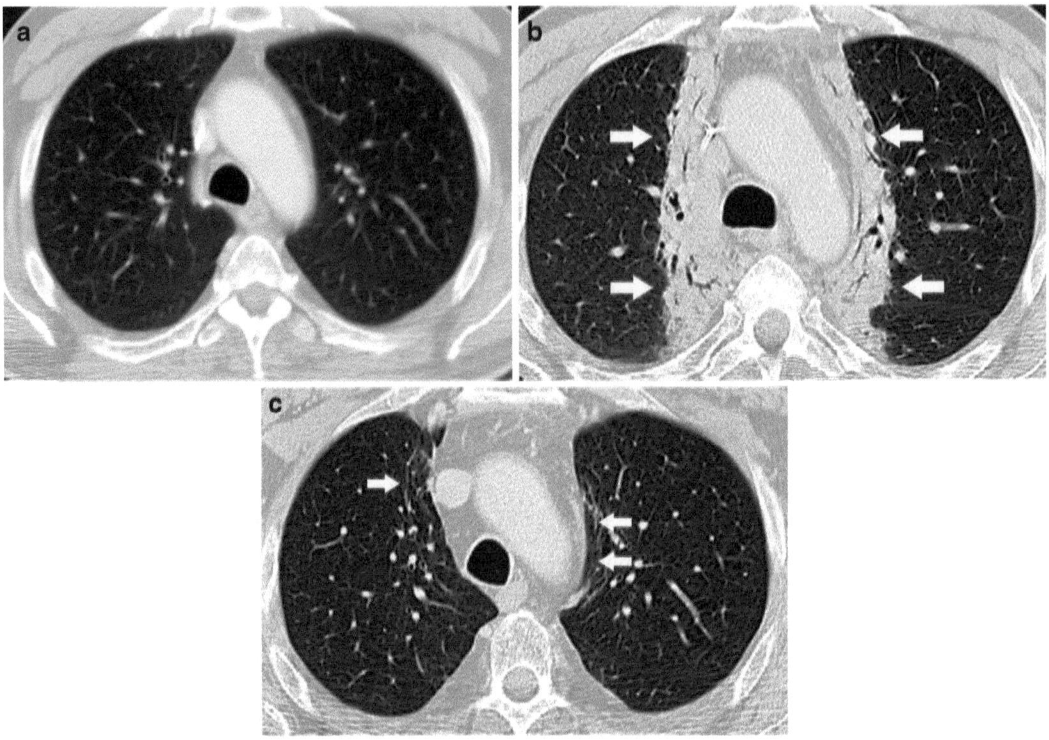

Fig. 13.1 Recall radiation pneumonitis developing after chemotherapy in a patient who received mediastinal radiation 2 years earlier for non-Hodgkin lymphoma. (**a**) Image from CT scan before chemotherapy shows normal lung. (**b**) Image from CT scan obtained 2 weeks after chemotherapy depicts consolidation in both upper lobes with sharp lateral margins (*arrows*) corresponding to the radiation field. (**c**) CT scan image 4 weeks after chemotherapy shows partial clearing with residual reticulation (*arrows*)

common from 35 to 40 Gy and almost inevitable above that [3]. Fractionation of doses, as is the usual practice, greatly reduces the biologic impact of radiation therapy and is the dominant factor in determining the late effects of radiation [1].

The volume of lung tissue irradiated is related to the size of the radiation field, and lung injury mostly occurs within this field. In the treatment of lung carcinoma, about 25–33 % of the lung is usually included in the field. Sometimes a larger tumor requires a larger field. Whereas radiating the entirety of both lungs with 30 Gy or more is nearly always fatal [4], the same dose or even a higher one administered to a smaller portion of one lung may not cause symptoms.

Many chemotherapeutic agents are themselves toxic to the lungs. Certain cytotoxic drugs, such as vincristine, bleomycin, mitomycin, and cyclophosphamide, can accentuate the effects of radiation [5], sometimes resulting in a synergistic response, especially bleomycin [6]. Dactinomycin and doxorubicin, while not toxic to the lungs, also heighten the effects of radiation [7, 8]. "Recall" radiation pneumonitis is the recurrence of pneumonitis in a radiation field following the administration of doxorubicin or dactinomycin, even years after radiation therapy (Fig. 13.1) [8, 9].

Development of symptomatic radiation pneumonitis from occult radiation-induced lung injury following withdrawal of corticosteroid therapy after lung radiation has been described [4, 10, 11].

Finally, underlying lung disease may be an important factor in the clinical impact of radiation-induced lung injury. Emphysema, pneumoconiosis, and remote tuberculosis may promote radiation fibrosis. Other processes that result in increased mass of lung tissue per unit volume, such as consolidated pneumonia and asbestos exposure, may lead to increased lung injury as more tissue is included in the radiation field [4, 12]. However, other lung diseases, such as chronic bronchitis, do not promote radiation injury [13].

Pathology

Radiation pneumopathy is the pathologic term comprising radiation pneumonitis and radiation fibrosis [4]. During the first 24–48 h following radiation to the lungs, the lymphoid follicles degenerate. Bronchial mucosa becomes edematous and hyperemic with leukocytic infiltration of the bronchial wall.

Acute radiation pneumonitis develops 1–6 months following therapy and is characterized by thickening of the alveolar septa by edema and round cell infiltration, hyperplasia and desquamation of alveolar lining cells, fibrinous alveolar exudation leading to hyaline membrane formation, endothelial damage with engorgement and thrombus formation, and arteritis. A variable degree of interstitial and alveolar fibrosis may develop.

Radiation pneumonitis is an early inflammatory reaction characterized histologically by diffuse alveolar damage. Proteinaceous material accumulates in the alveolar air spaces, and hyaline membranes develop in the respiratory bronchioles and alveolar ducts. Initially, the interstitium of the lung becomes thickened by edema and capillary congestion followed by infiltrations by fibroblasts and deposition of loose connective tissue. The inflammatory cellular infiltrate is usually minimal. The type II pneumocytes become hyperplastic [14].

Radiation fibrosis consists primarily of fibrosis of the air spaces and interstitium. Elastic fibers are increased in number and are fragmented. Lung architecture becomes distorted. Proliferation of myofibroblasts and deposition of connective tissue lead to intimal thickening of blood vessels [15].

Clinical Features

Patients rarely have pulmonary symptoms immediately following radiation therapy to the chest. Radiation pneumonitis usually develops 1–3 months following completion of a course of radiation therapy, reflecting the low mitotic rate of cells in the lung parenchyma.

Symptoms may precede radiographic abnormalities [12]. Dyspnea is most common, and other symptoms include cough with or without blood-tinged sputum. Frank hemoptysis is rare. Fever is uncommon and is usually mild. One series of 29 patients with radiation pneumonitis reported dyspnea in 28 (93 %), cough in 17 (58 %), and fever in 2 (7 %) [16]. Patients often have a mild to moderate polymorphonuclear leukocytosis and an elevated erythrocyte sedimentation rate [1]. In general, the earlier the onset of symptoms, the more severe the injury and the more protracted the clinical course. When only a small volume of lung is damaged, symptoms may be absent. A larger volume of damage can lead to severe respiratory insufficiency, cor pulmonale, and even death [1].

Radiation fibrosis describes the clinical syndrome resulting from chronic radiation-induced lung damage and usually occurs 6–24 months following radiation therapy, with the fibrotic process usually stabilizing in 1 or 2 years. Patients need not have experienced acute pneumonitis, and some patients with radiographic evidence of radiation fibrosis are asymptomatic. When symptoms occur, dyspnea is the most common. Chronic pulmonary insufficiency can develop in cases of severe radiation fibrosis or with severe underlying pulmonary disease. Chronic right heart failure may ensue from chronic pulmonary arterial hypertension [10, 17].

Imaging

Radiography and CT are the primary imaging tools used to evaluate patients following radiation therapy. CT is more sensitive than chest radiography for depicting radiation-induced lung injury [18].

Radiation Pneumonitis and Fibrosis

Findings of acute radiation pneumonitis usually are evident on the chest radiograph about 8 weeks

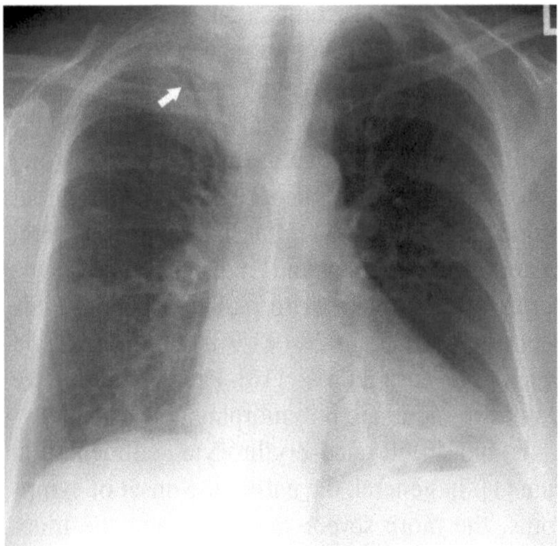

Fig. 13.2 Radiation pneumonitis. PA radiograph shows consolidation (*arrow*) in the right upper lobe

following completion of therapy with doses of 40 Gy (Fig. 13.2). With every 10 Gy increment in dose, radiographic abnormalities develop approximately 1 week earlier [19].

The abnormalities of radiation pneumonitis on the chest radiograph are usually limited to the radiation field. Sometimes the shape of the port is clearly visible with straight margins crossing normal anatomic boundaries such as pulmonary fissures. Whereas the areas of affected lung may be clearly depicted on the frontal radiograph, the abnormalities may extend uniformly from front to back on the lateral radiograph because of the orientation of the radiated lung in the sagittal plane (Fig. 13.3).

The earliest radiographic manifestations of acute radiation pneumonitis on the chest radiograph include a diffuse haze in the irradiated lung with indistinctness of the pulmonary vessels [20, 21]. Patchy lung consolidation may develop, becoming more confluent. Volume loss is common, presumably the result of surfactant depletion and resultant atelectasis. Pleural effusion is uncommon [22], but a small effusion is sometimes detected on CT.

CT can demonstrate acute radiation pneumonitis several weeks before it becomes visible on radiographs [23]. Patchy ground-glass opacity and denser consolidation develop in the radiation field and become more confluent over time (Fig. 13.4).

As the acute radiation-induced lung injury gradually progresses to radiation fibrosis, the abnormalities change on both CT scans and chest radiographs. On the chest radiograph, the affected lung loses volume, and the normal bronchovascular architecture becomes obliterated (Fig. 13.5). Fibrotic bands often extend from the periphery of the affected lung to the hilum. In milder cases of radiation fibrosis, the only radiographic manifestations may be mild elevation of one or both hila, retraction of pulmonary vessels, or pleural thickening (Fig. 13.6) [19]. CT shows dense consolidation or bands of fibrosis conforming to the radiation field, with associated volume loss, architectural distortion, and traction bronchiectasis.

Occasionally, patchy lung consolidation may develop outside the radiation port and can involve both lungs, usually 6 weeks to 10 months following completion of therapy. Biopsy in some cases has shown organizing pneumonia [24, 25].

Three-dimensional (3D) conformal and intensity-modulated radiation therapy (IMRT), two forms of stereotactic body radiation therapy (SBRT), are techniques that permit delivery of higher doses to the target lesion while minimizing injury to adjacent tissue. Both use computer analysis of 3D imaging data sets, usually helical CT, to plan and deliver radiation therapy [26–28]. Because of the numerous overlapping radiation ports employed by these techniques, the radiographic and CT appearances of radiation-induced lung injury may be unusual (Fig. 13.7).

Koenig et al. [29] described three patterns of radiation fibrosis on CT following 3D conformal therapy in a series of 19 patients. Five patients (26.3 %) had radiation fibrosis similar to that occurring with conventional therapy. Mass-like fibrosis at the site of the original tumor occurred in 8 patients (42.1 %), and linear scar developed at the site of the irradiated tumor in 6 patients (31.6 %).

Kimura et al. [30], in a study of 45 patients with 52 lung cancers, described three similar patterns of radiation fibrosis, with 32 lesions (61.5 %) having a modified conventional pattern,

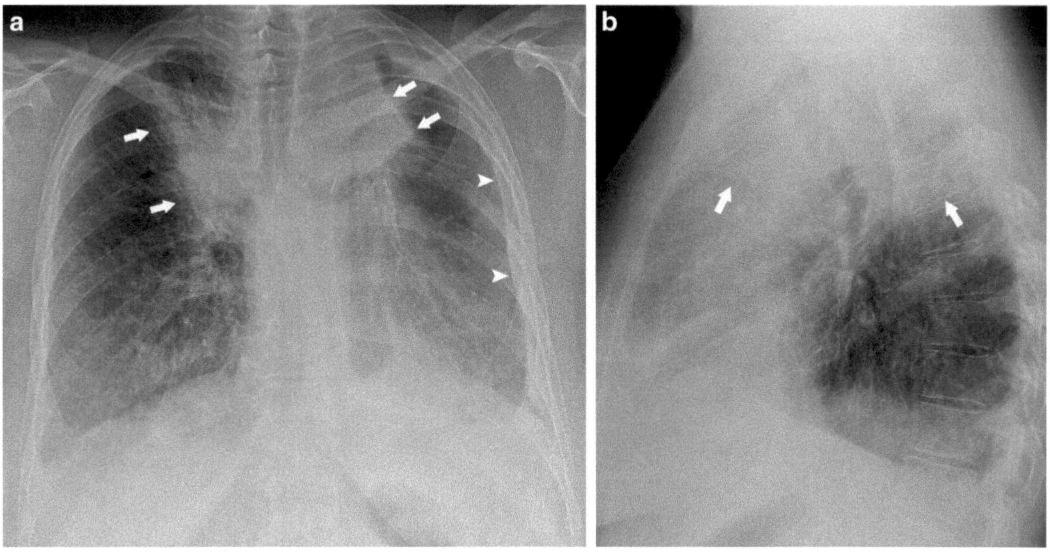

Fig. 13.3 Bilateral radiation fibrosis. (**a**) PA chest radiograph shows extensive bilateral fibrosis with sharp lateral margins (*arrows*). Traction from this lung fibrosis has caused thickening of the extrapleural fat stripe (*arrowheads*) lateral to the left lung. (**b**) Lateral chest radiograph depicts upper lung fibrosis with sharp inferior margins (*arrows*)

9 (17.3 %) having mass-like fibrosis, and 11 (21.2 %) having a scar-like pattern. Additionally, they reported five patterns of acute radiation pneumonitis on CT. Twenty lesions (38.5 %) had diffuse consolidation, 8 (15.4 %) had patchy consolidation and ground-glass opacity, 6 (11.5 %) had diffuse ground-glass opacity, 1 (2.0 %) had patchy ground-glass opacity, and 17 (32.6 %) had no visible abnormality. Ten of the 17 (58.8 %) lesions showing no evidence of acute radiation pneumonitis went on to develop the scar-like pattern of radiation fibrosis. Two patients with a scar-like pattern of radiation fibrosis and two patients with a mass-like pattern of radiation fibrosis had local recurrences of carcinoma characterized by increasing size of the lung abnormality.

In the first month following SBRT, the lung appears normal on CT. About 3–6 months after SBRT, diffuse or patchy lung consolidation in the high-dose region and diffuse or patchy ground-glass opacity in the low-dose region may develop, reflecting acute radiation pneumonitis. About 6–9 months after SBRT, acute radiation pneumonitis manifesting as diffuse or patchy lung consolidation may progress into more solid consolidation as radiation fibrosis ensues. In the absence of tumor recurrence (Fig. 13.8), these abnormalities will stabilize 1 or 2 years after SBRT.

Other Complications

Pulmonary Necrosis

Pulmonary necrosis is an uncommon, severe, late complication of adjuvant radiation therapy following surgery for lung carcinoma. It occurs after treatment with high doses of radiation, and a bronchopleural fistula can develop [31].

Organizing Pneumonia

Organizing pneumonia following radiation therapy has been described in patients receiving adjuvant therapy for breast carcinoma [31]. Initially consolidation or ground-glass opacity develops subpleurally in irradiated lung and then progresses in a characteristic migratory pattern to areas of nonirradiated lung (Fig. 13.9). Only two cases of organizing pneumonia following radiation therapy for lung carcinoma have been reported [32, 33]. Patients usually present with nonproductive cough,

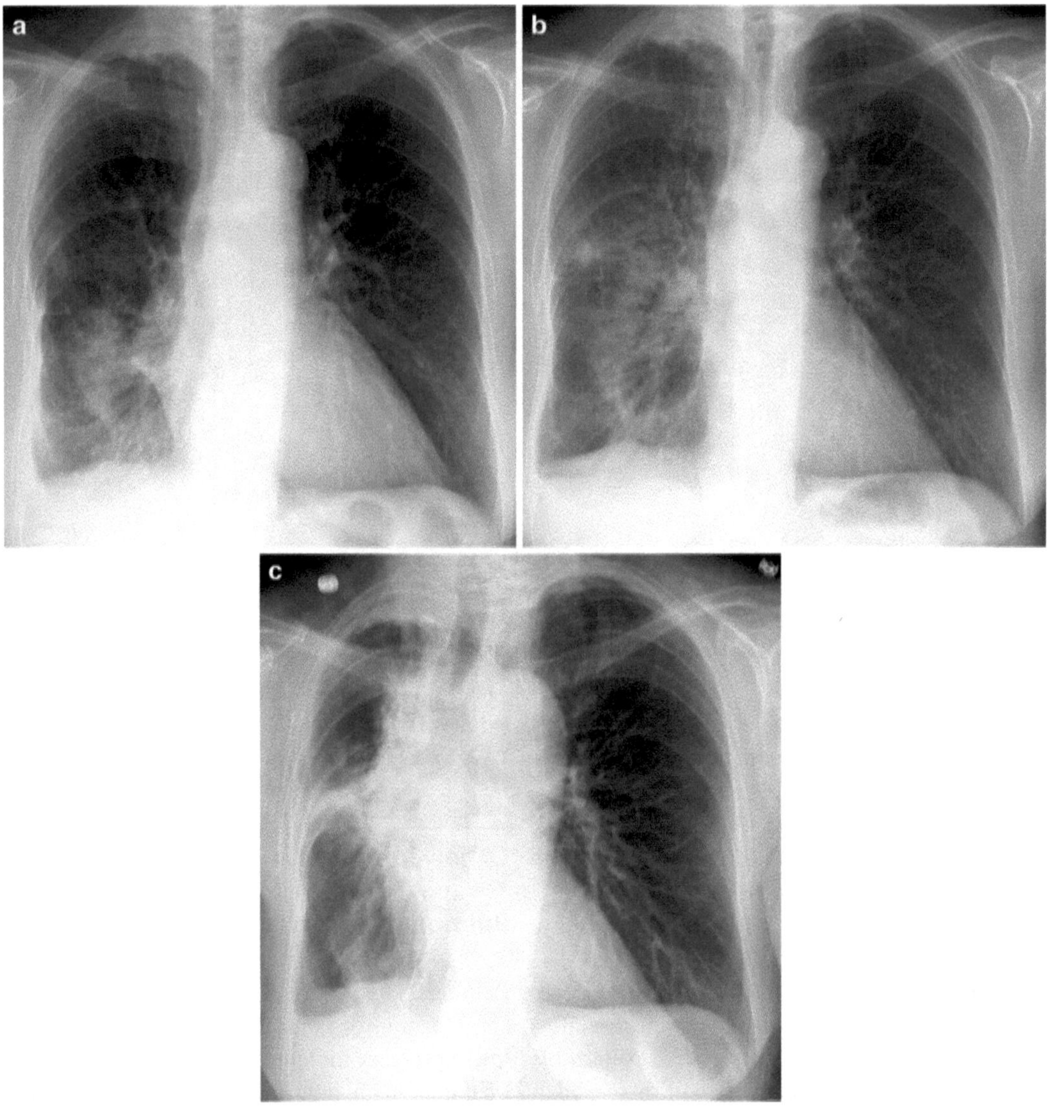

Fig. 13.4 Progressive radiation fibrosis in a patient with lung carcinoma. (**a–c**) Sequential PA chest radiographs over a 1-year period show progressive radiation fibrosis in the right lung

mild dyspnea, and low-grade fever and symptoms and radiographic abnormalities respond well to corticosteroid therapy.

Bronchial Stenosis

Direct bronchial injury occurs sporadically following both external beam radiation therapy and endobronchial brachytherapy for lung carcinoma. Following high-dose-rate endobronchial radiation therapy, approximately 10 % of patients developed bronchial stenosis (Fig. 13.10) [34]. One series of 103 patients treated twice daily with doses ranging from 70.8 to 86.4 Gy had rates of bronchial stenosis of 7 % at 1 year and 38 % at 4 years. Lower doses (74 Gy) had rates of 4 % and higher (86 Gy) had 25 % [35].

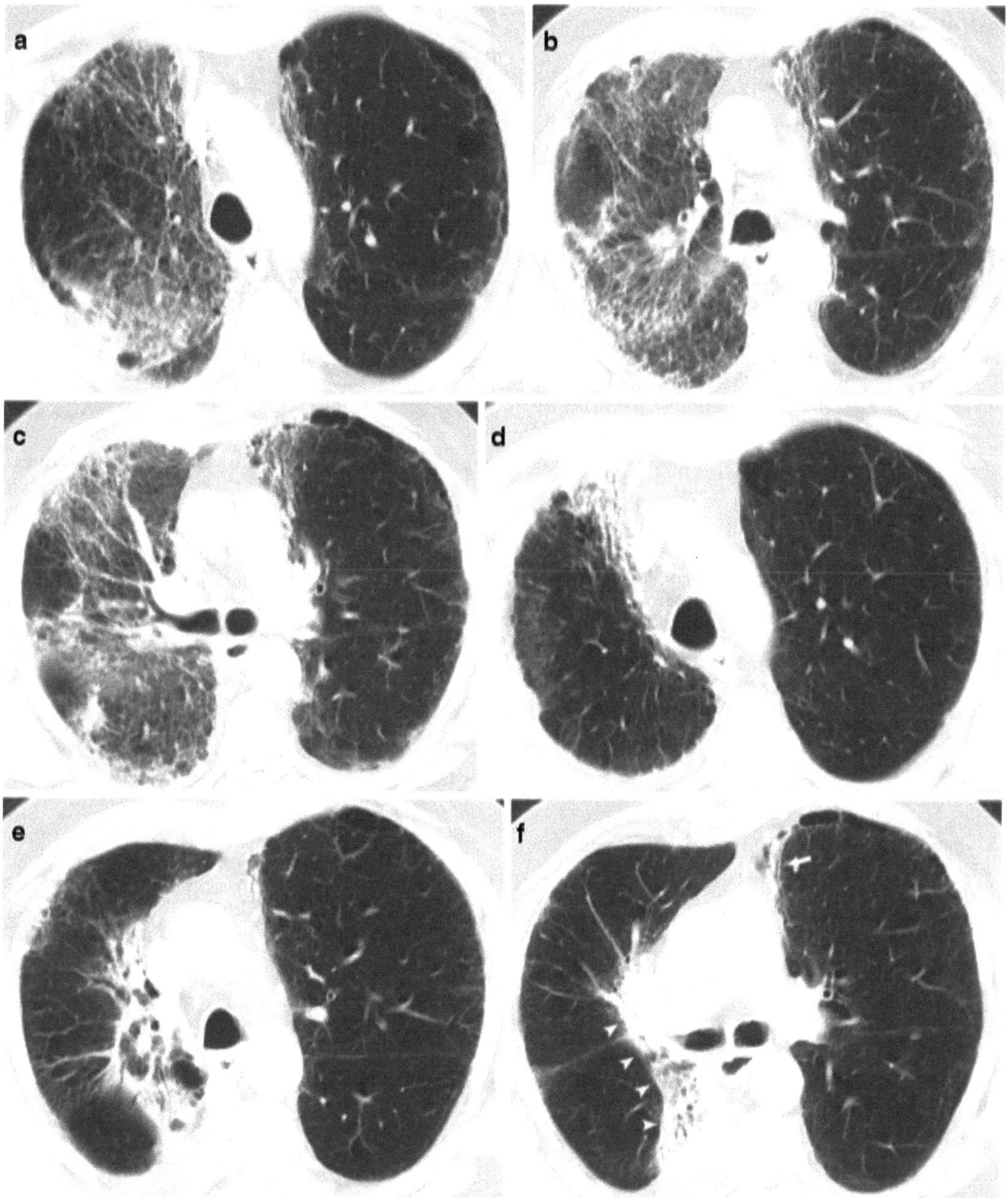

Fig. 13.5 Progressive radiation pneumonitis in a patient with lung carcinoma. (**a–c**) Images from CT scan show patchy ground-glass opacity and reticulation predominantly in the right lung. (**d–f**) Images from CT scan 6 months later show development of consolidation in the medial right lung with a sharp lateral margin crossing the major fissure (*arrowheads*). Mild consolidation has developed anteriorly in the left upper lobe (*arrow*). Ground-glass opacity has resolved

Pleural Effusion

A small pleural effusion may develop following radiation therapy, usually in conjunction with acute radiation pneumonitis and resolving as radiation pneumonitis resolves. Persistent or enlarging pleural effusion despite resolution of pneumonitis is suggestive recurrence or metastasis of tumor.

Esophageal Injury

The esophagus may be within the radiation field in patients being treated for lung cancer. Esophageal dysmotility or stricture may develop [36]. Dysmotility usually occurs 4–12 weeks following radiation therapy [37]. Strictures, while uncommon, usually develop within 3–18 months, most around 6 months. On esophagography, radiation-induced strictures usually have smooth, tapered margins but can be irregular (Fig. 13.11). A total dose of 50 Gy or more is usually required to cause stricture, and the rates increase with dose. Moreover, concomitant treatment with systemic chemotherapeutic agents, particularly doxorubicin, increases the risk of stricture formation even

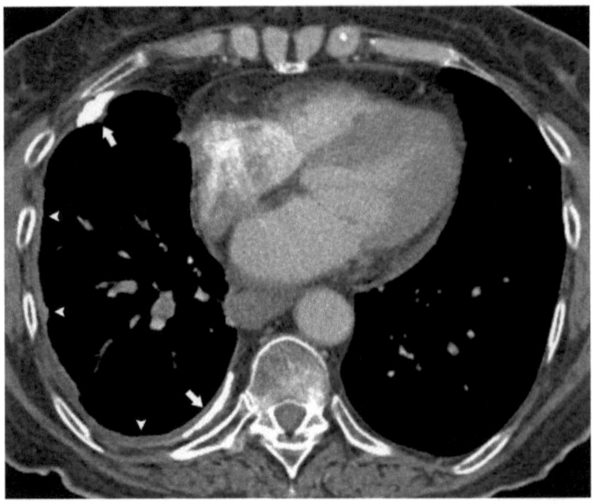

Fig. 13.6 Radiation-induced pleural thickening. Contrast-enhanced CT scan shows diffuse right pleural thickening (*arrowheads*) with calcification (*arrows*)

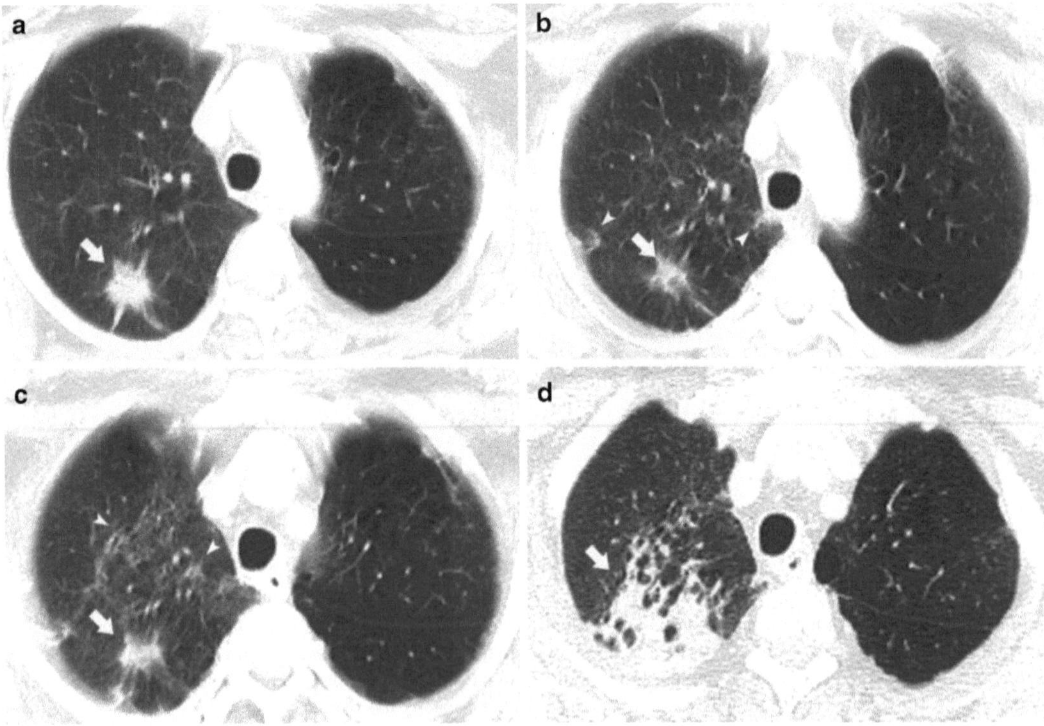

Fig. 13.7 Progressive radiation injury following stereotactic body radiation therapy (SBRT) for lung carcinoma. (**a**) Pretreatment CT scan shows spiculated right upper lobe nodule (*arrow*). (**b**) CT scan image 1 month following radiation therapy shows decrease in size of the right upper lobe nodule (*arrow*). Mild patchy lung consolidation has developed (*arrowheads*). (**c**) CT scan image 2 months following radiation therapy shows persistence of the right upper lobe nodule (*arrow*) and new patchy reticulation (*arrowheads*). (**d**) CT scan image 4 months following radiation therapy depicts extensive consolidation in the right upper lobe (*arrow*), obscuring the nodule

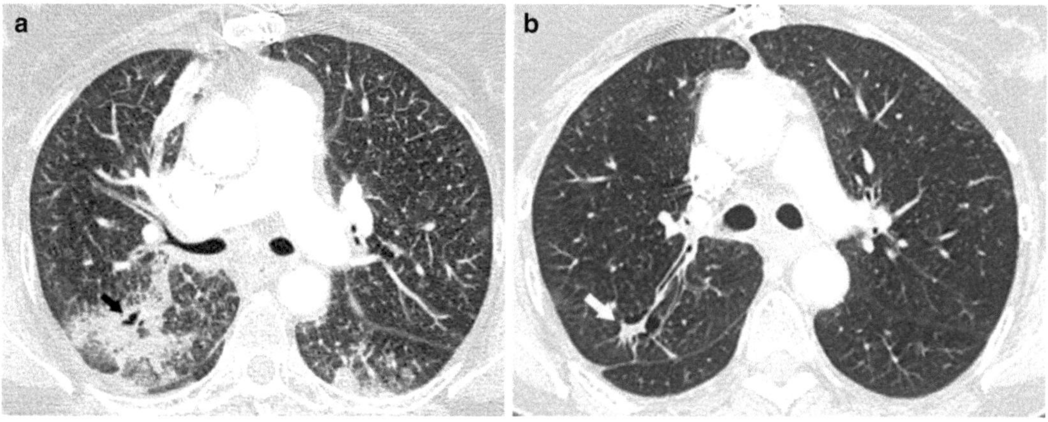

Fig. 13.8 Radiation pneumonitis and fibrosis following SBRT. (**a**) CT image shows radiation pneumonitis in the posterior segment of the right upper lobe surrounding and obscuring the lung carcinoma, which has central cavitation (*arrow*). (**b**) CT image 6 months later shows residual fibrosis (*arrow*)

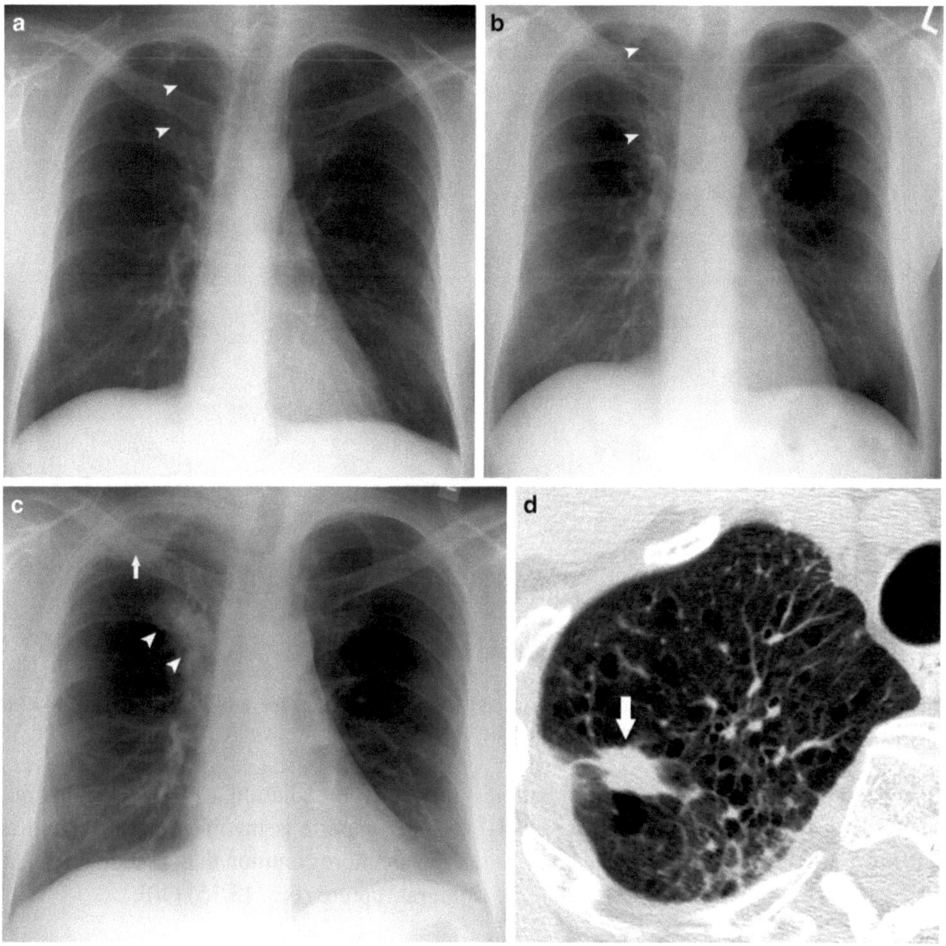

Fig. 13.9 Recurrent neoplasm following radiation therapy. (**a**) PA chest radiograph 1 year after radiation therapy shows mild reticulation in the right upper lobe (*arrowheads*). (**b**) PA chest radiograph 1 year later shows increased right upper lobe consolidation and reticulation (*arrowheads*). (**c**) PA chest radiograph 18 months after (**b**) shows new right upper lobe nodule (*arrow*) and right hilar lymphadenopathy (*arrowheads*). (**d**) CT scan confirms right upper lobe spiculated nodule (*arrow*), proven to represent recurrent lung carcinoma

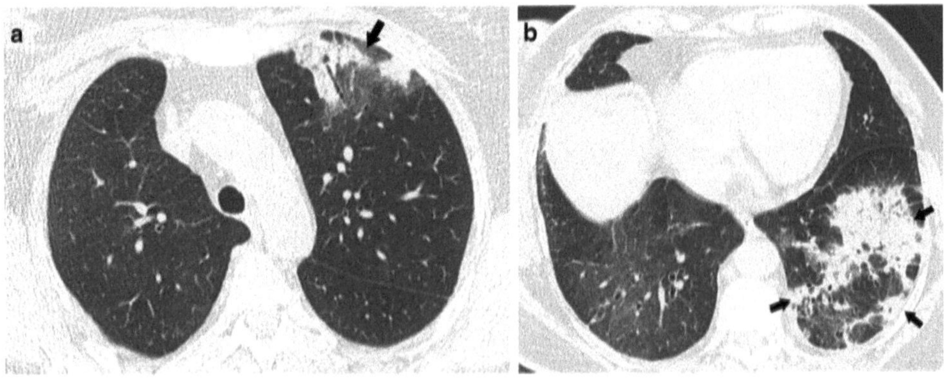

Fig. 13.10 Organizing pneumonia reaction following radiation therapy. (**a**) CT image at the level of the aortic arch shows perilobular and peribronchial consolidation in the left upper lobe (*arrow*). (**b**) CT image more caudad depicts patchy perilobular and peribronchial consolidation in the left lower lobe (*arrows*)

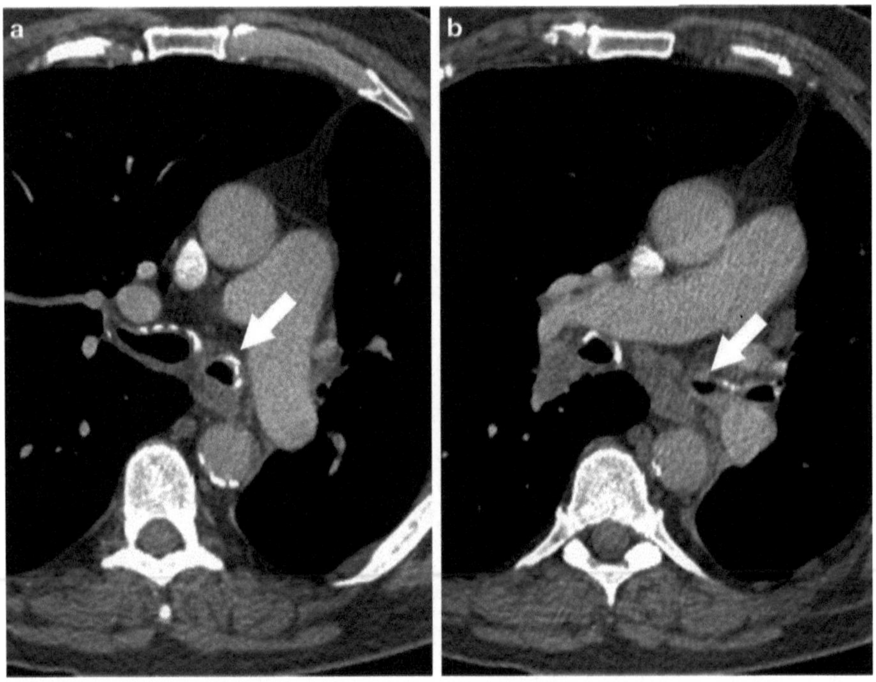

Fig. 13.11 Bronchial stenosis following mediastinal and left hilar radiation for lung carcinoma. (**a**, **b**) Contrast-enhanced CT scan images show narrowing of the left main bronchus (*arrows*) with mild mural thickening

with low radiation dose [38]. Severe radiation esophagitis (Fig. 13.12) may lead to fistula development (Fig. 13.13).

Vascular Injury

Stenosis of the superior vena cava is a rare complication developing years after radiation fibrosis (Fig. 13.14) [39]. Larger arteries can also be injured from radiation, usually when the mediastinum or axilla is involved. Stenosis and occlusion are more common than pseudoaneurysm and mural rupture (Fig. 13.15) [40].

Second Primary Neoplasm

A second primary neoplasm can arise as the result of radiation, usually within the radiation

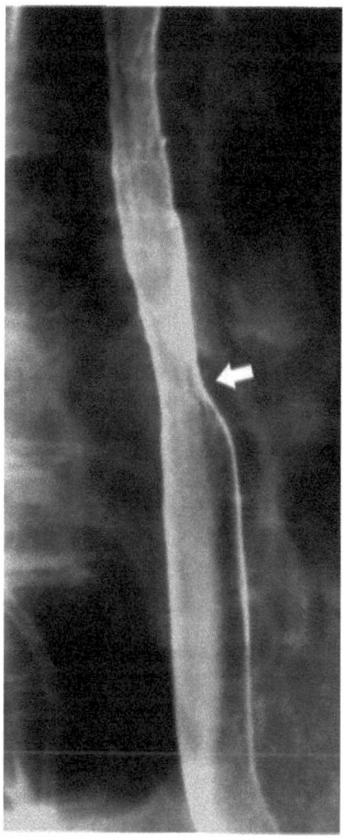

Fig. 13.12 Image from double-contrast esophagram shows long esophageal stricture with smooth transition to normal esophagus (*arrow*) (courtesy of Charles A. Rohrmann, M.D. Seattle, WA)

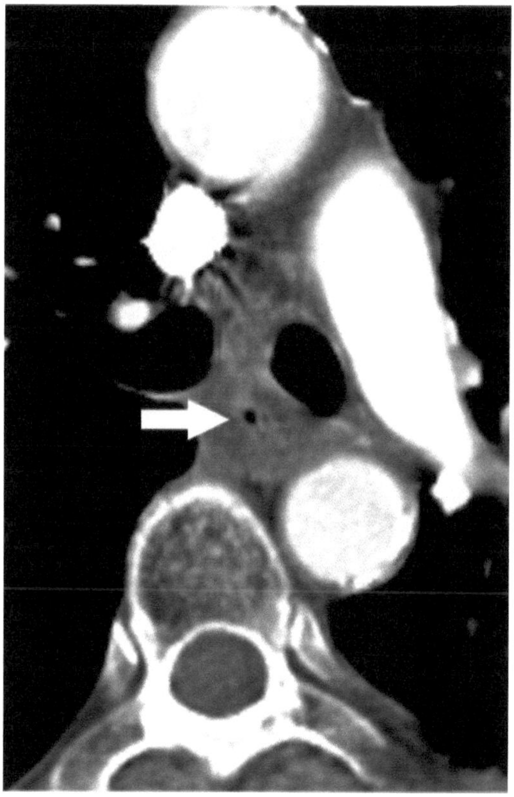

Fig. 13.13 Radiation esophagitis following mediastinal radiation for lung carcinoma. Contrast-enhanced CT image shows marked esophageal mural thickening with luminal narrowing (*arrow*)

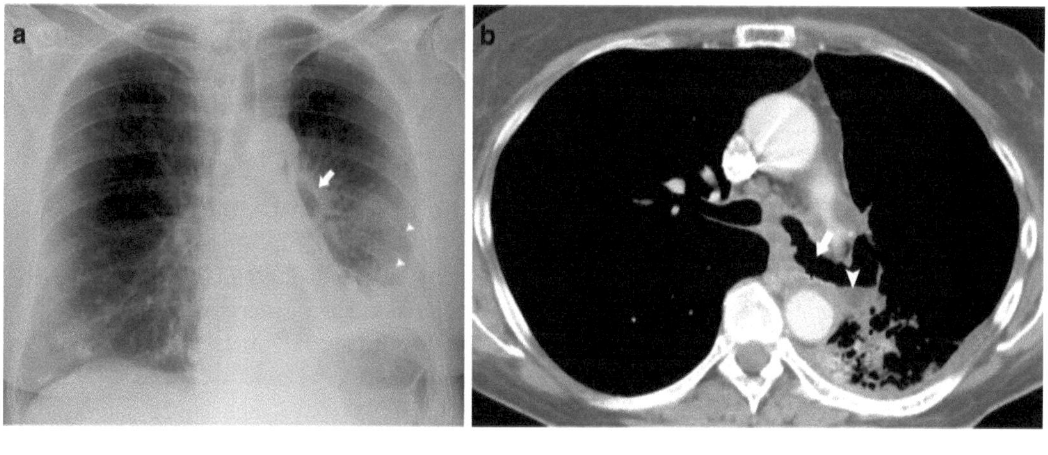

Fig. 13.14 Esophagobronchial fistula following radiation to the left chest for lung carcinoma. (**a**) AP chest radiograph shows abnormal gas collection (*arrow*) adjacent to the left hilum surrounded by patchy lung consolidation. Left pleural thickening is present (*arrowheads*). (**b**) Image from contrast-enhanced CT scan shows fistula (*arrow*) between left main bronchus and esophagus with contained fluid collection (*arrowhead*). Left lower lobe consolidation is present

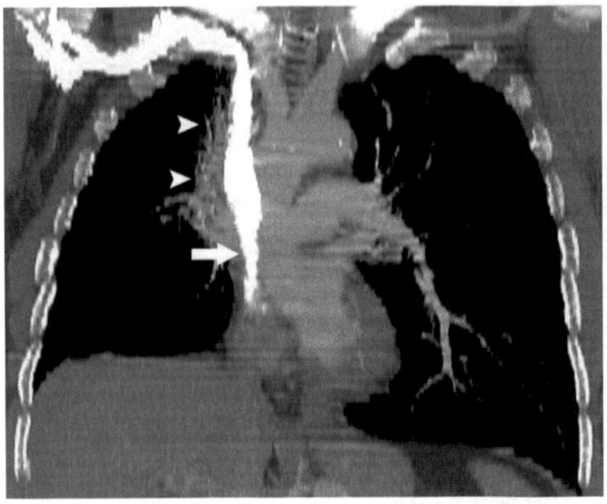

Fig. 13.15 Superior vena cava stenosis following radiation therapy for lung carcinoma. Coronal reconstruction from contrast-enhanced CT scan shows stenosis of the lower superior vena cava (*arrow*) and radiation fibrosis in the medial right upper lung (*arrowheads*)

field. The latency period is usually long, even greater than 10 years, with risk increasing over time. The major risk factors promoting a secondary tumor include age at treatment (highest for radiation during childhood), type of tissue in the field, and total dose [41]. Lower doses (<30 Gy) are associated with neoplasms of the central nervous system and thyroid, whereas higher doses are associated with sarcomas of the bone (Fig. 13.16) and soft tissues. Patients with genetic predispositions to malignancy and those treated with alkylating agents are also at increased risk of developing a second malignancy. Mesothelioma may occur anywhere from 5 to over 40 years following radiation therapy (median 13.5 years). Combined therapy using alkylating agents may also increase the risk of second malignancy.

Bones

Radiation damage to bones in the field may occur. Radiographic manifestations include atrophy, osteoporosis, and fragmentation (Fig. 13.17). Fractures may fail to heal, and osteonecrotic fragments usually become sclerotic. Dystrophic calcification may develop in the adjacent soft tissues [42–44].

Heart and Pericardium

Mediastinal radiation can affect the heart, leading to myocardial fibrosis or coronary arteritis with accelerated atherosclerosis [45–48]. The pericardium is more often affected than the heart itself. Pericarditis occurs in 2–6 % of patients following radiation to the mediastinum, almost always with doses over 40 Gy [49]. Typically, pericardial effusion develops 12–18 months after the completion of radiation. Chronic pericarditis occurs less commonly and usually more than 4 years after radiation therapy. Constrictive physiology develops in 15–20 % of these patients.

Other Imaging Modalities

Ventilation–Perfusion Scanning

Lung scans using 99m-technetium (^{99m}Tc)-labeled macroalbumin aggregates show decreased perfusion in lung tissue in the radiation field, and sometimes outside the field as well [18]. On CT scans, lung vessels peripheral to the radiation field may be narrowed and attenuated, presumably the result of diminished perfusion because of radiation-induced vasculitis and sclerosis. Single-photon emission computed tomography (SPECT) imaging can be used to generate a three-dimensional map of perfusion and ventilation defects. Perfusion defects are more common than ventilation defects.

Magnetic Resonance Imaging

The utility of magnetic resonance imaging (MRI) to image the lungs after radiation is limited. Radiation fibrosis has low signal intensity on both T1- and T2-weighted sequences [50], and most neoplasms have high signal intensity on T2-weighted images. However, acute radiation pneumonitis, pneumonia, and pulmonary hemorrhage can have signal intensity characteristics similar to neoplasm and can be mistaken for recurrent tumor. Enhancement following

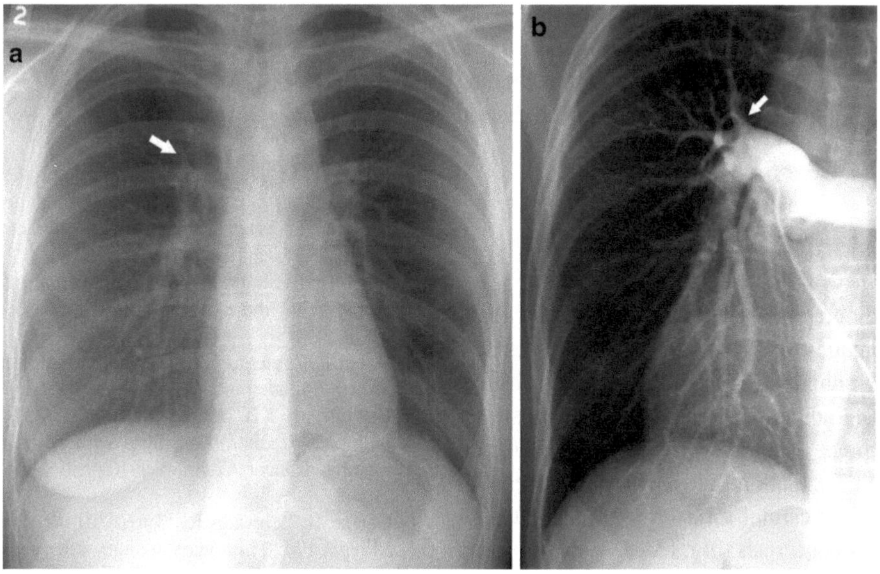

Fig. 13.16 Radiation arteritis. (**a**) PA radiograph shows attenuation of the right upper lobe pulmonary artery (*arrow*) with a paucity of vessels in the periphery. (**b**) Image from pulmonary angiogram confirms right upper lobe pulmonary artery stenosis (*arrow*) and diminished vascularity

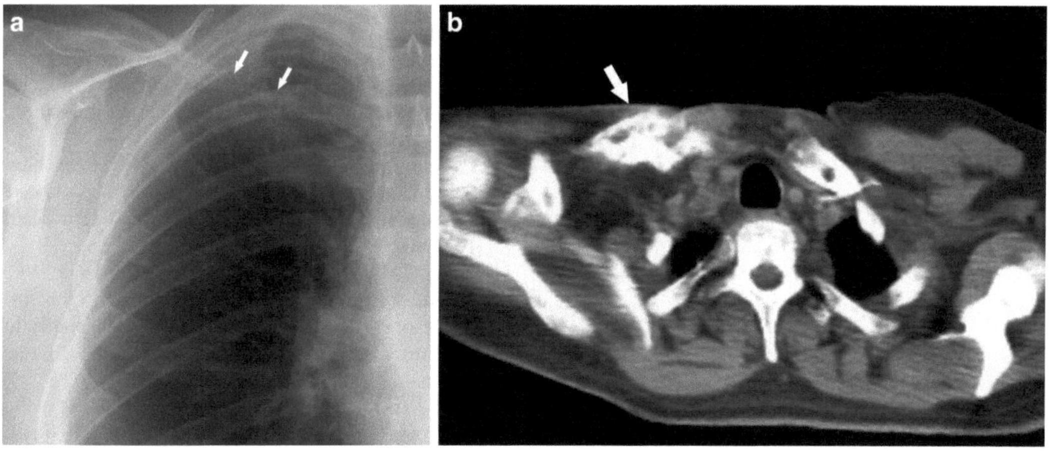

Fig. 13.17 Osteosarcoma developing 20 years after radiation therapy for Hodgkin lymphoma. (**a**) Coned-down PA chest radiograph shows a lytic lesion in the mid right clavicle (*arrows*). (**b**) Image from contrast-enhanced CT depicts a right clavicular mass with osteoid matrix (*arrow*)

intravenous administration of gadolinium–DTPA can occur with both radiation fibrosis and recurrent tumor [51].

FDG-PET

While most commonly used in the pretreatment evaluation of lung carcinoma, 2-[18F] fluoro-2-deoxy-D-glucose (^{18}FDG) positron emission tomography (PET) may also play a role in imaging patients following radiation therapy for lung carcinoma. ^{18}FDG-PET is more accurate than chest radiograph, CT, and MRI for distinguishing persistent or recurrent tumor from necrotic tumor and radiation fibrosis. Reported sensitivities and specificities range from 97 to 100 % and 62 to 100 %, respectively, with reported accuracies of 78 to 98 % [52–59]. Because acute radiation pneumonitis can result in a false-positive study, [18]FDG-PET should not be obtained until 4–5 months after completion of radiation therapy [53].

Conclusion

Chest radiography and CT are the primary imaging techniques for demonstrating the thoracic effects of radiation therapy. CT is more sensitive than chest radiography and better demonstrates complications such as early or mild radiation pneumonitis, radiation fibrosis, bronchial stenosis, pleural or pericardial effusion, vascular attenuation, and osteonecrosis (Fig. 13.18). Other imaging techniques, such as [18]FDG-PET, ventilation–perfusion scanning, and MRI, have evolving roles in assessing the pulmonary effects of radiation.

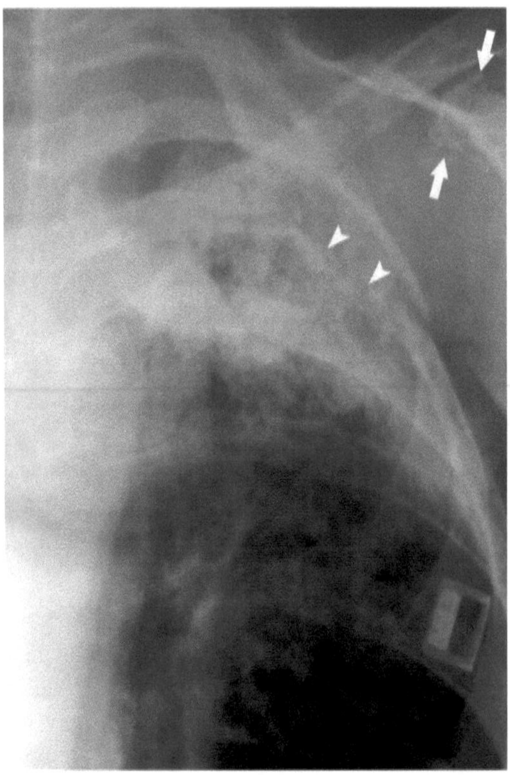

Fig. 13.18 Radiation osteonecrosis. Coned-down PA chest radiograph shows left upper lobe radiation fibrosis. The coracoid process of the scapula (*arrows*) and left fourth rib (*arrowheads*) are fragmented, and the other bones in the radiation field are sclerotic

References

1. Movsas B, Raffin TA, Epstein AH, Link Jr CJ. Pulmonary radiation injury. Chest. 1997;111(4):1061–76.
2. Roach III M, Gandara DR, Yuo HS, et al. Radiation pneumonitis following combined modality therapy for lung cancer: analysis of prognostic factors. J Clin Oncol. 1995;13(10):2606–12.
3. Libshitz HI, Southard ME. Complications of radiation therapy: the thorax. Semin Roentgenol. 1974;9(1):41–9.
4. Rubin P, Casseratt GW. Clinical radiation pathology. 3rd ed. Philadelphia: WB Saunders; 1968. p. 423–70.
5. Lamoureux KB. Increased clinically symptomatic pulmonary radiation reactions with adjuvant chemotherapy. Cancer Chemother Rep. 1974;58(5 Pt 1):705–8.
6. Catane R, Schwade JG, Turrisi III AT, Webber BL, Muggia FM. Pulmonary toxicity after radiation and bleomycin: a review. Int J Radiat Oncol Biol Phys. 1979;5(9):1513–8.
7. Cassady JR, Richter MP, Piro AJ, Jaffe N. Radiation-adriamycin interactions: preliminary clinical observations. Cancer. 1975;36(3):946–9.
8. Ma LD, Taylor GA, Wharam MD, Wiley JM. "Recall" pneumonitis: adriamycin potentiation of radiation pneumonitis in two children. Radiology. 1993;187(2):465–7.
9. Son YH, Kapp DS. Esophago-pulmonary toxicity from concomitant use of adriamycin and irradiation. Conn Med. 1981;45(12):755–9.
10. Castellino RA, Glatstein E, Turbow MM, Rosenberg S, Kaplan HS. Latent radiation injury of lungs or heart activated by steroid withdrawal. Ann Intern Med. 1974;80(5):593–9.
11. Parris TM, Knight JG, Hess CE, Constable WC. Severe radiation pneumonitis precipitated by withdrawal of corticosteroids: a diagnostic and therapeutic dilemma. AJR Am J Roentgenol. 1979;132(2):284–6.
12. Fried JR, Goldberg H. Post-irradiation changes in the lungs and thorax. AJR Am J Roentgenol. 1940;43:877–95.
13. Gillam PMS, Heaf PJD, Hoffbrand BI, Hilton G. Chronic bronchitis and radiotherapy of the lung. Lancet. 1964;1(7348):1245–8.
14. Fajardo LF, Berthrong M. Radiation injury in surgical pathology. Part I. Am J Surg Pathol. 1978;2(2):159–99.
15. Wilkinson MJ, Maclennan KA. Vascular changes in irradiated lungs: a morphometric study. J Pathol. 1989;158(3):229–32.
16. Perry MC, Eaton WL, Propert KJ, et al. Chemotherapy with or without radiation therapy in limited small-cell carcinoma of the lung. N Engl J Med. 1987;316(15):912–8.
17. Stone DJ, Schwartz MJ, Green RA. Fatal pulmonary insufficiency due to radiation effect upon the lung. Am J Med. 1956;21(2):211–26.

18. Bell J, McGivern D, Bullimore J, Hill J, Davies ER, Goddard P. Diagnostic imaging of post-irradiation changes in the chest. Clin Radiol. 1988;39(2):109–19.
19. Libshitz HI. Radiation changes in the lung. Semin Roentgenol. 1993;28(4):303–20.
20. Davis SD, Yankelevitz DF, Henschke CI. Radiation effects on the lung: clinical features, pathology, and imaging findings. AJR Am J Roentgenol. 1992;159:1157–64.
21. Logan PM. Thoracic manifestations of external beam radiotherapy. AJR Am J Roentgenol. 1998;171(3):569–77.
22. Bachman AL, Macken K. Pleural effusions following supervoltage radiation for breast carcinoma. Radiology. 1959;72(5):699–709.
23. Ikezoe J, Morimoto S, Takashima S, Takeuchi N, Arisawa J, Kozuka T. Acute radiation-induced pulmonary injury: computed tomography evaluation. Semin Ultrasound CT MR. 1990;11(5):409–16.
24. Crestani B, Valeyre D, Roden S, Wallaert B, Dalphin JC, Cordier JF. Bronchiolitis obliterans organizing pneumonia syndrome primed by radiation therapy to the breast. The Groupe d'Etudes et de Recherche sur les Maladies Orphelines Pulmonaires (GERM"O"P). Am J Respir Crit Care Med. 1998;158(6):1929–35.
25. Takigawa N, Segawa Y, Saeki T, et al. Bronchiolitis obliterans organizing pneumonia syndrome in breast-conserving therapy for early breast cancer: radiation-induced lung toxicity. Int J Radiat Oncol Biol Phys. 2000;48(3):751–5.
26. Glatstein E. Intensity-modulated radiation therapy: the inverse, the converse, and the perverse. Semin Radiat Oncol. 2002;12(3):272–81.
27. Leibel SA, Fuks Z, Zelefsky MJ, et al. Intensity-modulated radiotherapy. Cancer J. 2002;8(2):164–76.
28. Patel RR, Mehta M. Three-dimensional conformal radiotherapy for lung cancer: promises and pitfalls. Curr Oncol Rep. 2002;4(4):347–53.
29. Koenig TR, Munden RF, Erasmus JJ, et al. Radiation injury of the lung after three-dimensional conformal radiation therapy. AJR Am J Roentgenol. 2002;178(6):1383–8.
30. Kimura T, Matsuura K, Murakami Y, et al. CT appearance of radiation injury of the lung and clinical symptoms after stereotactic body radiation therapy (SBRT) for lung cancers: are patients with pulmonary emphysema also candidates for SBRT for lung cancers? Int J Radiat Oncol Biol Phys. 2006;66(2):483–91.
31. Mesurolle B, Qanadli SD, Merad M, et al. Unusual radiologic findings in the thorax after radiation therapy. Radiographics. 2000;20(1):67–81.
32. Hamanishi T, Morimatu T, Oida K, et al. [Occurrence of BOOP outside radiation field after radiation therapy for small cell lung cancer]. Nihon Kokyuki Gakkai Zasshi. 2001;39(9):683–8.
33. Iijima M, Sakahara H. [Radiation pneumonitis resembling bronchiolitis obliterans organizing pneumonia after postoperative irradiation for lung cancer: a case report]. Nihon Igaku Hoshasen Gakkai Zasshi. 2003;63(6):332–3.
34. Speiser BL, Spratling L. Radiation bronchitis and stenosis secondary to high dose rate endobronchial irradiation. Int J Radiat Oncol Biol Phys. 1993;25(4):589–97.
35. Miller KL, Shafman TD, Anscher MS, et al. Bronchial stenosis: an underreported complication of high-dose external beam radiotherapy for lung cancer? Int J Radiat Oncol Biol Phys. 2005;61(1):64–9.
36. Goldstein HM, Rogers LF, Fletcher GH, Dodd GD. Radiological manifestations of radiation-induced injury to the normal upper gastrointestinal tract. Radiology. 1975;117(1):135–40.
37. Lepke RA, Libshitz HI. Radiation-induced injury of the esophagus. Radiology. 1983;148(2):375–8.
38. Coia LR, Myerson RJ, Tepper JE. Late effects of radiation therapy on the gastrointestinal tract. Int J Radiat Oncol Biol Phys. 1995;31(5):1213–36.
39. Van Putten JW, Schlosser NJ, Vujaskovic Z, Leest AH, Groen HJ. Superior vena cava obstruction caused by radiation induced venous fibrosis. Thorax. 2000;55(3):245–6.
40. Fajardo LF, Lee A. Rupture of major vessels after radiation. Cancer. 1975;36(3):904–13.
41. Meadows AT. Second tumours. Eur J Cancer. 2001;37(16):2074–9; discussion 2079–81.
42. Delanian S, Lefaix JL. [Mature bone radionecrosis: from recent physiopathological knowledge to an innovative therapeutic action]. Cancer Radiother. 2002;6(1):1–9.
43. Howland WJ, Loeffler RK, Starchman DE, Johnson RG. Postirradiation atrophic changes of bone and related complications. Radiology. 1975;117(3 Pt 1):677–85.
44. Rouanet P, Fabre JM, Tica V, Anaf V, Jozwick M, Pujol H. Chest wall reconstruction for radionecrosis after breast carcinoma therapy. Ann Plast Surg. 1995;34(5):465–70.
45. Annest LS, Anderson RP, Li W, Hafermann MD. Coronary artery disease following mediastinal radiation therapy. J Thorac Cardiovasc Surg. 1983;85(5):257–63.
46. Corn BW, Trock BJ, Goodman RL. Irradiation-related ischemic heart disease. J Clin Oncol. 1990;8(4):741–50.
47. Gutierrez CA, Just-Viera JO. Clinical spectrum of radiation induced pericarditis. Am Surg. 1983;49(2):113–5.
48. Vallebona A. Cardiac damage following therapeutic chest irradiation. Importance, evaluation and treatment. Minerva Cardioangiol. 2000;48(3):79–87.
49. Applefeld MM, Cole JF, Pollock SH, et al. The late appearance of chronic pericardial disease in patients treated by radiotherapy for Hodgkin's disease. Ann Intern Med. 1981;94(3):338–41.
50. Glazer HS, Lee JK, Levitt RG, et al. Radiation fibrosis: differentiation from recurrent tumor by MR imaging. Radiology. 1985;156(3):721–6.
51. Werthmuller WC, Schiebler ML, Whaley RA, Mauro MA, McCartney WH. Gadolinium-DTPA enhancement of lung radiation fibrosis. J Comput Assist Tomogr. 1989;13(6):946–8.

52. Duhaylongsod FG, Lowe VJ, Patz EF Jr, Vaughn AL, Coleman RE, Wolfe WG. Detection of primary and recurrent lung cancer by means of F-18 fluorodeoxy-glucose positron emission tomography (FDG PET). J Thorac Cardiovasc Surg. 1995;110(1):130–9; discussion 139–40.
53. Frank A, Lefkowitz D, Jaeger S, et al. Decision logic for retreatment of asymptomatic lung cancer recurrence based on positron emission tomography findings. Int J Radiat Oncol Biol Phys. 1995;32(5): 1495–512.
54. Ichiya Y, Kuwabara Y, Otsuka M, et al. Assessment of response to cancer therapy using fluorine-18-fluorodeoxyglucose and positron emission tomography. J Nucl Med. 1991;32(9):1655–60.
55. Inoue T, Kim EE, Komaki R, et al. Detecting recurrent or residual lung cancer with FDG-PET. J Nucl Med. 1995;36(5):788–93.
56. Kim EE, Chung SK, Haynie TP, et al. Differentiation of residual or recurrent tumors from post-treatment changes with F-18 FDG PET. Radiographics. 1992;12(2):269–79.
57. Kubota K, Yamada S, Ishiwata K, et al. Evaluation of the treatment response of lung cancer with positron emission tomography and L-[methyl-11C]methionine: a preliminary study. Eur J Nucl Med. 1993;20(6): 495–501.
58. Kubota K, Yamada S, Ishiwata K, Ito M, Ido T. Positron emission tomography for treatment evaluation and recurrence detection compared with CT in long-term follow-up cases of lung cancer. Clin Nucl Med. 1992;17(11):877–81.
59. Patz Jr EF, Lowe VJ, Hoffman JM, Paine SS, Harris LK, Goodman PC. Persistent or recurrent bronchogenic carcinoma: detection with PET and 2-[F-18]-2-deoxy-d-glucose. Radiology. 1994;191(2):379–82.

Imaging Following Treatment of Lung Cancer

14

Hiren J. Mehta and James G. Ravenel

Unfortunately, only approximately 20% of patients with newly diagnosed lung cancer will have localized disease and will be candidates for potentially curative treatment [1]. Of these patients eligible for curative intent therapy, a small fraction of patients either will refuse the treatment or will not be eligible for curative intent therapy secondary to their underlying medical comorbidities and/or their performance status. The rest will receive either a curative intent surgical resection or a curative intent radiation or some combination of curative intent chemotherapy and radiation therapy [2]. Patients who receive curative intent therapy need adequate follow-up imaging. The purpose of imaging in these patients is twofold. First is to identify and manage complications related to the curative intent therapy itself. These include managing postoperative complications of surgery, chemotherapy, and radiation therapy. Second is to measure the tumor to document response and to detect recurrences of the primary lung cancer and/or development of a new primary lung cancer early enough to allow potentially curative retreatment [3]. In the ensuing sections we discuss the role of imaging after each modality of curative intent therapy. Issues related to follow-up for palliative therapy of lung cancer are not discussed in this chapter.

H.J. Mehta, M.D. (✉)
Division of Pulmonary Medicine, Medical University of South Carolina, Charleston, SC 29425, USA
e-mail: mehtah@musc.edu

J.G. Ravenel, M.D.
Department of Radiology, Medical University of South Carolina, 96 Jonathan Lucas St, Room 211, P. O. Box 250322, Charleston, SC 29425, USA

Follow-Up Imaging for Complications of Therapy

Surgery

Unfortunately, complications following lung resection are relatively common occurring in up to 1/3 of patients who undergo complete pneumonectomy [4]. While many of these can be routinely managed, some may be life threatening. Complications that may be directly attributable to the pulmonary resection itself include persistent air in the pleural space, bronchial dehiscence/bronchopleural fistula, chylothorax, and torsion of the mediastinum, all of which can manifest within the first 3–6 months after the surgery [5]. Other complications include hydrostatic edema, aspiration, and infection.

Air leaks are common following lobar resection and should resolve within 7 days as the remaining lung fills the thoracic cavity. Risk factors for an air leak lasting greater than 7 days and requiring prolonged thoracostomy tube drainage include low postoperative predicted lung function, pleural adhesions, and extent of lung resection [6]. Following complete pneumonectomy, gas can remain in the pleural space for up to 6 months after resection. As long as the gas fluid

J.G. Ravenel (ed.), *Lung Cancer Imaging*, Contemporary Medical Imaging,
DOI 10.1007/978-1-60761-620-7_14, © Springer Science+Business Media New York 2013

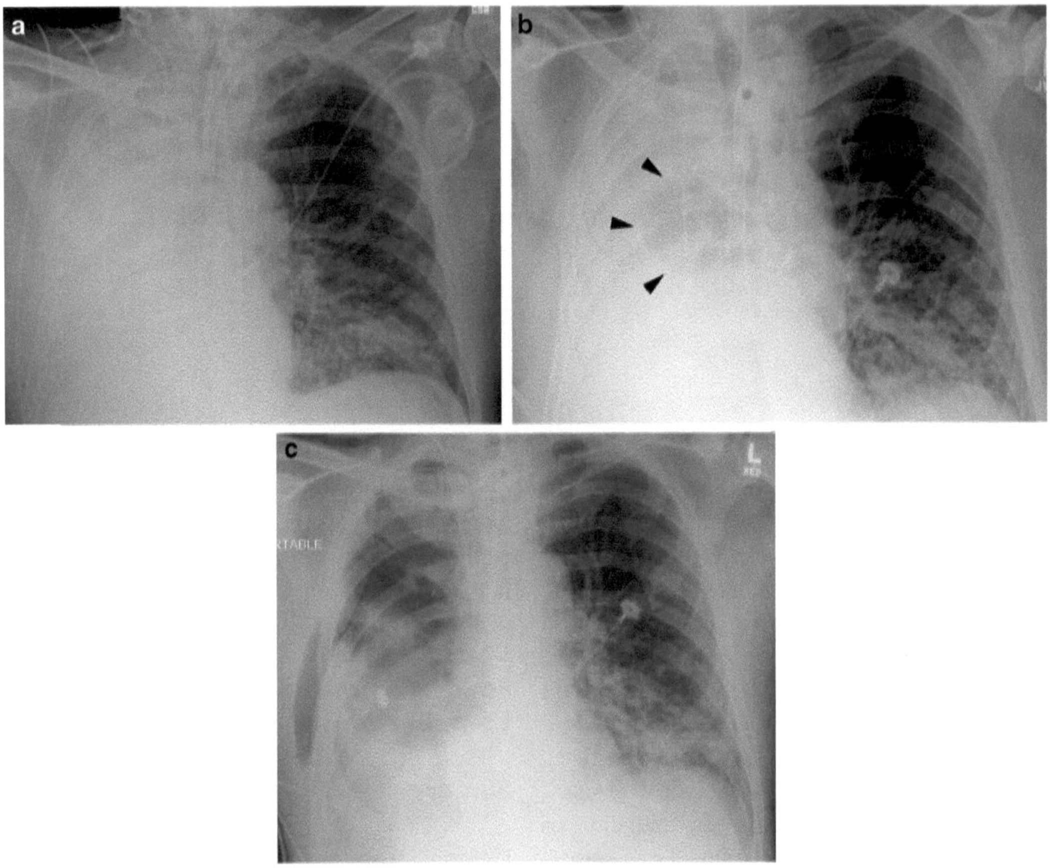

Fig. 14.1 Bronchopleural fistula. (**a**) Frontal radiograph on postoperative day 10 reveals complete filling in of the right pneumonectomy space. (**b**) Frontal radiograph on postoperative day 14 reveals circular lucency over the right pneumonectomy space (*arrowheads*). (**c**) Frontal radiograph on postoperative day 17 reveals near-complete replacement of fluid with ga in right pneumonectomy space

level is rising, there should not be immediate concern. A drop of greater than 2 cm of the gas fluid level, reappearance of gas in the pneumonectomy space, or persistence of gas fluid level past 6 months all suggest the diagnosis of a bronchopleural fistula [7] (Fig. 14.1). Chylothorax may be indistinguishable from other causes of pleural effusion although a rapid increase in fluid in the immediate postoperative period suggests the diagnosis which can be subsequently confirmed by pleural fluid analysis. Lung torsion is quite rare and may be quite difficult to diagnose. Often there is increasing density to the lung and an unusual orientation of the fissure may be visible. CT with contrast is often quite valuable in confirming the diagnosis by showing obstruction of the bronchus and pulmonary artery [5] (Fig. 14.2).

Nezu et al. showed that FEV1 is approximately 10–15% lower than preoperative values after a lobectomy and approximately 25–35% lower after a pneumonectomy [8]. Patients undergoing resection for localized lung cancer have significantly lower baseline quality of life when compared with the normal population, and resection causes further deterioration in quality of life, especially during the first 3–6 months after surgery. Symptom-directed imaging is recommended postoperatively in the first few months.

Radiation and Chemotherapy

Radiation pneumonitis and fibrosis are common complications post radiation therapy. Pulmonary

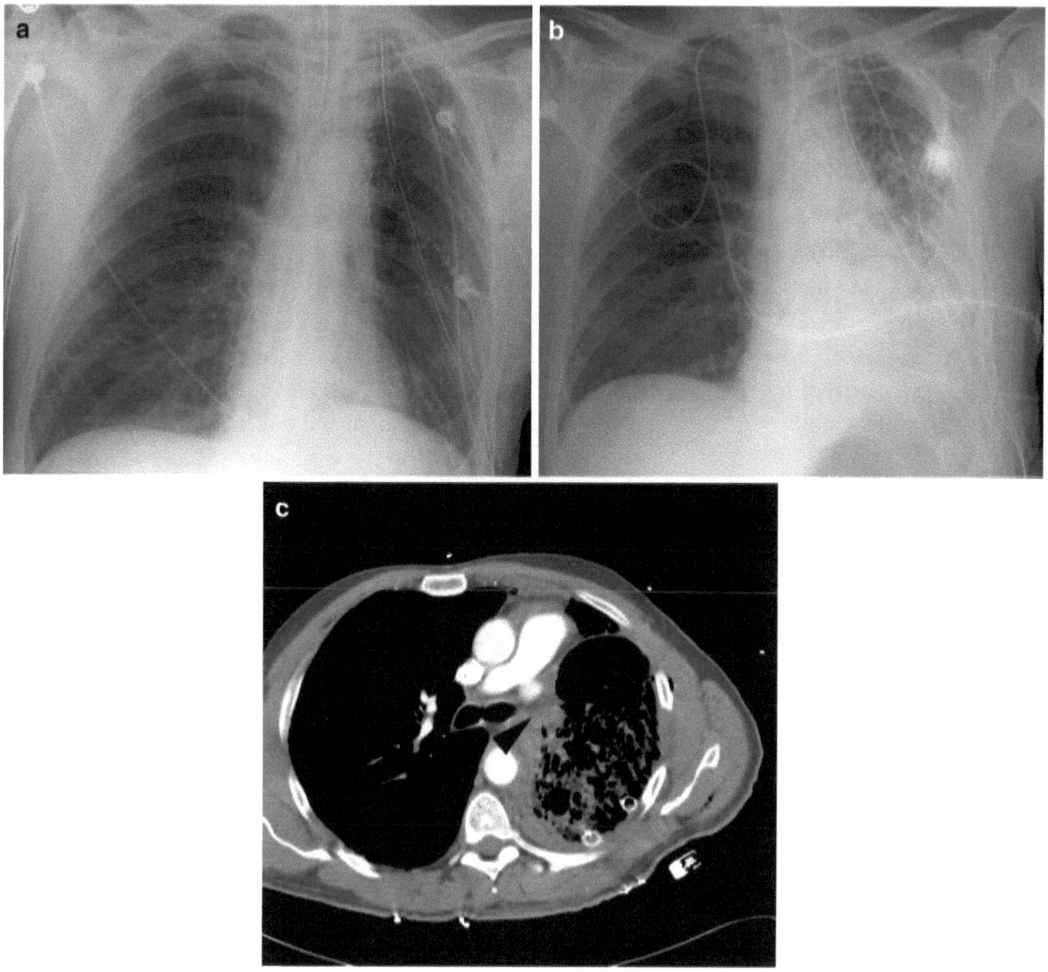

Fig. 14.2 Postoperative lobar torsion. (**a**) Frontal radiograph on postoperative day 1 following left upper lobectomy reveals expected aeration of the remaining left lower lobe. (**b**) Frontal radiograph on postoperative day 2 reveals rapidly progressive air-space opacities in the remaining left lung. (**c**) Contrast-enhanced axial CT image on postoperative day 2 reveals abrupt cutoff of the left pulmonary artery (*arrowhead*) and absence of blood flow to the left lower lobe consistent with infarction

radiation toxicity is related to the volume of lung irradiated, the cumulative dose effects of radiation-sensitizing agents, and undefined factors determining the biological predisposition of the patient. Acute radiation pneumonitis usually occurs within 3 months of treatment and in 3–4% of patients receiving curative intent radiation therapy for lung cancer [9, 10]. The most significant pulmonary toxicities of chemotherapy are drop in DLCO and drug-induced pneumonitis [11]. There are currently no guidelines or recommendations available to screen patients to identify these toxicities and the decision to obtain imaging is based on patients' presentation and at physicians' discretion.

Stereotactic body radiation therapy (SBRT) uses multiple convergent beams to deliver high-radiation doses to the tumor in 1–5 fractions. In a study by Timmerman et al. patients with inoperable non-small-cell lung cancer (NSCLC) who received SBRT had a survival rate of 55.8% at 3 years, high rates of local tumor control, and moderate treatment-related morbidity [12]. Very few studies have looked into the utility of CT/PET to follow patients post SBRT. The original RTOG 0236 trial used q3- and then q6-month CTs. PET scans were performed only if there was evidence of progression on CT. Several small non-randomized studies since then have looked into the utility of CT/PET and could not generate any consensus on the use of one modality over the other, nor on how to interpret the abnormal tests or on the timing of the tests [13–16]. A more thorough description of radiation-induced injury can be found in the next chapter.

Follow-Up Imaging for Surveillance and Recurrence

The purpose of imaging for surveillance is detection of disease recurrence and/or development of new primary disease [3]. While major societies include surveillance chest radiograph as part of follow-up recommendations [17–19], the hard evidence for this practice is somewhat difficult to find [20]. Some case series have reported that 68–100% of patients with metachronous lung cancers were asymptomatic and had the new primary lung cancer detected by radiographic methods, making the case for surveillance imaging [21, 22]. One prospective study of 192 patients with aggressive follow-up showed a better 3-year survival for asymptomatic recurrence detection (31% vs. 13%) and that 43% of asymptomatic recurrences could be treated surgically [23]. Several retrospective studies came to the separate conclusion that strict follow-up had little effect on mortality [24–28].

There are several reasons why surveillance chest imaging after curative intent therapy could have little effect on mortality. Although, 5-year recurrence rates of 20–39% have been reported following curative intent surgery for stage I lung cancer [29–36], most of these recurrences are distant metastases and the recurrences may be detected several years after the treatment [30, 32, 33]. Similar to the screened population setting, lead and length time bias make the relevance of the survival data unclear. Computed tomography (CT) surveillance can be likened to screening a high-risk population so that while anecdotal evidence may seem to support its use, there is no good data on which to recommend its use. In the absence of good evidence, most major society guidelines are developed by consensus of expert panels and not necessarily by more rigorous meta-analysis. Hence there is wide divergence among the guidelines regarding recommendations for chest imaging after curative intent therapy for lung cancer. Accordingly, American College of Chest Physicians (ACCP) recommends for patients treated with curative intent therapy, and those having adequate performance and pulmonary function, surveillance with a history, physical examination, and either chest X-ray (CXR) or CT chest every 6 months for 2 years and then annually [3]. The Association of Community Cancer Centers (ACCC) guidelines recommend routine CXR for surveillance. Guidelines from the American College of Radiology (ACR) recommend a postresection chest CT scan to establish a new baseline and then annually in addition to interval CXR every 2–4 months [37]. The guidelines from the National Comprehensive Cancer Network (NCCN) rely entirely on chest CT scanning for surveillance imaging with no role for CXR [38]. American Society of Clinical Oncology (ASCO) guidelines for NSCLC specifically state that there is no proven value for either chest radiograph (CXR) or CT in surveillance in management of these patients [39]. Table 14.1 summarizes major society guidelines.

There is considerable interest in using positron emission tomography (PET) scan for follow-up surveillance after curative intent therapy as it may be able to distinguish recurrent cancer from the parenchymal scarring, distortion of bronchovascular anatomy, pleural thickening, and mediastinal fibrosis commonly seen on conventional imaging after initial treatment [40]. PET has 96% sensitivity and 84% specificity for detecting recurrent lung cancer after treatment with surgery, chemotherapy, or radiotherapy [41–44]. However, the specificity of PET scan after definitive treatment is lower than at initial staging due to increased uptake on PET scan from inflammatory changes related to tumor necrosis and radiation pneumonitis [40]. Routine use of PET surveillance is not recommended by any of the

Table 14.1 Imaging recommendations for surveillance methods in patients with non-small-cell lung cancer (NSCLC) following curative intent therapy

		Imaging frequency		
Source of guidelines	Imaging modality	0–2 years	2–5 years	After 5 years
ACCP [3]	CXR or CT chest	6 monthly	Yearly	Yearly
ACCC [90]	CXR	3 monthly	6 monthly	Yearly
ACR [37]	CXR and CT chest	CXR 2–4 monthly and CT chest yearly	CXR 6 monthly and CT chest yearly	CXR yearly and CT chest yearly
NCCN [38]	CT chest	6 monthly	Yearly	Yearly
ASCO [39]	None	No imaging f/u	No imaging f/u	No imaging f/u

ACCP American College of Chest Physicians, *ACCC* Association of Community Cancer Centers, *ACR* American College of Radiology, *NCCN* National Comprehensive Cancer Network, *ASCO* American Society of Clinical Oncology, *CXR* chest X-ray, *CT* computed tomography

major societies as there are no data showing that incorporating PET scanning into a surveillance program improves either survival or quality of life following curative intent therapy.

Follow-Up Imaging Post Neoadjuvant Therapy

Induction chemotherapy may be employed in selected patients with mediastinal disease in order to render patients resectable for cure. Because of the inherent difficulties of repeat mediastinoscopy, PET has been evaluated as a means of restaging the mediastinum in 130 patients in four separate studies. Two reports which included a total of 49 patients had a combined accuracy of 95% [45, 46]. When compared directly to CT for all lymph nodes, accuracy was better for PET in one [47] and CT in the other [48]. PET response does however correlate to some degree with survival as those with follow-up standardized uptake value (SUV) less than 2.5 or decreased over 20% have improved time to disease progression and overall survival [49, 50]. The survival benefit with PET response in surgically treated patients was also seen after neoadjuvant chemotherapy [45, 51] and chemoradiotherapy [52, 53]; however, this finding is not universal across studies and several studies actually show a greater predictive value for CT-based anatomic measurements [54, 55]. Thus, similar to initial staging, the true value of PET/CT in the neoadjuvant setting is the selection of appropriate site and technique for re-biopsy and to avoid futile thoracotomy through the detection of clinically silent distant metastatic disease.

Follow-Up Imaging for Treatment Response

Assessment of the change in tumor burden is an important feature of the clinical evaluation of cancer therapeutics: both tumor shrinkage (objective response) and disease progression are useful endpoints in clinical practice and trials [56]. At the current time objective tumor response using imaging modalities carries with it a body of evidence greater than for any other biomarker supporting its utility as a measure of promising treatment effect in phase II screening trials [57–59]. Originally, tumor response in clinical trials was guided by the World Health Organization (WHO) and required bi-dimensional measurements. Several studies have looked at the use of unidimensional long axis measurements (Response Evaluation Criteria in Solid Tumors Group—RECIST) compared to bi-dimensional and volumetric measures of response. The RECIST criteria have been shown to be equivalent to WHO criteria and volumetric measurement in classification of response to therapy [60–63]. In one study 1,221 lung cancer patients in clinical trials were evaluated, and a 31% response rate was documented by using both RECIST and WHO criteria, with only one disagreement between stable disease and partial

Table 14.2 RECIST 1.1 [56] definitions of response in target lesions and target lymph nodes

	Target lesion	Target lymph nodes
Complete response (CR)	Disappearance of all target lesions	Reduction in short axis to <10 mm
Partial response (PR)	At least 30% decrease in the sum of diameters of target lesions from baseline	Same as PR for target lesion, but should include short-axis diameter of the nodes
Progressive disease (PD)	At least 20% increase in the sum of diameters of target lesions and an absolute increase of at least 5 mm from baseline	Same as PD for target lesion, but should include short-axis diameter of the nodes
Stable disease (SD)	Neither sufficient shrinkage to qualify for PR nor sufficient increase to qualify for PD	Same as SD for target lesion, but should include short-axis diameter of the nodes

response [62]. Thus, unidimensional long axis measurement using RECIST is the current standard for response in most clinical trials. The most recent RECIST 1.1 criteria definitions of complete response (CR), partial response (PR), progressive disease (PD), and stable disease (SD) in target lesion and lymph nodes are summarized in Table 14.2.

Optimal assessment of response, however, is dependent on the reproducibility of measurements. Perhaps more important than technique, reader variability may play a greater role in accuracy of response assessment [64, 65]. Inter- and intraobserver variations for initial tumor size are 10–15% and 5%, respectively [64, 66], with an impact on disease progression or response to a greater degree. Using RECIST criteria, inter- and intraobserver variability for progressive disease ranged from 21–48% (avg. 30%) to 3–15% (avg. 9%), respectively. Response was affected to a lesser degree, interobserver 3–27% (avg. 15%) and intraobserver 0–6% (avg. 4%) [66]. Thus, to the extent possible, the same scanning technique and interpreter should follow an individual case.

Automated volumetric imaging has the potential advantage of eliminating measurement variability through improved precision [67, 68]. Accuracy and precision can be best maintained by standardizing protocols including reconstruction interval, reconstruction kernel, and field of view [69]. As a practical matter, patient motion, respiration, and relationship to adjacent structures further degrade the accuracy of volumetric change to a much greater extent than the precision of the technique [70]. While studies comparing volumetry with RECIST have generally been favorable to volume assessment [71–73] (with the caveat that volumetric response has not been rigorously defined across studies), a study evaluating two dimensional measurements and semi-automated volume measurements on scans obtained the same day (no growth) showed similar degrees of variability (up to 20% variance) in size across all measurements [74]. Additionally, most studies only account for the volume of pulmonary lesions that can be adequately segmented and do not include all sites of tumor as called for by RECIST. Thus volumetry may not be an improvement over standard 2D measurements or an adequate tumor biomarker for therapeutic trials.

Regardless all anatomic response measurements are limited in scope particularly in the setting of targeted therapies that may (1) prolong survival without change in tumor size, (2) mischaracterize increased size due to tumor bleeding or edema (response to drug) as progression, or (3) fail to characterize new tumor tissue in a complex mass [75]. To this end physiologic or metabolic imaging may perform better as a biomarker of response/progression than anatomic analysis. FDG-PET may eventually provide additional data by following metabolic response via SUV determination.

The rationale for using metabolic response criteria is based on the concept that metabolic changes are likely to precede anatomic changes. In addition, FDG-PET may provide more accurate information in anatomically complex regions, in previously radiated tissues, and in assessment of response to targeted therapies. Evidence-based analysis is difficult owing to different image acquisition techniques, measurement technique, response criteria, and difficulty in quantifying response in low SUV tumors [76]. In general, it has been shown that prognosis is improved and survival enhanced in subjects with a decrease in SUV following therapy [49, 77–80]. Ultimately, the utility of a metabolic response approach will require agreed-upon criteria that can be reproduced across many sites. Two such methodologies have been proposed [81, 82].

A corollary to this approach is the use of PET/CT to provide earlier information on response following a single cycle of chemotherapy. The rationale for this approach is that it will eventually allow for more rapid assessment of disease response and the earlier discontinuation of ineffective treatment. The proof of this concept can be seen in a small study of 5 patients treated with gefitinib. As early as 2 days after treatment, a change in SUVmax could be identified and this change correlated with metabolic response at 4 weeks [83]. A similar result was obtained in a time course evaluation of PET/CT changes where long-term responders could be seen in as early as 1 week and SUVmax continued to decrease at 3 weeks [80] and from a study that showed that after one cycle of chemotherapy, a reduction in SUV by 20% correlated with overall tumor response by RECIST criteria [49]. Still unknown is whether a change in therapy at these early time points would result in benefit to nonresponders.

The SUVs have limited value in the prediction of malignancy, compared to inflammatory or infectious lesion. However, once malignancy has been established, SUV may have a role in assessing prognosis and guiding management. SUV appears to correlate with tumor doubling time [84]. Furthermore, survival for surgically managed T1 tumors with SUV <7 had a 2-year survival of 86% vs. 60% for SUV >7 [85]. Patients with a "false-negative" PET scan most often have T1N0 lesions with a good long-term survival [86]. In practice, follow-up ideally should occur at least 4 weeks after chemotherapy to avoid an early "false-negative" assessment of therapeutic response due to the inflammatory response from cellular apoptosis that may result in residual activity at the site of the lesion [87]. Further complicating the role of SUV is the fact that different machines, reconstruction algorithms, and forms of attenuation correction will impact the measured SUV, even for the identical lesion [88]. Therefore accurate interpretation of SUV as a marker of therapeutic response requires that the same techniques be applied meticulously and consistently to individual patients.

Conflicting data exists as to whether the measure of metabolic activity in mediastinal nodes is useful in following response. While 18F-FDG PET is sensitive for the detection of residual disease in the primary tumor, it is less than optimal in restaging the mediastinum [89], and reports of four studies show an overall accuracy ranging from 50 to 95% [46–48]. One study revealed an unacceptably high false-positive and false-negative rate, with positive predictive value for 18F-FDG PET of 16% (same as CT) [48].

A key question considered by the RECIST Working Group in developing RECIST 1.1 was whether it was appropriate to move from anatomic unidimensional assessment of tumor burden to either volumetric anatomical assessment or functional assessment with PET or MRI. They concluded that, at present, there is not sufficient standardization or evidence to abandon anatomical assessment of tumor burden. The only exception to this is in the use of FDG-PET imaging as an adjunct to determination of progression [56].

Conclusion

Successful follow-up of patients with lung cancer requires an understanding of the purpose and goals of imaging, the effects of the various treatments used, and careful/reproducible measurement techniques. There is still a gap between what is known and what is being done regarding the optimal timing and types of imaging procedures requiring further research to define evidence-based appropriate and cost-effective follow-up.

References

1. Mountain CF. Revisions in the International System for Staging Lung Cancer. Chest. 1997;111(6):1710–7.
2. Virgo KS, Johnson FE, Naunheim KS. Follow-up of patients with thoracic malignancies. Surg Oncol Clin N Am. 1999;8(2):355–69.

3. Colice GL, Unger M, Rubins J, American College of Chest Physicians. Follow-up and surveillance of the lung cancer patient following curative intent therapy: ACCP evidence-based clinical practice guideline (2nd edition). Chest. 2007;132(3 Suppl):355S–67S.
4. Pool KL, Munden RF, Vaporciyan A, O'Sullivan PJ. Radiographic imaging features of thoracic complications after pneumonectomy in oncologic patients. Eur J Radiol. 2012;81(1):165–72.
5. Kim EA, Lee KS, Shim YM, et al. Radiographic and CT findings in complications following pulmonary resection. Radiographics. 2002;22(1):67–86.
6. Brunelli A, Monteverde M, Borri A, Salati M, Marasco RD, Fianchini A. Predictors of prolonged air leak after pulmonary lobectomy. Ann Thorac Surg. 2004;77(4):1205–10; discussion 1210.
7. Chae EJ, Seo JB, Kim SY, et al. Radiographic and CT findings of thoracic complications after pneumonectomy. Radiographics. 2006;26(5):1449–68.
8. Nezu K, Kushibe K, Tojo T, Takahama M, Kitamura S. Recovery and limitation of exercise capacity after lung resection for lung cancer. Chest. 1998;113(6):1511–6.
9. Cox JD, Pajak TF, Marcial VA, et al. Dose–response for local control with hyperfractionated radiation therapy in advanced carcinomas of the upper aerodigestive tracts: preliminary report of radiation therapy oncology group protocol 83–13. Int J Radiat Oncol Biol Phys. 1990;18(3):515–21.
10. Abratt RP, Morgan GW. Lung toxicity following chest irradiation in patients with lung cancer. Lung Cancer. 2002;35(2):103–9.
11. Leo F, Solli P, Spaggiari L, et al. Respiratory function changes after chemotherapy: an additional risk for postoperative respiratory complications? Ann Thorac Surg. 2004;77(1):260–5; discussion 5.
12. Timmerman R, Paulus R, Galvin J, et al. Stereotactic body radiation therapy for inoperable early stage lung cancer. JAMA. 2010;303(11):1070–6.
13. Ishimori T, Saga T, Nagata Y, et al. 18F-FDG and 11C-methionine PET for evaluation of treatment response of lung cancer after stereotactic radiotherapy. Ann Nucl Med. 2004;18(8):669–74.
14. Henderson MA, Hoopes DJ, Fletcher JW, et al. A pilot trial of serial 18F-fluorodeoxyglucose positron emission tomography in patients with medically inoperable stage I non-small-cell lung cancer treated with hypofractionated stereotactic body radiotherapy. Int J Radiat Oncol Biol Phys. 2010;76(3):789–95.
15. Hoopes DJ, Tann M, Fletcher JW, et al. FDG-PET and stereotactic body radiotherapy (SBRT) for stage I non-small-cell lung cancer. Lung Cancer. 2007;56(2):229–34.
16. Feigenberg SJ, Lango M, Nicolaou N, Ridge JA. Intensity-modulated radiotherapy for early larynx cancer: is there a role? Int J Radiat Oncol Biol Phys. 2007;68(1):2–3.
17. Sause WT, Byhardt RW, Curran Jr WJ, et al. Follow-up of non-small cell lung cancer. American College of Radiology. ACR Appropriateness Criteria. Radiology. 2000;215(Suppl):1363–72.
18. Smith TJ. Evidence-based follow-up of lung cancer patients. Semin Oncol. 2003;30(3):361–8.
19. Ettinger DS, Cox JD, Ginsberg RJ, et al. NCCN Non-Small-Cell Lung Cancer Practice Guidelines. The National Comprehensive Cancer Network. Oncology (Williston Park). 1996;10(11 Suppl):81–111.
20. Colice GL, Rubins J, Unger M, American College of Chest Physicians. Follow-up and surveillance of the lung cancer patient following curative-intent therapy. Chest. 2003;123(1 Suppl):272S–83S.
21. Adebonojo SA, Moritz DM, Danby CA. The results of modern surgical therapy for multiple primary lung cancers. Chest. 1997;112(3):693–701.
22. Antakli T, Schaefer RF, Rutherford JE, Read RC. Second primary lung cancer. Ann Thorac Surg. 1995;59(4):863–6; discussion 867.
23. Westeel V, Choma D, Clément F, et al. Relevance of an intensive postoperative follow-up after surgery for non-small cell lung cancer. Ann Thorac Surg. 2000; 70(4):1185–90.
24. Virgo KS, McKirgan LW, Caputo MC, et al. Post-treatment management options for patients with lung cancer. Ann Surg. 1995;222(6):700–10.
25. Walsh GL, O'Connor M, Willis KM, et al. Is follow-up of lung cancer patients after resection medically indicated and cost-effective? Ann Thorac Surg. 1995;60(6):1563–70; discussion 1570–2.
26. Younes RN, Gross JL, Deheinzelin D. Follow-up in lung cancer: how often and for what purpose? Chest. 1999;115(6):1494–9.
27. Sohn HJ, Yang YJ, Ryu JS, et al. [18F]Fluorothymidine positron emission tomography before and 7 days after gefitinib treatment predicts response in patients with advanced adenocarcinoma of the lung. Clin Cancer Res. 2008;14(22):7423–9.
28. Gilbert S, Reid KR, Lam MY, Petsikas D. Who should follow up lung cancer patients after operation? Ann Thorac Surg. 2000;69(6):1696–700.
29. Immerman SC, Vanecko RM, Fry WA, Head LR, Shields TW. Site of recurrence in patients with stages I and II carcinoma of the lung resected for cure. Ann Thorac Surg. 1981;32(1):23–7.
30. Pairolero PC, Williams DE, Bergstralh EJ, Piehler JM, Bernatz PE, Payne WS. Postsurgical stage I bronchogenic carcinoma: morbid implications of recurrent disease. Ann Thorac Surg. 1984;38(4):331–8.
31. Iascone C, DeMeester TR, Albertucci M, Little AG, Golomb HM. Local recurrence of resectable non-oat cell carcinoma of the lung. A warning against conservative treatment for N0 and N1 disease. Cancer. 1986;57(3):471–6.
32. Martini N, Bains MS, Burt ME, et al. Incidence of local recurrence and second primary tumors in resected stage I lung cancer. J Thorac Cardiovasc Surg. 1995;109(1):120–9.
33. Harpole Jr DH, Herndon II JE, Wolfe WG, Iglehart JD, Marks JR. A prognostic model of recurrence and

death in stage I non-small cell lung cancer utilizing presentation, histopathology, and oncoprotein expression. Cancer Res. 1995;55(1):51–6.
34. Thomas P, Rubinstein L. Cancer recurrence after resection: T1 N0 non-small cell lung cancer. Lung Cancer Study Group. Ann Thorac Surg. 1990;49(2):242–6; discussion 246–7.
35. Thomas Jr PA, Rubinstein L. Malignant disease appearing late after operation for T1 N0 non-small-cell lung cancer. The Lung Cancer Study Group. J Thorac Cardiovasc Surg. 1993;106(6):1053–8.
36. Baldini EH, DeCamp Jr MM, Katz MS, et al. Patterns of recurrence and outcome for patients with clinical stage II non-small-cell lung cancer. Am J Clin Oncol. 1999;22(1):8–14.
37. Follow-up of non-small cell lung cancer: American College of Radiology appropriateness criteria; 2005. http://www.google.com/url?sa=t&rct=j&q=&esrc=s&source=web&cd=1&ved=0CD8QFjAA&url=http%3A%2F%2Fwww.acr.org%2F~%2Fmedia%2F632D81E7C9094D6E87EE4F601179C44A.pdf&ei=7HjcUM3jLpPh0wGj0YDQCQ&usg=AFQjCNFZX2iXzXmCDXdFLQf_0E6pKj0CCw&bvm=bv.1355534169,d.dmQ
38. National Comprehensive Cancer Network. Practice guidelines for non-small cell lung cancer. Rockledge, PA. National Comprehensive Cancer Network; 2000. http://www.nccn.org/network/business_insights/flash_updates/flash_update_information.asp?FlashID=32
39. Pfister DG, Johnson DH, Azzoli CG, et al. American Society of Clinical Oncology treatment of unresectable non-small-cell lung cancer guideline: update 2003. J Clin Oncol. 2004;22(2):330–53.
40. Bruzzi JF, Munden RF. PET/CT imaging of lung cancer. J Thorac Imaging. 2006;21(2):123–36.
41. Patz Jr EF, Lowe VJ, Hoffman JM, Paine SS, Harris LK, Goodman PC. Persistent or recurrent bronchogenic carcinoma: detection with PET and 2-[F-18]-2-deoxy-d-glucose. Radiology. 1994;191(2):379–82.
42. Inoue T, Kim EE, Komaki R, et al. Detecting recurrent or residual lung cancer with FDG-PET. J Nucl Med. 1995;36(5):788–93.
43. Duhaylongsod FG, Lowe VJ, Patz Jr EF, Vaughn AL, Coleman RE, Wolfe WG. Detection of primary and recurrent lung cancer by means of F-18 fluorodeoxyglucose positron emission tomography (FDG PET). J Thorac Cardiovasc Surg. 1995;110(1):130–9; discussion 139–40.
44. Hellwig D, Gröschel A, Graeter TP, et al. Diagnostic performance and prognostic impact of FDG-PET in suspected recurrence of surgically treated non-small cell lung cancer. Eur J Nucl Med Mol Imaging. 2006;33(1):13–21.
45. Vansteenkiste JF, Stroobants SG, De Leyn PR, Dupont PJ, Verbeken EK. Potential use of FDG-PET scan after induction chemotherapy in surgically staged IIIa-N2 non-small-cell lung cancer: a prospective pilot study. The Leuven Lung Cancer Group. Ann Oncol. 1998;9(11):1193–8.
46. Cerfolio RJ, Ojha B, Mukherjee S, Pask AH, Bass CS, Katholi CR. Positron emission tomography scanning with 2-fluoro-2-deoxy-d-glucose as a predictor of response of neoadjuvant treatment for non-small cell carcinoma. J Thorac Cardiovasc Surg. 2003;125(4):938–44.
47. Akhurst T, Downey RJ, Ginsberg MS, et al. An initial experience with FDG-PET in the imaging of residual disease after induction therapy for lung cancer. Ann Thorac Surg. 2002;73(1):259–64; discussion 264–6.
48. Port JL, Kent MS, Korst RJ, Keresztes R, Levin MA, Altorki NK. Positron emission tomography scanning poorly predicts response to preoperative chemotherapy in non-small cell lung cancer. Ann Thorac Surg. 2004;77(1):254–9; discussion 259.
49. Weber WA, Petersen V, Schmidt B, et al. Positron emission tomography in non-small-cell lung cancer: prediction of response to chemotherapy by quantitative assessment of glucose use. J Clin Oncol. 2003;21(14):2651–7.
50. Patz Jr EF, Connolly J, Herndon J. Prognostic value of thoracic FDG PET imaging after treatment for non-small cell lung cancer. AJR Am J Roentgenol. 2000;174(3):769–74.
51. Hoekstra CJ, Stroobants SG, Smit EF, et al. Prognostic relevance of response evaluation using [18F]-2-fluoro-2-deoxy-D-glucose positron emission tomography in patients with locally advanced non-small-cell lung cancer. J Clin Oncol. 2005;23(33):8362–70.
52. Eschmann SM, Friedel G, Paulsen F, et al. Repeat 18F-FDG PET for monitoring neoadjuvant chemotherapy in patients with stage III non-small cell lung cancer. Lung Cancer. 2007;55(2):165–71.
53. Hellwig D, Graeter TP, Ukena D, Georg T, Kirsch CM, Schäfers HJ. Value of F-18-fluorodeoxyglucose positron emission tomography after induction therapy of locally advanced bronchogenic carcinoma. J Thorac Cardiovasc Surg. 2004;128(6):892–9.
54. Pottgen C, Levegrun S, Theegarten D, et al. Value of 18F-fluoro-2-deoxy-D-glucose-positron emission tomography/computed tomography in non-small-cell lung cancer for prediction of pathologic response and times to relapse after neoadjuvant chemoradiotherapy. Clin Cancer Res. 2006;12(1):97–106.
55. Tanvetyanon T, Eikman EA, Sommers E, Robinson L, Boulware D, Bepler G. Computed tomography response, but not positron emission tomography scan response, predicts survival after neoadjuvant chemotherapy for resectable non-small-cell lung cancer. J Clin Oncol. 2008;26(28):4610–6.
56. Eisenhauer EA, Therasse P, Bogaerts J, et al. New response evaluation criteria in solid tumours: revised RECIST guideline (version 1.1). Eur J Cancer. 2009;45(2):228–47.
57. Paesmans M, Sculier JP, Libert P, et al. Response to chemotherapy has predictive value for further survival of patients with advanced non-small cell lung cancer: 10 years experience of the European Lung Cancer Working Party. Eur J Cancer. 1997;33(14):2326–32.

58. Buyse M, Thirion P, Carlson RW, Burzykowski T, Molenberghs G, Piedbois P. Relation between tumour response to first-line chemotherapy and survival in advanced colorectal cancer: a meta-analysis. Meta-Analysis Group in Cancer. Lancet. 2000;356(9227):373–8.
59. El-Maraghi RH, Eisenhauer EA. Review of phase II trial designs used in studies of molecular targeted agents: outcomes and predictors of success in phase III. J Clin Oncol. 2008;26(8):1346–54.
60. Sohaib SA, Turner B, Hanson JA, Farquharson M, Oliver RT, Reznek RH. CT assessment of tumour response to treatment: comparison of linear, cross-sectional and volumetric measures of tumour size. Br J Radiol. 2000;73(875):1178–84.
61. Watanabe H, Yamamoto S, Kunitoh H, et al. Tumor response to chemotherapy: the validity and reproducibility of RECIST guidelines in NSCLC patients. Cancer Sci. 2003;94(11):1015–20.
62. Therasse P, Arbuck SG, Eisenhauer EA, et al. New guidelines to evaluate the response to treatment in solid tumors. European Organization for Research and Treatment of Cancer, National Cancer Institute of the United States, National Cancer Institute of Canada. J Natl Cancer Inst. 2000;92(3):205–16.
63. James K, Eisenhauer E, Christian M, et al. Measuring response in solid tumors: unidimensional versus bidimensional measurement. J Natl Cancer Inst. 1999;91(6):523–8.
64. Erasmus JJ, Gladish GW, Broemeling L, et al. Interobserver and intraobserver variability in measurement of non-small-cell carcinoma lung lesions: implications for assessment of tumor response. J Clin Oncol. 2003;21(3):2574–82.
65. Revel MP, Bissery A, Bienvenu M, Aycard L, Lefort C, Frija G. Are two-dimensional CT measurements of small noncalcified pulmonary nodules reliable? Radiology. 2004;231(2):453–8.
66. Hopper KD, Kasales CJ, Van Slyke MA, Schwartz TA, TenHave TR, Jozefiak JA. Analysis of interobserver and intraobserver variability in CT tumor measurements. AJR Am J Roentgenol. 1996;167(4):851–4.
67. Petrou M, Quint LE, Nan B, Baker LH. Pulmonary nodule volumetric measurement variability as a function of CT slice thickness and nodule morphology. AJR Am J Roentgenol. 2007;188(2):306–12.
68. Revel MP, Lefort C, Bissery A, et al. Pulmonary nodules: preliminary experience with three-dimensional evaluation. Radiology. 2004;231(2):459–66.
69. Ravenel JG, Leue WM, Nietert PJ, Miller JV, Taylor KK, Silvestri GA. Pulmonary nodule volume: effects of reconstruction parameters on automated measurements—a phantom study. Radiology. 2008;247(2):400–8.
70. Gavrielides MA, Kinnard LM, Myers KJ, Petrick N. Noncalcified lung nodules: volumetric assessment with thoracic CT. Radiology. 2009;251(1):26–37.
71. Marten K, Auer F, Schmidt S, Kohl G, Rummeny EJ, Engelke C. Inadequacy of manual measurements compared to automated CT volumetry in assessment of treatment response of pulmonary metastases using RECIST criteria. Eur Radiol. 2006;16(4):781–90.
72. Tran LN, Brown MS, Goldin JG, et al. Comparison of treatment response classifications between unidimensional, bidimensional, and volumetric measurements of metastatic lung lesions on chest computed tomography. Acad Radiol. 2004;11(12):1355–60.
73. Zhao B, Schwartz LH, Moskowitz CS, Ginsberg MS, Rizvi NA, Kris MG. Lung cancer: computerized quantification of tumor response—initial results. Radiology. 2006;241(3):892–8.
74. Zhao B, James LP, Moskowitz CS, et al. Evaluating variability in tumor measurements from same-day repeat CT scans of patients with non-small cell lung cancer. Radiology. 2009;252(1):263–72.
75. Shankar LK, Van den Abbeele A, Yap J, Benjamin R, Scheutze S, Fitzgerald TJ. Considerations for the use of imaging tools for phase II treatment trials in oncology. Clin Cancer Res. 2009;15(6):1891–7.
76. Hicks RJ. Role of 18F-FDG PET in assessment of response in non-small cell lung cancer. J Nucl Med. 2009;50 Suppl 1:31S–42S.
77. de Geus-Oei LF, van der Heijden HF, Visser EP, et al. Chemotherapy response evaluation with 18F-FDG PET in patients with non-small cell lung cancer. J Nucl Med. 2007;48(10):1592–8.
78. Mac Manus MP, Hicks RJ. PET scanning in lung cancer: current status and future directions. Semin Surg Oncol. 2003;21(3):149–55.
79. Mac Manus MP, Hicks RJ, Matthews JP, Wirth A, Rischin D, Ball DL. Metabolic (FDG-PET) response after radical radiotherapy/chemoradiotherapy for non-small cell lung cancer correlates with patterns of failure. Lung Cancer. 2005;49(1):95–108.
80. Nahmias C, Hanna WT, Wahl LM, Long MJ, Hubner KF, Townsend DW. Time course of early response to chemotherapy in non-small cell lung cancer patients with 18F-FDG PET/CT. J Nucl Med. 2007;48(5):744–51.
81. Wahl RL, Jacene H, Kasamon Y, Lodge MA. From RECIST to PERCIST: evolving considerations for PET response criteria in solid tumors. J Nucl Med. 2009;50 Suppl 1:122S–50S.
82. Young H, Baum R, Cremerius U, et al. Measurement of clinical and subclinical tumour response using [18F]-fluorodeoxyglucose and positron emission tomography: review and 1999 EORTC recommendations. European Organization for Research and Treatment of Cancer (EORTC) PET Study Group. Eur J Cancer. 1999;35(13):1773–82.
83. Sunaga N, Oriuchi N, Kaira K, et al. Usefulness of FDG-PET for early prediction of the response to gefitinib in non-small cell lung cancer. Lung Cancer. 2008;59(2):203–10.
84. Vesselle H, Schmidt RA, Pugsley JM, et al. Lung cancer proliferation correlates with [F-18]

fluorodeoxyglucose uptake by positron emission tomography. Clin Cancer Res. 2000;6(10):3837–44.
85. Vansteenkiste JF, Stroobants SG, Dupont PJ, et al. Prognostic importance of the standardized uptake value on (18)F-fluoro-2-deoxy-glucose-positron emission tomography scan in non-small-cell lung cancer: an analysis of 125 cases. Leuven Lung Cancer Group. J Clin Oncol. 1999;17(10):3201–6.
86. Cheran SK, Nielsen ND, Patz Jr EF. False-negative findings for primary lung tumors on FDG positron emission tomography: staging and prognostic implications. AJR Am J Roentgenol. 2004;182(5):1129–32.
87. Weber WA. Use of PET for monitoring cancer therapy and for predicting outcome. J Nucl Med. 2005;46(6):983–95.
88. Schoder H, Erdi YE, Chao K, Gonen M, Larson SM, Yeung HW. Clinical implications of different image reconstruction parameters for interpretation of whole-body PET studies in cancer patients. J Nucl Med. 2004;45(4):559–66.
89. Van Schil P. The restaging issue. Lung Cancer. 2003;42 Suppl 1:S39–45.
90. Association of Community Cancer Centers. Oncology patient management guidelines, version 3.0. Rockville, MD; 2000. http://accc-cancer.org/

Chemotherapy-Related Lung Injury

15

Kristopher W. Cummings and Sanjeev Bhalla

As advances are made in the treatment of lung cancer with new chemotherapeutic regimens and agents, heightened awareness must be paid to the potential for drug-related lung injury. It has been estimated that up to 10 % of patients receiving chemotherapy have resulting pulmonary toxicities [1]. However, making the diagnosis of chemotherapy-induced lung injury is challenging, as it is nearly always a diagnosis of exclusion. The presenting symptoms are frequently nonspecific, including progressive dyspnea, cough, and often fever. Depending on the specific drug, injury can manifest anywhere from days to years after first administration and be dose-dependent or independent. Infection, in this immunocompromised patient population, is often at the forefront of clinical consideration as it is common and can have identical radiographic and clinical presentations (Fig. 15.1). Early detection of drug-related injury is critical as in many cases complete recovery will occur with removal of the offending agent. The combination of a high level of clinical suspicion, radiographic findings, and pathologic abnormalities all play a role in establishing a diagnosis of chemotherapy-related lung injury (Fig. 15.2).

Unfortunately, the understanding of drug-related lung injury and its causes is limited. This is attributable to many factors, including under-reporting of reactions, limited clinical studies of newer agents, the inherent difficulty in establishing the diagnosis, and lack of information regarding the differences in pharmacokinetic behavior in individual patients. Pathologically, oxidative injury, direct cytotoxic damage, intracellular phospholipid deposition, and immune-mediated injury have all been recognized in the process of drug-related lung damage [2]. In terms of clinical and radiographic presentations, chemotherapy-induced lung injury can be divided into five major categories: diffuse alveolar damage (DAD), nonspecific interstitial pneumonia, organizing pneumonia, eosinophilic pneumonia, and pulmonary hemorrhage. These will be discussed individually, followed by a brief discussion of the major chemotherapeutic agents used in the treatment of lung cancer, focusing on pulmonary complications.

K.W. Cummings, M.D. • S. Bhalla, M.D. (✉)
Department of Radiology, Barnes-Jewish Hospital, 510 South Kingshighway, St. Louis, MO 63110, USA
e-mail: bhallas@mir.wustl.edu

Diffuse Alveolar Damage

Diffuse alveolar damage (DAD) is the histological manifestation of the clinical syndrome adult respiratory distress syndrome (Fig. 15.3). A myriad of causes for DAD exist with sepsis, infection, and aspiration among the more common. Resulting from cytotoxic injury to the alveolar capillary walls, this entity can be the result of chemotherapeutic drug exposure. In the acute stage, the wall disruption results in filling of alveoli with an inflammatory exudate. Chronically,

J.G. Ravenel (ed.), *Lung Cancer Imaging*, Contemporary Medical Imaging,
DOI 10.1007/978-1-60761-620-7_15,

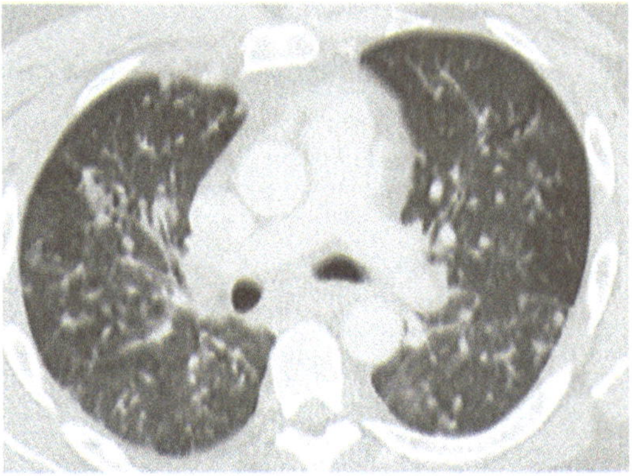

Fig. 15.1 Nodular infiltrate in a patient treated for lung cancer. This 61-year-old patient was treated with Iressa (gefitinib) for bronchioloalveolar carcinoma. The predominant CT pattern is random nodules. Understanding that this is not a typical appearance of chemotherapy-related lung injury allows the radiologist to offer an alternative explanation for the patient's shortness of breath. In this case, the diagnosis was granulomatous infection from histoplasmosis

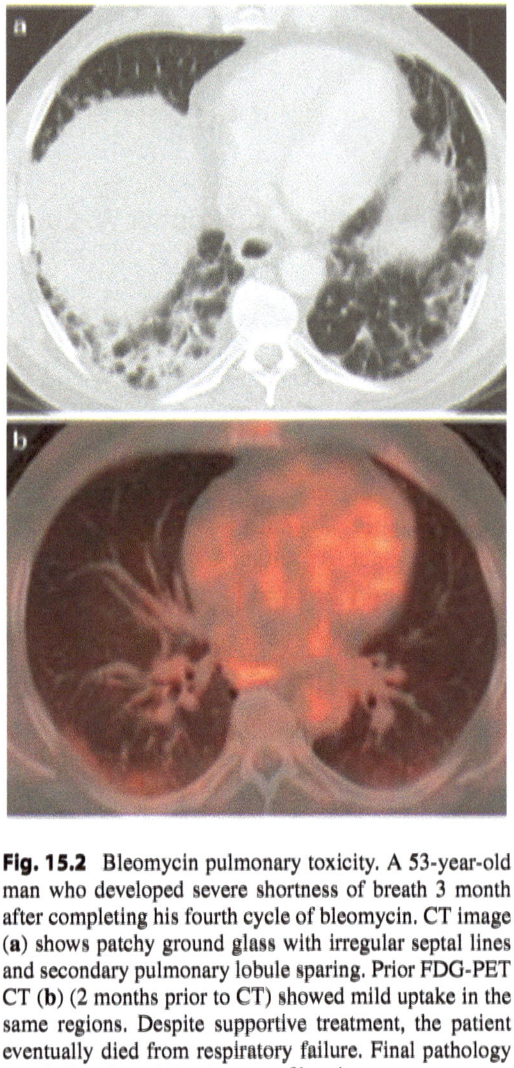

Fig. 15.2 Bleomycin pulmonary toxicity. A 53-year-old man who developed severe shortness of breath 3 month after completing his fourth cycle of bleomycin. CT image (**a**) shows patchy ground glass with irregular septal lines and secondary pulmonary lobule sparing. Prior FDG-PET CT (**b**) (2 months prior to CT) showed mild uptake in the same regions. Despite supportive treatment, the patient eventually died from respiratory failure. Final pathology was in keeping with pulmonary fibrosis

this results in fibroblast proliferation and subsequent fibrosis.

When this acute lung injury occurs, patients present with severe dyspnea, arterial hypoxemia, and respiratory failure. Mortality rates for DAD are estimated to approach 60 % [3]. While radiographs may initially be normal, there is rapid development of diffuse consolidation. On CT, basilar predominant consolidation and ground glass opacities are seen. An anterior-posterior lung attenuation gradient has also been described with denser consolidation seen in the dependent portion of the lungs [3]. In the late reparative stages, fibrosis, architectural distortion, and traction bronchiectasis are seen. Unlike in usual interstitial pneumonia, the fibrosis in DAD is typically nonprogressive and may even show improvement over time [4].

Nonspecific Interstitial Pneumonia

Representing the most common form of interstitial lung disease related to drug exposure [4], nonspecific interstitial pneumonia is a category used to classify diseases not meeting criteria for usual interstitial pneumonia or desquamative interstitial pneumonia. Patients typically present with subacute to chronic dyspnea and cough. Histologically, the disease is temporally homogeneous and encompasses a spectrum of abnormalities ranging from cellular infiltration of the interstitium to fibrosis. Radiographically, ground glass opacities and septal line thickening in a basilar peripheral pattern are seen (Fig. 15.4).

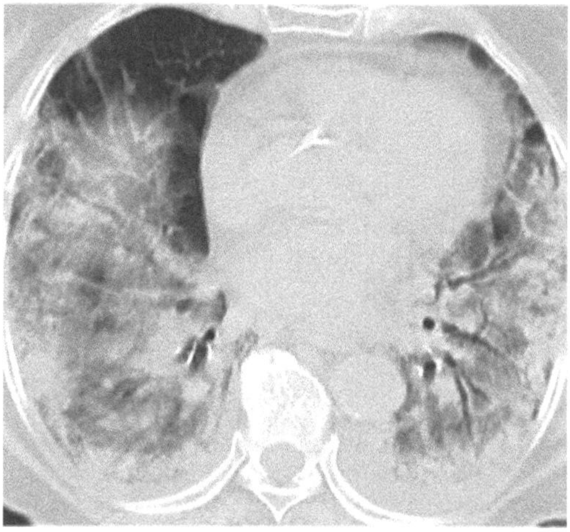

Fig. 15.3 Cytosine arabinoside diffuse alveolar damage. An 80-year-old woman who had received cytosine arabinoside. CT images show diffuse, bilateral ground glass opacities and mild bronchiectasis. Pathology showed changes of diffuse alveolar damage and cultures were negative

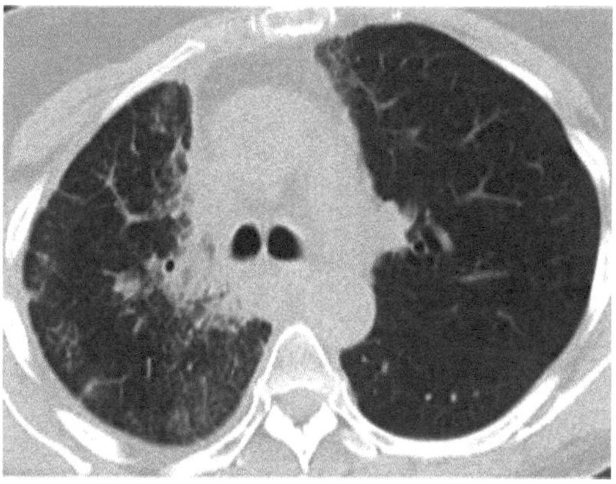

Fig. 15.5 Organizing pneumonia in the setting of a platinum-based agent and paclitaxel. A 62-year-old woman who had received cisplatin and paclitaxel for non-small cell lung cancer. Increasing ground glass was noted in the radiation field for which the patient underwent biopsy. Pathology demonstrated features of organizing pneumonia

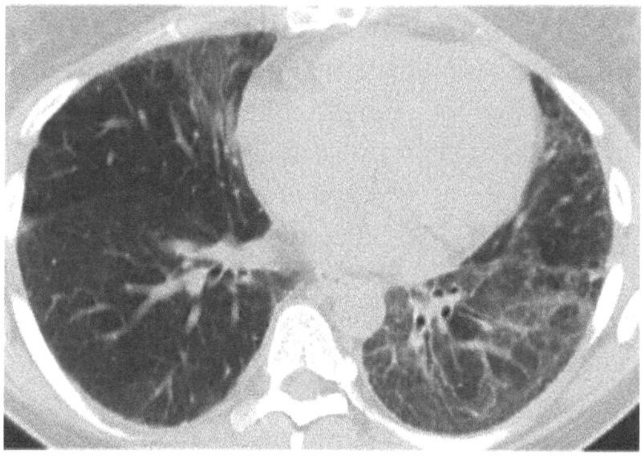

Fig. 15.4 Nonspecific interstitial pneumonitis (NSIP) from topotecan. A 68-year-old man who had progressive dyspnea after receiving treatment with topotecan. CT image shows asymmetric ground glass with subtle reticulation. Bronchoalveolar lavage was unrevealing and patient underwent biopsy which was most in keeping with NSIP

Organizing Pneumonia

Organizing pneumonia can be seen in the setting of many underlying lung diseases, including drug toxicities, or can be idiopathic or cryptogenic. Patients typically present subacutely with nonspecific symptoms such as nonproductive cough, dyspnea, or low-grade fevers. Histologically, there is plugging of the distal respiratory bronchioles and alveolar ducts with organizing connective tissue. There is notable absence of fibrosis, honeycombing, or architectural distortion of the lung unless it is superimposed on other underlying diseases. Radiographically, organizing pneumonia is seen as peripheral and/or peribronchovascular foci of consolidation or ground glass opacities (Figs. 15.5 and 15.6).

Eosinophilic Pneumonia

Eosinophilic lung disease occurs when eosinophils are recruited to the lung interstitium as a result of an immunologic response. When drug-induced, this form of pulmonary disease takes several different clinical forms. In simple pulmonary eosinophilia or Loffler's syndrome, patients are either asymptomatic or present with minimal complaints such as cough (Fig. 15.7). Patchy,

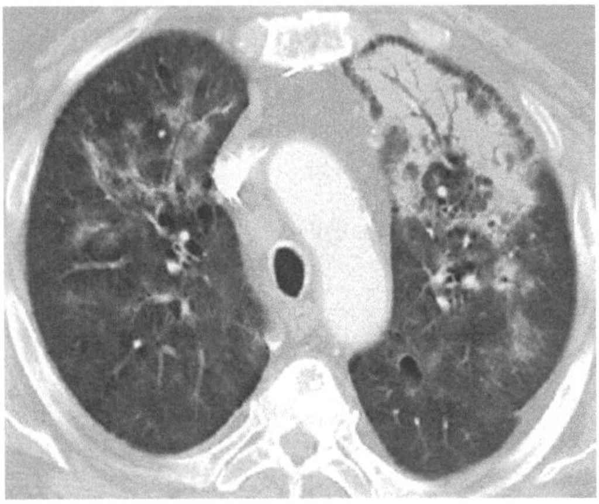

Fig. 15.6 Organizing pneumonia after mitomycin-C. A 70-year-old man who developed mild shortness of breath after mitomycin-C therapy. CT shows a more characteristic appearance of organizing pneumonia with peripheral, upper lobe consolidation. Paraseptal emphysema was also present which prevented the consolidation from completely abutting the pleura

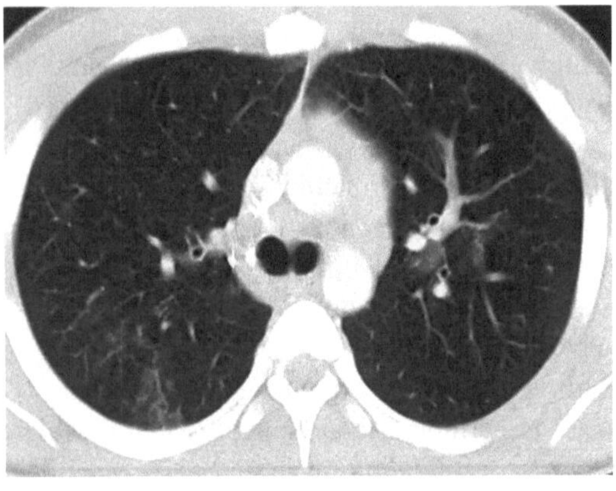

Fig. 15.7 Chronic eosinophilic pneumonia after cyclophosphamide therapy. This 29-year-old man presented with a nonproductive cough after his second cycle of cyclophoshamide therapy and received a CT examination after an abnormal chest radiograph. CT showed upper lobe predominant ground glass opacities. On bronchoscopic biopsy, findings were in keeping with chronic eosinophilic pneumonia and organizing pneumonia

migratory pulmonary infiltrates are seen, usually in the setting of peripheral blood eosinophilia. Other patients present with chronic cough or dyspnea and have peripheral often linear areas of consolidation indicative of chronic eosinophilic pneumonia. Acute eosinophilic pneumonia presents with rapidly progressing hypoxemia and respiratory failure. In this form of disease, interstitial infiltrates progress to alveolar consolidation (Fig. 15.8).

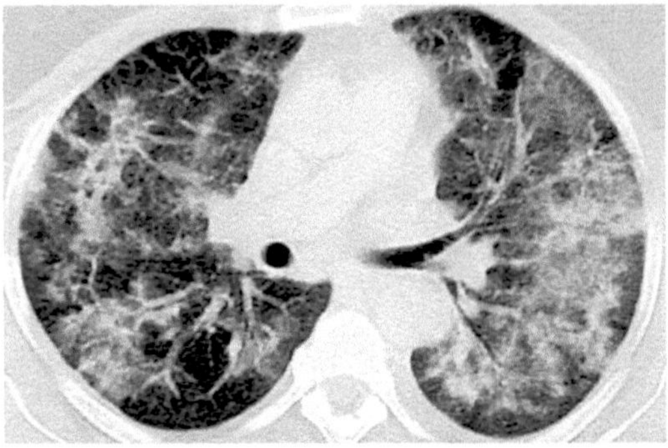

Fig. 15.8 Acute eosinophilic pneumonia after paclitaxel. This 48-year-old woman presented in acute respiratory distress after one cycle of paclitaxel. Bronchoscopic alveolar lavage was rich with eosinophils. Patient was treated with steroids and recovered uneventfully

Making the diagnosis of drug-induced eosinophilic lung disease is difficult. Other causes, such as parasitic or fungal infections, must be excluded. An appropriate time course for development of signs and symptoms with respect to initiation of drug therapy must be present. Elevated eosinophil counts in the peripheral blood, bronchoalveolar lavage fluid, or tissue samples should be present. In most cases, discontinuing drug therapy will result in resolution of symptoms and radiographic abnormalities. Frequently steroids are given, especially in acute eosinophilic pneumonia, to hasten clinical improvement [5].

Pulmonary Hemorrhage

Diffuse alveolar hemorrhage is another rare form of drug-induced pulmonary injury. Clinically, patients present with hemoptysis, anemia, and/or have hemorrhagic bronchoalveolar lavage fluid. This pulmonary injury can occur as a result of a hypersensitivity (immunologic) reaction, a small vessel pulmonary capillaritis, or secondary to drugs that interfere with the coagulation cascade [6]. Patients present either acutely or subacutely

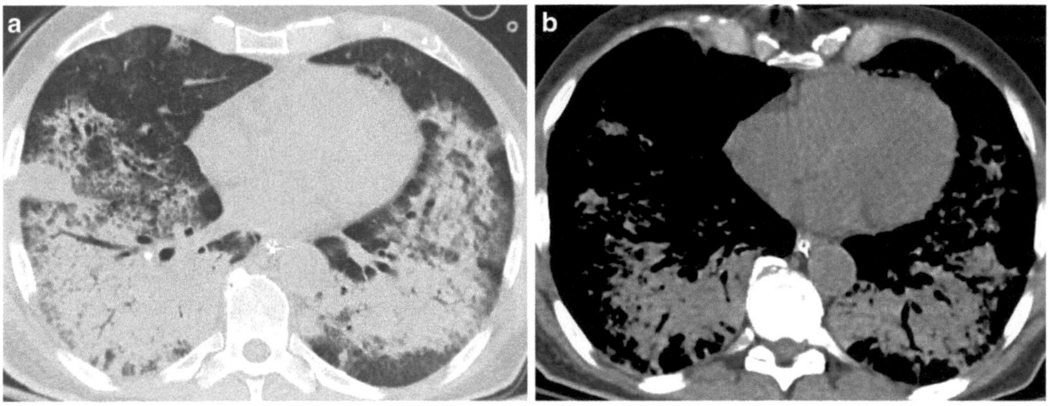

Fig. 15.9 Pulmonary hemorrhage after vinblastine and mitomycin-C therapy. A 49-year-old man with severe shortness of breath after completing his first cycle of vinblastine and mitomycin-C. Bronchoscopy showed diffuse pulmonary hemorrhage. The hemorrhagic nature of the consolidation better seen on the lung window (**a**) might be suggested by the slightly high attenuation on the soft tissue window (**b**)

with anemia and frequently with hemoptysis. On CT, diffuse ground glass opacities and areas of consolidation are seen (Fig. 15.9).

Specific Drugs

Platinum-Based Agents

Platinum-based chemotherapeutic agents work by covalently binding and cross-linking DNA strands in order to prevent cell replication. Cisplatin and carboplatin are widely used second-generation chemotherapeutic agents in the treatment of lung cancer, especially non-small cell lung cancer. The risk of significant pulmonary toxicity is considered less than 1 % [7]. The major toxicity associated with cisplatin is nephrotoxicity and that of carboplatin myelosuppression [8].

Alkylating Agents

Through a different biochemical interaction with DNA, alkylating agents also prevent the replication of DNA and thus cell replication. While cyclophosphamide has been a widely used first-generation agent, ifosfamide is a second-generation agent that is increasingly being used in lung cancer treatment. Systemic damaging effects occur as a result of toxic drug metabolites produced in the liver and to a lesser degree in the lung. These agents are considered to have a 1–5 % chance of significant pulmonary toxicity [7]. Due to its earlier widespread use in the treatment of various malignancies and vasculitides, the risk of pulmonary toxicity with cyclophosphamide is well known. Both an early acute pneumonitis and a late, progressive fibrosis have been described (Fig. 15.7) [9]. Patients with early onset pneumonitis usually present with cough, dyspnea, and fever within the first 6 months of treatment and radiographically have ground glass opacities and septal line thickening (a noncardiogenic pulmonary edema pattern) (Fig. 15.10) which usually resolves upon discontinuing the drug. The late-onset fibrosis can occur years after treatment with cyclophosphamide and results radiographically in an upper lobe predominate peripheral fibrosis without honeycombing which is progressive and usually unresponsive to steroids and/or discontinuation of the drug. Histologically, this late stage fibrosis is most commonly a result of DAD [4].

Another well-known complication of ifosfamide and cyclophosphamide therapy is hemorrhagic cystitis. This can range from a mild hematuria to life-threatening hemorrhage. The use of higher individual doses, higher cumulative doses, and the use of ifosfamide all increase the risk for this complication [10]. To reduce the risk of hemorrhagic cystitis, patients are given mesna,

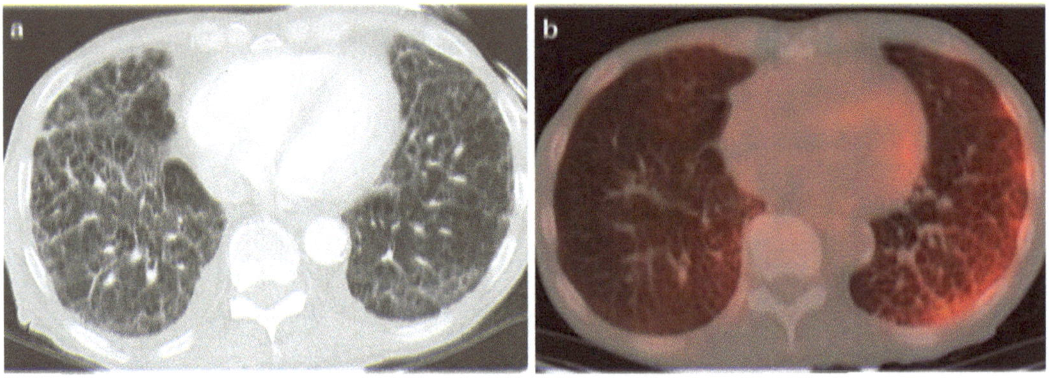

Fig. 15.10 Cyclophosphamide-related pulmonary injury. A 71-year-old man who developed severe shortness of breath after completing two cycles of cyclophosphamide therapy. CT images (**a**) of the lungs shows diffuse septal line thickening with patchy ground glass and small effusions. Subsequent FDG-PET CT (**b**) showed moderate uptake throughout the lungs. Transbronchial biopsy and cultures excluded infection. Findings were believed to be secondary to cytoxan therapy and improved with supportive therapy

a compound that is excreted into the urine and binds the harmful toxic metabolites of cyclophosphamide and ifosfamide.

Taxanes

Taxane medications work by preventing the normal disassembly of tubulin, preventing cells from undergoing mitosis. Considered third-generation lung cancer chemotherapeutic agents, paclitaxel and docetaxel are newer agents whose risk of pulmonary toxicity has been estimated as moderate (1–5 %) [7]. The most frequently reported pulmonary injury is a hypersensitivity pneumonitis [11]. Pathologically, this can present as an acute eosinophilic pneumonia and/or DAD (Fig. 15.8). As taxanes are considered radiation sensitizers, concomitant or antecedent radiation may increase the risk of pulmonary toxicity (Fig. 15.5) [12].

Antimetabolites

A pyrimidine analog that hastens cell death by incorporating into DNA, gemcitabine is an antimetabolite chemotherapeutic agent that has been shown to be highly active against non-small cell lung cancer. Three forms of pulmonary toxicity have been described [1]. An acute, self-limited dyspnea has been reported in up to 10 % of patients within hours to days after drug exposure [13]. A hypersensitivity reaction with bronchospasm is more uncommon. A form of toxicity has also been reported which can rapidly progress to respiratory insufficiency. In this form, the radiographic appearance is one resembling a DAD pattern with progressive pulmonary consolidation and ground glass opacities (Fig. 15.11).

Topoisomerase Inhibitors

By interfering with enzymes required for DNA maintenance, topoisomerase inhibitors can exert antitumor activity. Irinotecan, topotecan, and etoposide have been used in the treatment of non-small and small cell lung cancers. Serious pulmonary toxicity has been reported to occur in approximately 0.4 % of patients treated with irinotecan [14]. Bronchiolitis, nonspecific interstitial pneumonia, and DAD have all been reported with exposure to topotecan (Fig. 15.4) [15].

Vinca Alkaloids

By interfering with microtubule function, vinca alkaloids disrupt cell division and exert antitumor activity. Vinblastine and vinorelbine are examples of this type of medication and are felt to

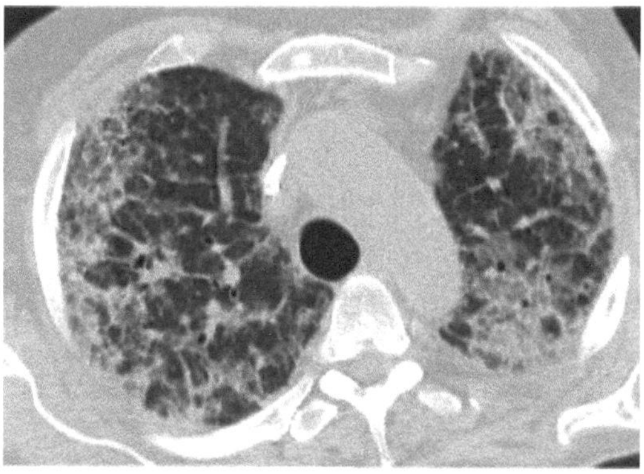

Fig. 15.11 Gemcitabine pulmonary toxicity. A 61-year-old man who had completed gemcitabine therapy and developed shortness of breath. Despite antibiotic therapy, his symptoms progressed. Pathology was in keeping with diffuse alveolar damage believed to be secondary to his drug therapy

uncommonly cause pulmonary toxicity. Reports of patients receiving these medications and developing pulmonary injury have been used in combination with other agents, such as mitomycin-C which is known to have pulmonary toxicity [16].

Antibiotics

Mitomycin-C is an antineoplastic antibiotic derived from *Streptomyces caespitosus* which cross-links DNA strands preventing DNA synthesis. While the major serious toxicity is related to myelosuppression, pulmonary toxicity has been estimated to occur between 3 and 12 % of patients [17, 18]. Acute bronchospasm, organizing pneumonia, acute pneumonitis, DAD, and nonspecific interstitial pneumonia have all been reported with exposure to this medication (Fig. 15.6). In addition, there have been reports of the development of a hemolytic uremic syndrome which can result in noncardiogenic pulmonary edema (Fig. 15.9) [19]. A large percentage of these patients developed DAD.

Targeted Agents

Tyrosine kinase inhibitors are a class of drugs that interferes with signaling related to the epidermal growth factor receptor. Gefitinib (Iressa) was first in class and had been used in patients with advanced non-small cell lung cancer who have failed to respond to standard regimens. A pattern of DAD has been associated with this drug in several case reports [20]. The effect seems to be related to class of drugs as a similar interstitial lung disease has been seen with erlotinib (Tarceva), although at a relatively decreased frequency [21]. The vascular endothelial growth factor (VEGF) inhibitor bevacizumab (Avastin) has been associated with hemoptysis, pulmonary hemorrhage, and pulmonary embolism [22].

Summary

Chemotherapy-related lung injury is a well-recognized phenomenon. Pathologically, pulmonary injury is seen as DAD, nonspecific interstitial pneumonia, organizing pneumonia, eosinophilic pneumonia, and/or pulmonary hemorrhage. Establishing the diagnosis requires a high level of clinical suspicion, exclusion of infectious causes, an appropriate exposure history and time course, and often supportive evidence from radiologic and histopathologic studies, as the presenting signs and symptoms are usually nonspecific. Early detection is critical, as drug cessation with or without steroid administration can often reverse deleterious effects.

References

1. Limper AH. Chemotherapy-induced lung disease. Clin Chest Med. 2004;25(1):53–64.
2. Limper AH. Drug-induced lung injury. In: Mason RJ, Broaddus VC, Murray JF, Nadel JA, editors. Murray and Nadel's textbook of respiratory medicine. 4th ed. Philadelphia: Elsevier Saunders; 2005. p. 1888–908.
3. McAdams HP, Rosado-de-Christenson ML, Wehunt WD, Fishback NF. The alphabet soup revisited: the chronic interstitial pneumonias in the 1990s. Radiographics. 1996;16(5):1009–33.
4. Erasmus JJ, McAdams HP, Rossi SE. High-resolution CT of drug-induced lung disease. Radiol Clin North Am. 2002;40(1):61–72.
5. Allen JD. Drug-induced eosinophilic lung disease. Clin Chest Med. 2004;25(1):77–88.
6. Schwarz MI, Fontenot AP. Drug-induced diffuse alveolar hemorrhage syndromes and vasculitis. Clin Chest Med. 2004;25(1):133–40.

7. Machtay M. Pulmonary complications of anti-cancer treatment. In: Abeloff M, Armitage J, Niederhuber J, Kastan M, McKenna WG, editors. Clinical oncology. 3rd ed. Philadelphia: Elsevier Churchill Livingston; 2004. p. 1237–47.
8. Stinchcombe TE, Socinski MA. General aspects of chemotherapy. In: Detterbeck FC, Rivera MP, Socinski M, Rosenman J, editors. Diagnosis and treatment of lung cancer. 1st ed. Philadelphia: WB Saunders; 2001. p. 162–73.
9. Malik SW, Myers JL, DeRemee RA, Specks U. Lung toxicity with cyclophosphamide use: two distinct patterns. Am J Respir Crit Care Med. 1996;154(6 Pt 1): 1851–6.
10. Brade WP, Herdrich K, Varini M. Ifosfamide: pharmacology, safety and therapeutic potential. Cancer Treat Rev. 1985;12(1):1–47.
11. Wang GS, Yang KY, Perng RP. Life-threatening hypersensitivity pneumonitis induced by docetaxel (taxotere). Br J Cancer. 2001;85(9):1247–50.
12. Reckzeh B, Merte H, Pflüger KH, Pfab R, Wolf M, Havemann K. Severe lymphocytopenia and interstitial pneumonia in patients treated with paclitaxel and simultaneous radiotherapy for non-small cell lung cancer. J Clin Oncol. 1996;14(4):1071–6.
13. Nelson R, Tarasoff P. Dyspnea with gemcitabine is commonly seen, often disease related, transient, and rarely severe. Eur J Cancer. 1995;31(A):S197–8.
14. Madarnas Y, Webster P, Shorter AM, Bjarnason GA. Irinotecan-associated pulmonary toxicity. Anticancer Drugs. 2000;11:709–13.
15. Maitland ML, Wilcox R, Hogarth DK, et al. Diffuse alveolar damage after a single dose of topotecan in a patient with pulmonary fibrosis and small cell lung cancer. Lung Cancer. 2006;54(2):243–5.
16. Rao SX, Ramaswamy G, Levin M, McCravey JW. Fatal acute respiratory failure after vinblastine-mitomycin therapy in lung carcinoma. Arch Intern Med. 1985;145(10):1905–7.
17. Castro M, Veeder MH, Mailliard JA, Tazelaar HD, Jett JR. A prospective study of pulmonary function in patients receiving mitomycin. Chest. 1996;109(4): 939–44.
18. Linette DC, McGee KH, McFarland JA. Mitomycin-induced pulmonary toxicity: case report and review of the literature. Ann Pharmacother. 1992;26(4): 481–4.
19. Sheldon R, Slaughter D. A syndrome of microangiopathic hemolytic anemia, renal impairment, and pulmonary edema in chemotherapy-treated patients with adenocarcinoma. Cancer. 1986;58(7):1428–36.
20. Cohen MH, Williams GA, Sridhara R, Chen G, Pazdur R. FDA drug approval summary: gefitinib (ZD1839)(Iressa) tablets. Oncologist. 2003;8(4):303–6.
21. ter Heine R, van den Bosch RTA, Schaefer-Prokop CM, et al. Fatal interstitial lung disease associated with high erlotonib and metabolite levels. A case report and a review of the literature. Lung Cancer. 2012;75(3):391–7.
22. Barber NA, Ganti AK. Pulmonary toxicities from targeted therapies: a review. Target Oncol. 2011;6(4): 235–43.

Index

J.G. Ravenel (ed.), *Lung Cancer Imaging*, Contemporary Medical Imaging,
DOI 10.1007/978-1-60761-620-7,

MIX
Papier aus verantwortungsvollen Quellen
Paper from responsible sources
FSC® C105338

If you have any concerns about our products,
you can contact us on
ProductSafety@springernature.com

In case Publisher is established outside the EU,
the EU authorized representative is:
Springer Nature Customer Service Center GmbH
Europaplatz 3, 69115 Heidelberg, Germany

Printed by Libri Plureos GmbH
in Hamburg, Germany